Philosophical Issues in Psychiatry III

International Perspectives in Philosophy and Psychiatry
Series editors: Bill (K.W.M.) Fulford, Lisa Bortolotti, Matthew Broome, Katherine Morris, John Z. Sadler, and Giovanni Stanghellini

VOLUMES IN THE SERIES:

Portrait of the Psychiatrist as a Young Man
The Early Writing and Work of R.D. Laing, 1927–1960
Beveridge

Mind, Meaning, and Mental Disorder 2e
Bolton and Hill

What is Mental Disorder?
Bolton

Delusions and Other Irrational Beliefs
Bortolotti

Postpsychiatry
Bracken and Thomas

Philosophy, Psychoanalysis, and the A-Rational Mind
Brakel

Unconscious Knowing and Other Essays in Psycho-Philosophical Analysis
Brakel

Psychiatry as Cognitive Neuroscience
Broome and Bortolotti (eds.)

Free Will and Responsibility: A Guide for Practitioners
Callender

Reconceiving Schizophrenia
Chung, Fulford, and Graham (eds.)

Darwin and Psychiatry
De Block and Adriaens (eds.)

Oxford Handbook of Philosophy and Psychiatry
Fulford, Davies, Gipps, Graham, Sadler, Stanghellini, and Thornton (eds.)

Nature and Narrative
An Introduction to the New Philosophy of Psychiatry
Fulford, Morris, Sadler, and Stanghellini (eds.)

Oxford Textbook of Philosophy and Psychiatry
Fulford, Thornton, and Graham (eds.)

The Mind and its Discontents
Gillett

Is evidence-based psychiatry ethical?
Gupta

Thinking Through Dementia
Hughes

Dementia
Mind, Meaning, and the Person
Hughes, Louw, and Sabat (eds.)

Talking Cures and Placebo Effects
Jopling

Philosophical Issues in Psychiatry II
Nosology
Kendler and Parnas

Philosophical Issues in Psychiatry III
The Nature and Sources of Historical Change
Kendler and Parnas

Discursive Perspectives in Therapeutic Practice
Lock and Strong (eds.)

Schizophrenia and the Fate of the Self
Lysaker and Lysaker

Responsibility and Psychopathy
Malatesti and McMillan

Body-Subjects and Disordered Minds
Matthews

Rationality and Compulsion
Applying Action Theory to Psychiatry
Nordenfelt

Philosophical Perspectives on Technology and Psychiatry
Phillips (ed.)

The Metaphor of Mental Illness
Pickering

Mapping the Edges and the In-between
Potter

Trauma, Truth, and Reconciliation
Healing Damaged Relationships
Potter (ed.)

The Philosophy of Psychiatry
A Companion
Radden

The Virtuous Psychiatrist
Radden and Sadler

Addiction and Weakness of Will
Radoilska

Autonomy and Mental Disorder
Radoilska (ed.)

Feelings of Being
Ratcliffe

Recovery of People with Mental Illness
Philosophical and Related Perspectives
Rudnick (ed.)

Values and Psychiatric Diagnosis
Sadler

Disembodied Spirits and Deanimated Bodies
The Psychopathology of Common Sense
Stanghellini

One Century of Karl Jaspers' General Psychopathology
Stanghellini and Fuchs

Emotions and Personhood
Stanghellini and Rosfort

Essential Philosophy of Psychiatry
Thornton

Empirical Ethics in Psychiatry
Widdershoven, McMillan, Hope, and Van der Scheer (eds.)

The Sublime Object of Psychiatry
Schizophrenia in Clinical and Cultural Theory
Woods

Alternative Perspectives on Psychiatric Validation
DSM, ICD, RDoC, and Beyond
Zachar, Stoyanov, Aragona, and Jablensky

Philosophical Issues in Psychiatry III
The Nature and Sources of Historical Change

Edited by

Kenneth S. Kendler, M.D.
Rachel Brown Banks Distinguished Professor of Psychiatry
Professor of Human Genetics
Director, Virginia Institute for Psychiatric and Behavioral Genetics
Virginia Commonwealth University
Richmond, VA

Josef Parnas, M.D., Dr.Med.
Clinical Professor
University of Copenhagen
Psychiatric Center Hvidovre & Danish National Research Foundation's Center for Subjectivity Research
Copenhagen, Denmark

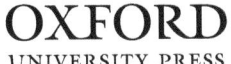

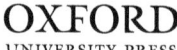
UNIVERSITY PRESS

Great Clarendon Street, Oxford, OX2 6DP,
United Kingdom

Oxford University Press is a department of the University of Oxford.
It furthers the University's objective of excellence in research, scholarship,
and education by publishing worldwide. Oxford is a registered trade mark of
Oxford University Press in the UK and in certain other countries

Chapters 1–40 and Chapter 42 © Oxford University Press 2015
Chapter 41 © Lippincott Williams & Willkins 2014

The moral rights of the authors have been asserted

First Edition published in 2015
Impression: 1

All rights reserved. No part of this publication may be reproduced, stored in
a retrieval system, or transmitted, in any form or by any means, without the
prior permission in writing of Oxford University Press, or as expressly permitted
by law, by licence or under terms agreed with the appropriate reprographics
rights organization. Enquiries concerning reproduction outside the scope of the
above should be sent to the Rights Department, Oxford University Press, at the
address above

You must not circulate this work in any other form
and you must impose this same condition on any acquirer

Published in the United States of America by Oxford University Press
198 Madison Avenue, New York, NY 10016, United States of America

British Library Cataloguing in Publication Data
Data available

Library of Congress Control Number: 2014940086

ISBN 978–0–19–872597–8

Printed and bound in Great Britain by
Clays Ltd., St Ives plc

Oxford University Press makes no representation, express or implied, that the
drug dosages in this book are correct. Readers must therefore always check
the product information and clinical procedures with the most up-to-date
published product information and data sheets provided by the manufacturers
and the most recent codes of conduct and safety regulations. The authors and
the publishers do not accept responsibility or legal liability for any errors in the
text or for the misuse or misapplication of material in this work. Except where
otherwise stated, drug dosages and recommendations are for the non-pregnant
adult who is not breast-feeding

Links to third party websites are provided by Oxford in good faith and
for information only. Oxford disclaims any responsibility for the materials
contained in any third party website referenced in this work.

Preface

The main chapters of this book began as talks given at a conference "Philosophical Issues in Psychiatry III: The Nature and Sources of Historical Change", held in Copenhagen, Denmark, on May 9–11, 2013. This conference was the third in a series of Copenhagen meetings on philosophical issues in psychiatry. The conference was sponsored by the Faculty of Health and Medical Sciences of the University of Copenhagen and the Center for Subjectivity Research, University of Copenhagen. The conference was organized and chaired by the editors of this volume, Kenneth S. Kendler, M.D. and Josef Parnas, M.D. The conference was from the outset conceived with the view toward subsequent publication.

We express our gratitude to the University of Copenhagen for their generous funding. We also thank Mrs. Merete Lynnerup for her friendly and stoic administrative help in preparing the meeting. Neither the conference nor its published volume would have materialized without indefatigable and engaged organizational and editorial assistance of Ms. Jill Opalesky. We also thank Mrs. Clarisse Sternberg for practical help during the conference.

We ended the preface to the first volume in this series as follows: "This project was, to use the philosophical term, emergent—in the end, the sum was much more than the individual parts." As with our previous edited books together, the two of us again feel this way about the present volume and hope that you, the readers, agree.

Table of Contents

List of Contributors *xiii*
Introduction: applying the tools of the history and philosophy of science to psychiatry *xv*
Kenneth S. Kendler

Part I Nature of historical change in science

Section 1 Objectivity and scientific change

1 Introduction to "Pluralism, incommensurability, and scientific change" *5*
Kenneth S. Kendler

2 Pluralism, incommensurability, and scientific change *7*
Helen E. Longino

3 For objective, value-laden, contextualist pluralism *20*
John Dupré

Section 2 Change in psychopathology

4 Introduction to "History and epistemology of psychopathology" *27*
Josef Parnas

5 History and epistemology of psychopathology *30*
German E. Berrios

6 Can hybridity overcome dualism? *51*
Helen E. Longino

Section 3 Scientific disagreement in the medical context

7 Introduction to "Expert disagreement and medical authority" *57*
Kenneth S. Kendler

8 Expert disagreement and medical authority *60*
Miriam Solomon

9 Trust, dissent, and decision vectors *73*
   Ian Hacking

Section 4 The social, the cultural, and psychiatric kinds

10 Introduction to "Varieties of social constructionism and the problem of progress in psychiatry" *83*
    Kenneth S. Kendler

11 Varieties of social constructionism and the problem of progress in psychiatry *85*
    Kenneth F. Schaffner and Kathryn Tabb

12 The role of cultural configurators in the formation of mental symptoms *107*
    German E. Berrios

Part II History of broad movements/structures within psychiatry

Section 5 The psychiatric history of the diencephalon

13 Introduction to "Biography of a brain structure: studying the diencephalon as an epistemic object" *121*
    Josef Parnas

14 Biography of a brain structure: studying the diencephalon as an epistemic object *123*
    Emilie Bovet

15 Some reflections on historiographic strategies for the neurosciences *140*
    Eric J. Engstrom

Section 6 The history of psychiatry as interdisciplinary history

16 Introduction to "On attitudes toward philosophy and psychology in German psychiatry, 1867–1917" *145*
    Kenneth S. Kendler

17 On attitudes toward philosophy and psychology in German psychiatry, 1867–1917 *149*
    Eric J. Engstrom

18 Interdisciplinarity versus compartmentalization: an eternal dilemma in psychiatry *165*
    Yuji Sato

Section 7 Psychiatry and psychoanalysis in the United States

19 Introduction to "The development of psychoanalysis in the context of American psychiatry" *171*
Kenneth S. Kendler

20 The development of psychoanalysis in the context of American psychiatry *173*
Robert Michels

21 Decline of psychoanalysis to the advantage of what? *180*
Josef Parnas

Section 8 The operational revolution

22 Introduction to "Psychiatry made easy: operation(al)ism and some of its consequences" *187*
Kenneth S. Kendler

23 Psychiatry made easy: operation(al)ism and some of its consequences *190*
Josef Parnas and Pierre Bovet

24 Hempel as a critic of Bridgman's operationalism: lessons for psychiatry from the history of science *213*
Kenneth F. Schaffner and Kathryn Tabb

Section 9 The evolution of genetic explanation in psychiatry

25 Introduction to "The nature of nature" *223*
Kenneth S. Kendler

26 The nature of nature *227*
Eric Turkheimer

27 Is it time for a "Copenhagen interpretation" in behavioral genetics? *245*
Peter Zachar

Section 10 Psychiatry and evolution

28 Introduction to "What can evolution tell us about the healthy mind?" *257*
Josef Parnas

29 What can evolution tell us about the healthy mind? *259*
John Dupré

30 What can history and social studies of sciences teach us about evolutionary psychiatry? *272*
Emilie Bovet

Part III Specific disorders from a historical perspective

Section 11 Schizophrenia and the dopamine hypothesis

31 Introduction to "Dopamine hypothesis of schizophrenia: an updated perspective" *281*
Josef Parnas

32 The dopamine hypothesis of schizophrenia: an updated perspective *283*
Kenneth S. Kendler

33 Why is the dopamine hypothesis of schizophrenia the only game in town? *295*
Miriam Solomon

Section 12 Conceptual status of depression today

34 Introduction to "Depression in a biopsychosocioeconomic context" *301*
Josef Parnas

35 Depression in a biopsychosocioeconomic context *302*
Yuji Sato

36 What do we want from a depression diagnosis? *319*
Eric Turkheimer

Section 13 The shaping of autism

37 Introduction to "On the ratio of science to activism in the shaping of autism" *325*
Josef Parnas

38 On the ratio of science to activism in the shaping of autism *326*
Ian Hacking

39 The shaping of autism and other psychiatric disorders: an alternative perspective *340*
Kenneth S. Kendler

Section 14 **The decision to include or exclude a diagnosis in psychiatric nosology: the case of premenstrual dysphoric disorder**

- **40** Introduction to "A DSM insiders' history of premenstrual dysphoric disorder" *349*
  Josef Parnas
- **41** A DSM insiders' history of premenstrual dysphoric disorder *350*
  Peter Zachar and Kenneth S. Kendler
- **42** The construction of a diagnosis is not a scientific issue *371*
  Robert Michels

  Index *373*

List of Contributors

Editors

Kenneth S. Kendler, M.D.
Rachel Brown Banks Distinguished
Professor of Psychiatry
Professor of Human Genetics
Director
Virginia Institute for Psychiatric and
Behavioral Genetics
Virginia Commonwealth University
Richmond, VA, USA

Chapter contributors

German E. Berrios, M.D.
Chair in the Epistemology of
Psychiatry
University of Cambridge
Cambridge
Emeritus Consultant
Neuropsychiatrist & Head of the
Department of Neuropsychiatry
Addenbrooke's Hospital
Cambridge
Life Fellow
Robinson College
University of Cambridge
Cambridge, UK

Emilie Bovet, Ph.D.
Senior Lecturer
Faculty of Political and Social Sciences
University of Lausanne
Research Associate
University Institute of Social and
Preventive Medicine, CHUV
University of Lausanne and
Research Associate
University of Health Sciences (HESAV)
Lausanne, Switzerland

Josef Parnas, M.D., Dr.Med.
Clinical Professor
University of Copenhagen
Psychiatric Center Hvidovre & Danish
National Research Foundation's
Center for Subjectivity Research
Copenhagen, Denmark

Pierre Bovet, M.D.
Professor
Department of Psychiatry
CHUV, University of Lausanne
Lausanne, Switzerland

John Dupré, Ph.D.
Director
Egenis, Centre for the Study of Life
Sciences and
Professor of Philosophy of Science
Department of Sociology, Philosophy,
and Anthropology
University of Exeter
Exeter, UK

Eric J. Engstrom, Ph.D.
Department of History
Humboldt University
Berlin, Germany

Ian Hacking, Ph.D.
Retired
Professeur honoraire Chaire de
philosophie et histoire des concepts
scientifique and
University Professor emeritus
Department of Philosophy
Collège de France and
University of Toronto
Toronto, Canada

Helen E. Longino, Ph.D.
Clarence Irving Lewis Professor in Philosophy
Philosophy Department
Stanford University
Standford, CA, USA

Robert Michels, M.D.
Walsh McDermott University Professor of Medicine
University Professor of Psychiatry
Weill Medical College of Cornell University and
Training and Supervising Analyst
Columbia University Center for Psychoanalytic Training and Research
New York, NY, USA

Yuji Sato, M.D., Ph.D.
Professor and Director
Centre for Clinical Research
Keio University School of Medicine
Tokyo, Japan

Kenneth F. Schaffner, Ph.D., M.D.
Distinguished University Professor
Department of History and Philosophy of Science
University of Pittsburgh
Pittsburgh, PA, USA

Miriam Solomon, Ph.D.
Professor and Department Chair
Philosophy Department
Temple University
Philadelphia, PA, USA

Kathryn Tabb, M.Phil., Ph.D. Candidate
Department of History and Philosophy of Science
University of Pittsburgh
Pittsburgh, PA, USA

Eric Turkheimer, Ph.D.
Professor of Psychology
Department of Psychology
University of Virginia
Charlottesville, VA, USA

Peter Zachar, Ph.D.
Professor of Psychology
Department of Psychology
Auburn University Montgomery
Montgomery, AL, USA

Introduction: applying the tools of the history and philosophy of science to psychiatry

Kenneth S. Kendler

> If the nature of the societies in which scientists live strongly influence both the hypotheses which they generate to explain the natural world as well as the reception of those hypotheses by other scientists, then one would expect this influence to be most clear-cut in those areas of science that bear most directly on human beings.
>
> (David Hull, 1990, p. 20)

The invitation to the contributors to this volume, which began as a meeting held in Copenhagen, Denmark, May 9–11, 2013, and sponsored by the Faculty of Health Sciences of the University of Copenhagen and the Danish National Research Foundation's Center for Subjectivity Research, included the following:

> An important question within the history and philosophy of science is the degree to which "progress" or "change" in science results from internal, largely empirically driven processes (e.g. new data or theories) versus arises as a result of a range of external influences including shifting cultural values, economic- and socio-political processes, other historical forces and the search for professional respect and authority. Psychiatry sits at the cross-roads of the biomedical science, the social sciences and the humanities. In being the one medical specialty that diagnoses and treats mental illness, it has been subject to major changes in the last 150 years. This conference seeks to understand the nature of the forces that have shaped these changes and especially how substantial "internal" advances in our knowledge of the nature and causes of psychiatric illness have interacted with a plethora of external forces that have impacted on the psychiatric profession.

More succinctly, the goals of that meeting and this volume could be summarized as "taking the conceptual frameworks developed in the burgeoning field of history and philosophy of science and applying them to the field of psychiatry." As suggested by the philosopher of biology, David Hull, in our introductory quote, psychiatry should be a rich field for inquiry for those who want to understand how internal and external forces impact on historical change in science as psychiatry is surely among those scientific fields "that bear most directly on human beings."

To accomplish this, we invited three types of individuals (some meeting more than one definition): (1) philosophers with expertise in the history and philosophy of science and an interest in things psychiatric, (2) psychiatrists and psychologists with interest and expertise in the history of their field and/or related philosophical issues, and (3) historians of psychiatry. We structured the meeting and this volume to encourage interactions among the participants. Each main chapter has both an introduction by one of the two organizers of the conference and editors of this volume (K.S. Kendler and J. Parnas), and a comment by another conference participant.

Writing on the history and philosophy of psychiatry is challenging because it requires a diverse set of skills and knowledge. Substantive knowledge of the discipline is needed. Good philosophers have said silly things about psychiatry for lack of that knowledge. But psychiatrists and psychologists have also written bad histories of their field for lack of historiographic and philosophical sophistication.

One way to produce high-quality work in the history and philosophy of psychiatry is from collaborations across the groups of authors represented in this book. We hope that a long-term effect of this conference will be to sow seeds for such future collaborative ventures. Such collaborations are critically facilitated by each group learning more about the language and concepts of the other. This, too, we hope is helped by this book.

Let me help to set the stage for this volume by reviewing the kinds of themes we hoped would be discussed in this meeting and volume. Psychiatry is a discipline that attracts an inordinate amount of social attention. When the rheumatologists or endocrinologists revise their diagnostic criteria, stories about controversies do not work their way into a prominent position in the general press. Psychiatry is also more sensitive to broad social trends than many other scientific disciplines. For example, it is probably safe to conclude that the broad changes in attitudes about gender orientation in Western society over the last 40 years has had a stronger impact on psychiatry in the United States than on other medical or biological disciplines, let alone on chemistry and physics. The last section in this volume reviews the history of premenstrual dysphoric disorder that is tied in to many themes, prominent among them being feminism and how it manifested itself in the fields of psychiatry and psychology over the last 30 years. As discussed by Ian Hacking in Chapter 38, we have witnessed in recent years an extraordinary rise of interest in autism and autism spectrum disorders such as Asperger's syndrome. In few other fields of medicine do affected individuals band together in support groups that sometimes explicitly deny the validity of their "illness status." At a broader level, general cultural trends have had major impacts on psychiatry. How much was the rise of psychoanalysis in the United States influenced by the broad "can-do" optimism about the flexibility of human nature that characterized post-World War II American society? How has the popular turn toward genetics stimulated by the sequencing of the human genome (and manifest by the ever-present iconic DNA double helix) impacted on societal attitudes toward the genetic component of mental illness that has been increasingly shown? How have broad cultural differences in the intellectual life of the United States and Europe contributed to differences in our views about the scientific, diagnostic, and philosophical underpinnings of psychiatry?

A number of these issues are concentrated in debates about the boundaries of mental illness. We have seen such issues reverberate through political, cultural, and social commentaries on whether, or ever, homosexuality, attention deficit hyperactivity disorder (ADHD), and autism should be seen as disorders. Schaffner and Tabb explore aspects of this problem in Chapter 11 in this volume. The question of whether grieving individuals who meet criteria for major depression should or should not be considered ill was discussed in the editorial pages of leading US newspapers. Having sat in many meetings of the Board of Trustees of the American Psychiatric Association (APA) as they tried to weave their way through the multiple controversies surrounding the fifth edition of the *Diagnostic and Statistical Manual of Mental Disorders* (DSM-5), I can attest to their concern about how psychiatric issues were playing out in the general media. So the influence goes both ways.

Other important nonempirical influences on psychiatry occur in its role within the field of medicine. Psychiatry is a low-prestige discipline. In the United States, our pay is near the bottom along with other specialties such as pediatrics and family practice that provide largely "cognitive care" (that is, talk to patients and write prescriptions) rather than doing procedures. Organized psychiatry is constantly vigilant to ensure that our professional space is not encroached upon by our near neighbors—psychologists—who in the United States frequently request prescription privileges. The increasing role of neuroscience in the self-image of psychiatry has raised other boundary problems. Should we merge with neurology and all become "applied neuroscientists?"

Subdisciplines within psychiatry fight vehemently for dominance as manifested by faculty appointments, chairmanships, and grant funding. Social psychiatry, once a vibrant force within American psychiatry, has all but disappeared (although remaining more active in other countries such as the United Kingdom). As Michels reviews in Chapter 20, within the last 75 years, we have seen the rise of psychoanalysis to almost complete dominance of academic psychiatry in the United States and then fall precipitously in status and power within American psychiatry associated with the rise of the biological psychiatric paradigm.

And then there are the economic forces. Psychiatric drugs are typically major money-makers for the large pharmaceutical companies (aka "big pharma"). They have had a range of important influences on the field including conducting critical drug trials but also attempting, in ways that range from appropriate to far less savory, to influence psychiatrists' behavior. The field has struggled with developing a more balanced and ethically defensible relationship with big pharma. In the United States, mental health care is funded at a much lower level than general medicine or surgery. Psychotherapy in particular is poorly reimbursed and this has provided a strong financial incentive for psychiatrists to move toward a psychopharmacologic style of practice with 15-minute "med-checks" substituting for the more traditional 50-minute psychotherapy hour. This has impacted on training with a turning away from the richness of the descriptive psychiatric tradition and psychotherapy toward the menu-driven world of the DSM criteria and pharmacological decision trees.

As we noted above, the nature and developments of psychiatric nosology are another area rich for philosophical and historical analysis given the intriguing mix of empirical, professional, and social/cultural forces at work. The operationalization of diagnostic criteria—so central to psychiatric research and practice, first in the United States and later in most other places of the world—is the subject of Chapter 23 by Parnas and P. Bovet in this volume. In Chapter 17, Engstrom reviews the career of Kraepelin, undoubtedly the most influential of psychiatric nosologists, and suggests that the portrayal in late twentieth-century psychiatry of his nosologic approach is quite inaccurate.

This conference was planned just as the DSM-5 juggernaut was winding down. This process of the DSM revision—called by the APA four times from 1980 to the present—is an historical event that ripples across the field of psychiatry and out into the general public. A similar process, still ongoing, is also undertaken by the World Health Organization to revise the International Classification of Diseases. The structure of these revisions and the degree to which social forces, clinical opinion, historical precedent, and empirical findings impact on the nature is a subject ripe for conceptual analysis. We see one example of that in Chapter 41 of this volume on premenstrual dysphoric disorder by Zachar and Kendler.

Moving from external to internal influences on the field of psychiatry, we have seen a range of changes in the sciences that undergird the increasingly diverse fields of psychiatric research. In just the last 20 years, stunning advances have been made in the techniques of clinical and systems neuroscience (e.g., functional magnetic resonance imaging) and basic molecular neuroscience. The world of molecular genetics has exploded with rapidly developing lab methods for genotyping and sequencing. New statistical and bioinformatics methods are being published weekly in an attempt to keep up with the deluge of new data. Major breakthroughs are starting to occur in gene finding for psychiatric disorders like schizophrenia and autism. Whole new areas of expression analysis and epigenetics have recently emerged. We have also seen, albeit at a slower pace, important advances in the social sciences relevant to psychiatry including neuropsychology, developmental psychopathology, personality psychology, social epidemiology, survey research, and psychometrics. We have seen the emergence of the "trialist"—the expert in conducting clinical trials of both drug and psychotherapies. Far too often in the past has it been declared that discovering the causes and cures of psychiatric disorders is "right around the corner." I have no intention of making such a claim. But internal scientific developments have surely been powerful engines for change in psychiatric science and we are beginning to see with a much slower time frame an impact on psychiatric practice.

These developments have not been without their tensions. The rise of the fields of molecular and systems neuroscience in psychiatry have been accompanied by a resurgence of reductionist fervor (that has visited the field of psychiatry a number of times in its history). The director of the US National Institute of Mental Health has shifted funding away from epidemiology and social science approaches toward molecular neurobiology. Finding the proper balance between the attraction of molecular science and the emergent nature of a number of key features of psychiatric illness has proven difficult.

Before closing, let me add a short personal story here in which I struggled with the key question: "What is science?" As a working psychiatric researcher who has, in mid to late career, awoken to the many philosophical issues of our field, I would have characterized myself in my early career as a naïve internalist. Had I been asked the question that began this essay, I would then have replied something like: "Of course, we should only pay attention to our empirical results. External social and political processes are irrelevant at best and pernicious at worst. To keep our unsullied scientific virtues, we should ignore them entirely." Now that I am older and perhaps wiser, I realize this position is impossible to sustain. All sorts of external factors impact on both the science and the practice of psychiatry. These are empirical facts. My prescriptive position—as I might interact with a young postdoctoral fellow—is hopefully more nuanced as well. I might say: "You cannot ignore National Institutes of Health funding priorities, upcoming changes in the DSM criteria, or, what is 'hot' in our field now. But while being practical, try to follow your scientific passion and listen to your data. Read widely and thoughtfully. Our goal, after all, is to try to understand the causes of these terrible disorders and grants are a means to that end, not the goal in themselves."

We hope that you find this volume stimulating and worthy of rereading. Our hope is that through your reading you will experience the synergism we have tried to build into this volume—that reading one chapter or comment will stimulate you to think in a new way about an earlier piece. As editors, we find the intellectual issues raised here fascinating and of deep relevance both to our own chosen field of psychiatry and to the broader enterprise of the "history and philosophy of science." We hope that you share in our excitement.

Reference

Hull, D.L. (1990). *Science as a Process: An Evolutionary Account of the Social and Conceptual Development of Science (Science and Its Conceptual Foundations series)*. Chicago, IL: University of Chicago Press.

Part I
Nature of historical change in science

Section 1
Objectivity and scientific change

Chapter 1

Introduction to "Pluralism, incommensurability, and scientific change"

Kenneth S. Kendler

The purpose of this conference was to gather philosophers, historians, and philosophically oriented psychiatrists and psychologists to discuss the nature of historical change in psychiatry. In the first chapter presented, Helen Longino lucidly sets the stage for what is to follow by making a critical distinction between two versions of this question—what I might call—the empirical and the proscriptive, or "normative." That is, we want to know how internal and external forces have impacted on historical change in psychiatry, and we want to ponder the deeper question of how *should* internal and external factors influence the development of our field. The normative question has a subtext that Longino articulates as follows: "What responses to internal versus external factors does our/my philosophical account of scientific knowledge make intelligible?"

In the main portion of her chapter, she reviews three major philosophical views of science and articulates how each would understand the nature of scientific change. For the first of these schools—the logical empiricists (aka logical positivists)—scientific knowledge is viewed as cumulative and progressive. Science itself produces knowledge that is objective and value-free. In terms of our question, the logical empiricists would be "internalists" all the way. As she cogently notes: "External concerns contaminate the scientific process. To permit them to enter into or to affect scientific processes is to abandon science for something else." This is a "purist" view of the scientific enterprise.

The second viewpoint—which she terms "holism"—reflects the perspective largely developed by Kuhn wherein scientific theories were inherent unities with interdependent rather than separable subunits. She focuses on the key concept of the theory-ladenness of meaning. This viewpoint was developed largely from a study of the history of science as exemplified in Kuhn's *The Structure of Scientific Revolutions* (Chalmers 1999). This holistic school has a very different view of historical change in science. As Kuhn articulated, we typically have slow incremental change over long periods of time in "normal science" working out the implications of given research paradigms. These long periods are then interrupted by more dramatic scientific revolutions where the rules of science and the associated world view shifts dramatically and a new paradigm is established. This perspective on scientific change departs from the strict internalist view of the logical empiricists. Change in science is produced by a whole range of empirical and social factors, often closely intertwined. As Longino notes, several different views of this holistic approach developed post Kuhn and included a more radical social constructivist view that would emphasize the central role of external factors as well as anarchic views of Feyerabend, who felt that in science "anything goes." Kuhn himself was more conservative, emphasizing a key set of scientific values that reflects an internalist perspective such as simplicity, accuracy, and explanatory power.

The third viewpoint that she reviews, which she calls "contextualism," treads a middle ground between the first two positions. This approach, she emphasizes, assumes that scientific change can occur in a wide array of ways from different motivations. General rules don't apply very well. Individual episodes of change are often *"context specific."* The Kuhnian "punctualist" model of change is seen as too restrictive. Instead, change goes on all the time in various forms. As she writes: "It can be prompted by new data, changes in cognitive needs, changes in scientific instrumentation, whether imaging tools, experimental devices, or the interview and questionnaire schedules of behavioral sciences, critical interaction within the community, or encounters with new approaches." In this viewpoint of science, the scientific enterprise is sometimes largely internal in nature but at other times will have been heavily influenced by external or contextual processes. She writes: "Philosophers and historians must engage in case-by-case analysis to determine if, what, and how social, political, and cultural values or interests have played a role in any given episode of change or adoption of approach."

Most readers will, I suspect, see the contextualist viewpoint as most appropriate for the field of psychiatry. This chapter provides a quite useful framework for what is to come later in this volume. It also illustrates how understanding the nature of change in a field as complex as psychiatry inevitably involves foundational questions about the nature of the scientific enterprise itself. It is the richness of these questions that motivated us to hold this conference in the first place.

Reference

Chalmers, A.F. (1999). *What is This Thing Called Science? An Assessment of the Nature and Status of Science and its Methods* (3rd ed.). Indianapolis, IN: Hackett Publishing Co.

Chapter 2
Pluralism, incommensurability, and scientific change

Helen E. Longino

2.1 Introduction

This chapter articulates three of the major philosophical approaches to scientific knowledge that underlie scientists' self-understandings and ground the things they are inclined to say about their practice. These approaches (logical empiricism, holism, and contextualism) offer different readings of the history of science and hence of the processes of scientific change as well as of the nature of diversity in science. Change is a response to some kind of novelty, so diversity is a precursor to change.

Kenneth Kendler, in his invitation to participants, posed a specific question about scientific change to the conferees:

> How [does] a field of working scientists respond to internal scientific advances versus external social, cultural, and political forces[?]

Here it is important to distinguish between two forms of the question. One is an empirical, sociological question:

> How in fact do [or have] communities of scientific researchers respond[ed] to such developments?

Historians, sociologists, and anthropologists of the sciences have offered a variety of responses to this empirical question, depending both on the details of the particular cases on which they focus and on the general philosophical approach to knowledge they adopt. The more philosophical versions of the question are either normative or analytic. The normative version is:

> How should communities respond to internal versus external factors?

Responses to this version of the question tend to presuppose an answer to this more analytic question:

> What responses to internal versus external factors does our/my philosophical account of scientific knowledge make intelligible?

Given the dependence of both the empirical and the normative understanding of the question on a philosophical view about the nature of scientific knowledge and/or inquiry, a review of the primary approaches that have been influential in recent decades seems in order.

I will focus on three philosophical approaches that offer sharply different assessments of the nature of scientific change as well as of diversity in the sciences: logical empiricism, holism, and contextualism. Each of these comes in both monist and pluralist flavors, which inflect their analyses of the nature of change and diversity. For each I will outline its relevant general features, its views of scientific change/diversity, its treatment of one example of behavioral research, and its recommendations with respect to Kenneth Kendler's question concerning internal and external factors. As a source of examples that give some content to the otherwise highly abstract notions to be invoked, I will rely on contemporary scientific research on aggression.[1] While aggression is not directly a psychiatric concept, the variety of approaches to its study overlap considerably with approaches to etiology in psychiatry, making it a suitable proxy for concepts that might be more controversial.

Recent aggression research shows change and diversity in

1. Conceptualization of its object: aggression is susceptible to various kinds of operationalization (that is, specification of measurable phenomena thought to be components of or signs of aggression) using tools from hospital, census, or criminal justice databases to questionnaires to self- and other-report. Different kinds of distinction (impulsive versus nonimpulsive, physical versus verbal, defensive versus instinctual) are also found in the literature.
2. Views of etiology: psychosocial, quantitative genetic, molecular genetic, neurological, interactive.
3. Valence: aggression has been studied as a factor in social dominance and leadership as well as in antisociality, criminality, and violence. As one it represents a trait to foster, as the other a trait to discourage.

2.2 Logical Empiricism

Logical empiricism is the version of empiricist epistemology that was originally developed by philosophers and philosophically minded scientists working in early twentieth-century Vienna and Berlin, and mid-twentieth-century Great Britain. It arrived in North America thanks to the forced exile or escape from Europe of Jews and intellectuals opposed to the Nazi Anschluss. Empiricism has a long history in philosophy, of course, having been developed as a systematic doctrine by the ancient Greeks. The twentieth-century *logical* empiricists, who included Rudolf Carnap, Moritz Schlick, Hans Reichenbach, and later Carl Hempel and Herbert Feigl, among others, were initially motivated to find ways to make sense of the changes in the content of scientific knowledge engendered by the replacement of

---

[1] The specific examples will be drawn from Longino (2013), a comparative epistemological, ontological, and social analysis of approaches to the investigation of human aggression and sexuality.

classical physics by relativity theory and quantum theory.[2] They also deplored the role metaphysics had played in nineteenth-century philosophy and social thought and were drawn to the formal systems of logic developed by Bertrand Russell and Gottlob Frege as tools for the systematization of science. It is their emphasis on the latter that gives this version of empiricism the designation "logical." Statements of scientific theories were held to be translatable into the notation of first-order logic thus facilitating representation of relations among scientific statements as logical ones, such as implication, consistency, inconsistency, or contradiction. This in turn enables a stricter, more regimented, interpretation of the empiricist commitment. In this regard, the logical empiricists first posited the necessity of a universal observation language (UOL). This is not a distinct language in the sense that English and Italian are distinct languages, but a specification of what will count as the basic units of observation and the terms that will refer to such units. There was debate about whether these units should be understood as sense data or as physical objects. What mattered is that there be such a set of terms specified as the basic nonlogical units of the formal system in terms of which all other terms could be defined. This permits articulation of the empiricist criterion of significance (articulated by David Hume in the eighteenth century):

1. All meaningful statements are either analytic or synthetic (either reducible to logical truths or expressive of actual or possible facts), and
2. A synthetic statement (expressive of actual or possible facts) is cognitively meaningful if and only if it is testable in sensory experience as that is representable in the UOL.

The logical systematization also permitted a more rigorous articulation of the empiricist view of theory or hypothesis justification. This is articulated in terms of confirmation. While there are refinements designed to eliminate empty justifications, confirmation of scientific claims consists fundamentally in ascertaining the truth of observation statements (expressible in the UOL) deducible from those claims. This is given form as the "hypothetico-deductivist" picture of scientific reasoning: articulate a hypothesis and specify its observable consequences (H → O, where H is a hypothesis, and O is a set of observation statements that will be true if H is true), then determine if the observations statements are true. This is given logical form as follows (again, this is the abstract form which received various refinements to exclude empty justifications):

$(H \rightarrow O) + (O_1, O_2, O_3, O_4, O_5, \ldots O_n)$ confirms H[3]
$(H \rightarrow O) + \text{not-}O_1$ (or $\text{not-}O_2$, or …) falsifies H.[4]

---

[2] See the essays in Giere and Richardson (1996) and in Hardcastle and Richardson (2003) for historical perspectives on the principal proponents of logical empiricism.

[3] See Hempel (1945) for a more precise articulation of the logical empiricist confirmation relation. The objections developed later hold for it as well.

[4] Karl Popper, whose work was admired by a great many scientists, emphasized falsification, and interpreted the criterion of significance in terms of falsifiability of claims (Popper 1963).

The activity of philosophers of science ought to be "rational reconstruction," that is, the organization of a theory into a deductive system, possibly an axiomatic system, all of whose terms are either in the UOL or defined in terms of the UOL, and all of whose statements are part of the deductive system, related to one another by the formal relations of implication or consistency. This enables the assessment of a theory via testing for consistency, testing of its observational consequences, and the elimination of those elements that cannot be tied down to the observational content of the theory.

Scientific change is theory change either by expansion or replacement. Theory change as replacement involves rejection of what is false/disconfirmed (or nonsense) in a prior theory and absorption of what is true/confirmed through its derivation from the principles of the new, replacing, theory. For example, relativity theory's replacement of classical physics involved rejection as false of claims about a luminiferous ether and rejection as nonempirical of claims of an absolute space and absolute time, but retention of the observation statements that were part of classical physics and their new derivation from the principles of relativity. The term given by logical empiricists to this kind of theory change was "reduction." In reduction, the meanings (of components of UOL) remain constant, and the pool of observational data constitutes a stable resource (changing only by expansion) against which to test all hypotheses.

Scientific knowledge, on this view, is cumulative and linearly progressive. Furthermore, a popular picture of scientific inquiry and knowledge as objective, value-free, and rational is spelled out in logical empiricist terms, and ratified by its formalization. This was a cold war picture of science as the source of knowledge of natural processes objectively arrived at which could then be put to human uses. It is also a conception of science bequeathed by the coiner of the term "positivist," August Comte. In this informal version, it is the view that all meaningful questions can be answered by empirical, scientific research, and that what is important is the accumulation of facts.

A logical empiricist approach to aggression research would require a specification of behavioral concepts in the UOL, that is, an operationalization that permits measurement of behavior, whether as episode or as disposition. Similarly, it would require a specification of the putative etiological factors in UOL, again an operationalization that permits precise measurement. Once the empirical concepts are thus tied down, it would be possible to identify observationally and/or experimentally the confirmed empirical generalizations. For example:

> N% of individuals experiencing abuse in childhood engage in aggressive behavior in young adulthood (where "abuse" and "aggressive behavior" have been given definitions in UOL).

Or:

> The brains of M% of individuals incarcerated for violent criminal offenses show reduced limbic area processing in PET scans compared to those of individuals incarcerated for nonviolent offenses.

How one proceeds from there is prescribed differently by the monist and pluralist flavors. The monist will either: (1) seek to identify the (causal) hypothesis/es that best fit/s the data, that is, the established empirical generalizations; or (2) seek to identify the (causal) hypothesis/es that fit/s the data and is/are potentially reducible to a theory at a lower (or more encompassing) level of explanation or of generality. The pluralist (e.g., a Carnap) would note that each rational reconstruction requires specification of a linguistic framework. The choice of such a framework (in which theoretical terms are defined in a UOL) is a pragmatic one leading to tolerance of multiple frameworks.

With its emphasis on the observable, logical empiricism was for a long time identified with behaviorism in psychology, but this identification presupposes that only behavioral concepts are susceptible to operational definitions, whereas nothing stands in the way of giving definitions in the UOL of nonbehavioral concepts, even of nonobservational concepts. The rub, of course, is that on the strict logical empiricist view, there is nothing more to the meaning of any term but its observational content as that is describable in the terms of the UOL.

As for the question Kenneth Kendler asked us all to consider, the logical empiricist offers a normative response: working scientists (and nonscientists) should respond only to internal developments, such as new data. External concerns contaminate the scientific process. To permit them to enter into or to affect scientific processes is to abandon science for something else.

Although it offered a powerful conception of empirical knowledge, logical empiricism encountered several insuperable problems. The first was internal: it simply was not possible to articulate the empiricist criterion of significance in a way that rules in the meaningful statements of scientific theories and rules out the pseudostatements of metaphysics. Terms like "mass" and "momentum" had meanings that exceeded their purely observational content, and even more damaging, the criterion of significance itself could not pass its own test.[5] The second was external as historically literate philosophers of science revealed that the actual history and practice of science failed to conform to the logical empiricist picture.

2.3 Holism (and History)

No publication had greater impact on thinking about scientific knowledge in the second half of the twentieth century than did Thomas Kuhn's *Structure of Scientific Revolutions* (1962/1996). While Kuhn is best known, N. Russell Hanson (1958) and Paul Feyerabend (1963, 1975) also argued for the theses of theory-ladenness associated with Kuhn. Contrary to the logical empiricists' picture of the anchoring of meaning in sensory experience, the holists argued that meaning flowed from theory to observation, that what Kuhn called paradigms (a congeries of theoretical ideas, methodological understandings, specific methods, cognitive aims, and values) determined the structure and content both of a theory's observational and experimental practices and of the language in which to describe them and their

---

[5] Hempel (1965) details the fate of the empiricist criterion of significance.

outcomes. Theories could only be understood as wholes, whose parts were interdependent rather than independent and modular.

The holists were persuaded to this view because of their studies of episodes in the history of science, especially the shifts from earth-centered to sun-centered astronomy, from Aristotelian physics to Newtonian, and then from Newtonian to relativity and quantum physics. As they read the record, successive theories, ostensibly about (at least some or much of) the same phenomena, made different and incompatible claims about the world. However, there is no straightforward way in which the successor theory either falsifies or reduces the ancestor theory, as expected in the logical empiricist view. Moreover, users of the ancestor were able to satisfy their cognitive needs by using the ancestor (until they couldn't). Astronomers were able to predict eclipses and the earth-centered astronomy remained perfectly satisfactory for navigation, for example.

Because language changed as theories changed, there could be no UOL. So while successive theories about the same phenomena were held to be incompatible—they could not both be true—they were also incommensurable—they could not be empirically evaluated vis-à-vis one another. In the transition from Aristotelian to Newtonian physics, and then later in the transition from classical physics to relativity theory, superficially shared terms like "matter", "mass," "energy, "time," and "space" changed their meaning. Incommensurability was at least threefold: (1) conceptual in that concepts borrowed from an earlier theory were seldom employed in the same way in the later theory, leading to misunderstanding between the two schools; (2) evaluative, in that what counted as a problem and what counted as an acceptable solution varied between them; and (3) experiential, in that adherents of different theories inhabit different worlds. As Kuhn (1996, p. 4) summed it up, "what differentiated these various schools was not failure of method [...] but what we shall come to call their incommensurable ways of seeing the world and of practicing science in it."

The emergence of holism in history and philosophy of science coincided with the distrust of authority fostered in the political ferment of the 1960s. Even though he disavowed such implications, in an ironic twist, Kuhn's book became the standard bearer for a popular counter-picture of science as nonobjective, value-laden (or value-susceptible), and nonrational. That this picture seemed to emerge from case histories gave it legitimacy and it was taken up and elaborated by humanists, social scientists, and by some philosophers dissatisfied by logical empiricist picture. The sociologists of science who came to be known as social constructivists took their inspiration from Kuhn, and the compelling nature of the historical analysis underlying the holist picture turned many philosophers to the defense of the rationality of science against what they perceived as a charge of irrationality.[6]

---

[6] For an early phase of the debate, see Lakatos and Musgrave (1970). This original divergence can be seen as the grounds of the "science wars" that characterized science studies in the 1990s.

Scientific change on the holist view is change of paradigm. According to Kuhn's version of holism, history reveals cycles of revolutionary and what he called normal science. Normal science, carried out under the auspices of a generally accepted paradigm (constituted of world view, methods and standards, typical problems, typical solutions, characteristic concepts), is disrupted by anomalies. Anomalies are experimental outcomes or observations that cannot be accommodated in the prevailing paradigm. While one or two can safely be ignored, the accumulation of anomalies inspires alternatives to the dominant paradigm. Eventually, one dominates and the activities of normal science resume under auspices of the new hegemonic paradigm (which involves a new world view, new meanings, and so forth). While there is progress within a paradigm as a theory becomes increasingly articulated with observations and measurement, science is neither cumulative nor progressive across revolutions.

A holist view of aggression research would treat each approach, whether successive or synchronic, as part of a paradigm: for example, genetic, psychosocial, neurobiological, integrative, and so on. These would be viewed as incommensurable: no shared language, even when terms seem identical. Here one might cite the expression "environment" which has different meanings in psychosocial approaches versus genetic approaches. In quantitative genetic approaches, environment is measured indirectly by reference to phenotypes and familial relatedness; in psychosocial approaches, environment is measured more directly: parental behavior and attitudes, features of the school environment, and so on. Monists and holists will have different prescriptions for diversity. Monist holists (of whom Kuhn is an example) will hold that normal science can only take place when one paradigm has achieved hegemonic status in the field. As long as there are multiple contesting paradigms, normal science is suspended. A pluralist holist (of whom Feyerabend is an example) will hold that insisting on a single paradigm stifles research. For the pluralist, more "paradigms" means more knowledge.

As for the question, "how [does] a field of working scientists respond to internal scientific advances versus external social, cultural, and political forces[?]," there are again several answers. Kuhn's social constructivist readers claimed that there is no in principle way to differentiate between these two types of input to scientific practice (Barnes and Bloor 1982; Shapin and Schaffer 1985). Kuhn himself, however, insisted that, continuous across paradigms and historical periods, there are values typical of science that, in abstract form, shape scientific responses to internal and external inputs. These include simplicity, accuracy, explanatory power, and others. While they may be interpreted and weighted differently in different paradigms, nevertheless the transparadigmatic adherence to these values, in the end, marks a scientific response from a nonscientific response (Kuhn 1977). The pluralist and epistemological anarchist Feyerabend, however, held that any rules (proscribing certain types of input) stifle science. Proscription of content of any kind is simply an exercise of unjustified power.

Holism also ran into problems. Many readers were concerned that holism made science deeply subjective and inaccessible to common norms of evaluation. One dimension of this problem is internal and has to do with the difficulty of making sense of the way theories could be both incompatible and incommensurable. Doesn't ascertaining incompatibility require some degree of commensurability? A second is more external in character and has to do with the psychological understanding of incommensurability and theory-ladenness promoted by the use of arguments from Gestalt psychology to illuminate theory-laden observation. This psychological approach underscores the subjectivist cast to the view and makes it hard to account for [what appear to be] instances of communication across paradigms.

One of the salutary effects of the emergence of the holist challenge was a turn away from the exclusively abstract models of the logical empiricists to analyses more grounded in actual science, either historical or contemporary. Philosophers attracted to either holism or logical empiricism engaged in various modifications of the views in efforts to overcome or sidestep the problems outlined. These efforts eventuated in a transformation in philosophy of science of the debates about knowledge between empiricists and holists into debates between instrumentalists (or antiscientific realists) and scientific realists about the referential character of scientific theories.[7]

2.4 Contextualism

The third major approach can be understood as weaving a line between logical empiricism and holism. It takes as a starting point an argument first advanced by the physicist and philosopher Pierre Duhem (1906/1954). Duhem pointed out that a theoretical hypothesis never directly implies the observational consequences that will serve to test it, but that assumptions are needed to establish the relevance of observational consequences to any given hypothesis. Thus the relation of confirmation or disconfirmation can never be represented as the formal one advanced by the logical empiricists (where $(H \to O) + O_1 \ldots O_n$, formally represents the confirmation relation for H and $(H \to O) + \text{not-}O_1 \ldots \text{not-}O_n$ represents the disconfirmation relation). Instead it must be represented as $((H + A) \to O) + O_1 \ldots O_n$. If researchers fail to observe any of O under circumstances when the hypothesis indicates they should be observed, one doesn't know whether the hypothesis (H) or the assumptions (A) are disconfirmed. When the relation between observation and hypothesis is thus mediated, observation is said to underdetermine hypothesis.

Duhem illustrated this argument, which has come to be known as the underdetermination argument, with examples from physics. Imagine a physicist testing the proposition that the vibration of a ray of light is parallel to the plane of polarization. S/he might set up conditions under which, if the proposition is

---

[7] For antirealist views modifying empiricism and holism respectively, see van Fraassen (1980) and Laudan (1981); for scientific realism, see Giere (1985) and Boyd (1983). "Instrumentalism" in this context refers to the view that scientific theories are instruments for prediction, not descriptions of reality.

true, alternating dark and light bands would be produced by intersecting rays of light. Duhem says that for this setup to constitute a genuine test, the physicist has to assume that "light consists of simple periodic vibrations, that these are normal to the light ray, that ... the mean kinetic energy of the vibratory motions is a measure of the intensity of the light ray" and so on. Similarly, in studies of behavior, researchers need to suppose that their measuring instruments (questionnaires, observation protocols, diagnostic criteria, and assay instruments) are adequate to capture variation in the phenomenon of interest, that responses to questionnaires of a particular kind are measures of dispositions to a particular behavior, and so on. The scope of this argument is quite general. There is, in general, a semantic gap between the statements articulating theoretical relations and the statements describing the data that can serve as evidence for those statements. We need only think about the difference in content between theoretical hypotheses in particle physics (about muons, pions, etc.) and the observations that serve as evidence (patterns in cloud chambers, or patterns in the ciphers imprinted on data tapes) or between hypotheses to the effect that a given behavioral disposition is the effect of certain hormonal exposures and statistical correlations of behavior and hormone exposure in a particular sample population (or set of such samples). The conclusion is that data alone cannot adjudicate among competing hypotheses/theories, because the assertions of hypotheses concern matters other than those described by the data statements. The relation between a theoretical hypothesis and evidence is always mediated by additional background assumptions, which form the context in which data acquire evidential relevance.

Contrary to logical empiricism, for contextualists, theoretical terms are independently meaningful, not defined in terms of a UOL. Contrary to holism, meanings can be retained across different theoretical frameworks. In the contextualist view, different background assumptions will assign different evidential relevance to the same data/observations. And, different theoretical approaches may make different data/observations evidentially relevant. There is no guarantee of a method that will, correctly followed, preserve scientific process/practice from influences of context, but at the same time, there is no insistence that all scientific change/judgment is influenced by context, or that there is some particular way in which it is so influenced. Philosophers and historians must engage in case-by-case analysis to determine if, what, and how social, political, and cultural values or interests have played a role in any given episode of change or adoption of approach.

Scientific change is, furthermore, multidimensional and ongoing, not an interruption to normal science, but the normal state of affairs. It can be prompted by new data, changes in cognitive needs, changes in scientific instrumentation, whether imaging tools, experimental devices, or the interview and questionnaire schedules of behavioral sciences, critical interaction within the community, or encounters with new approaches. Any of these types of change can prompt modification or abandonment of background assumptions. While the severity, pace, and abruptness of change may vary, on the contextualist view science is best understood as dynamic. The recent focus in philosophy on science as practice signals the shift to a more dynamic conception of scientific knowledge.[8] Monist contextualists anticipate the eventual identification of the right background assumptions that will both be correct and facilitate the arrival at the uniquely correct and ultimately unifiable set of theories of natural phenomena. Pluralist contextualists argue that there is no assumption-free method of determining the correct background assumptions, and that there may be phenomena that cannot be fully comprehended by means of a single theoretical approach. Instead full comprehension requires multiple approaches focused on different needs or answering to different questions about the same phenomena.[9]

When it comes to understanding aggression research, the contextualist view, which takes each approach on its own merits, notes that approaches investigating different etiologies may employ different or similar concepts; different or similar measuring strategies. For example, aggression and aggressive dispositions are measured using assessment tools that are shared across the approaches. The etiological factors studied and correlated with measured behavioral differences are, however, measured using tools that are proper to the etiological approach, whether that is quantitative behavior genetics, molecular behavior genetics, neurophysiology and anatomy, or the psychosocial approach that looks to social environmental factors.

For the contextualist, understanding evidential relations in these approaches requires identification of the background assumptions against which data (correlations of behaviors with putative etiological factors) acquire evidential relevance. For the monist, although she may not go so far as to dismiss the research as science for lack of a single hegemonic paradigm, the persistence of a diversity of approaches is nevertheless a problem that must be overcome before it is possible to talk about knowledge. There are two options for the monist here: either the "bon sens," or good sense, of the scientist that Duhem claimed would prevail, or a supposition that all but the correct assumption can be eliminated by more empirical research directed at the assumptions, rather than at the hypotheses directly. But, of course, the reason Duhem had to resort to "bon sens" is precisely that the empirical investigation of assumptions will itself be subject to the same underdetermination argument to which the empirical investigation of hypotheses is subject. And surely one scientist's good sense will not be identical to another's. Were a univocal good sense shared, there would not be as many debates within the sciences as there are.

The pluralist, on the other hand, can argue that critical discourse among members of a community weeds out many background assumptions, but not all. Plurality of approaches is a resource, not a hindrance. Refining and improving the methods of a given approach enables researchers to produce better knowledge

---

[8] Signaled by the founding of the Society for the Philosophy of Science in Practice in 2006.
[9] See Longino (2001).

within that particular framework but does not produce tools—either in the form of data or of methods—for cross-approach empirical evaluation. Behavior genetics and psychosocial approaches can each improve their measurement strategies, concepts, etc. but these internal improvements diminish the approaches' capacity for cross-approach comparative evaluation. On the contextualist view, there can be meaning commensurability in the sense that practitioners in one approach can understand the terms used in other approaches, but there is frequently *measurement* incommensurability, because measurement strategies in approaches investigating different etiological factors may be based on noncongruent representations of the causal field.[10] The complexity of a phenomenon, like human aggression, even when carefully operationalized, may mean plurality never resolves into a single comprehensive approach. This contextualist pluralism (or pluralistic contextualism) finds the identification of a scientific approach to psychological and behavioral phenomena exclusively with a biological approach such as behavior genetics or neurophysiology limiting and puzzling. As the survey of research on aggression shows, psychosocial and sociological approaches are just as scientific (e.g., involving rigorous measurement and careful statistical analysis) and contribute information and understanding not obtainable from the purely biological. Full understanding may require plurality.

Turning to Kenneth Kendler's question: "how [does] a field of working scientists respond to internal scientific advances versus external social, cultural, and political forces[?]" there is no single answer to the empirical question. This will depend on how "field" is understood and on the actual responses of individuals. But the contextualist will question the division into "advances" and "forces"; there may be social and other advances that prompt change of observational vocabulary, questions, and measurement strategy. One need only think of the changes that feminism, antiracism, and the movement for homosexual rights have induced in the medical and behavioral sciences, including psychiatry. As assumptions about gender differences, about race, and about sexual orientation were exposed as biased, those assumptions were abandoned, opening the way to different understandings of gendered, racialized, and sexual experience. And there may be internal advances that support change of social and other configurations, as research on stereotype threat and implicit bias promises to do. While none will countenance proclaiming as fact what is only wished for, contextualists acknowledge a more constructive role for interests and values in the complex practices of scientific inquiry than do other philosophical approaches. Furthermore, the contextualist claims that a contextualist understanding of inquiry is best situated to identify and expose to critical analysis those values and interests that may be embedded in the background assumptions of an approach.

Contextualism, like its predecessors, has challenges. If pluralism is the price that must be paid for saving objectivity and rationality, are objectivity and

---

[10] See Longino (2013).

rationality really saved? How does one place a boundary between what is context and what is contextualized? Addressing these questions lies in the future of contextualism.

2.5 Conclusion

It is tempting to blame commitments to a logical empiricist conception of scientific methodology for some of the ills of one's chosen science. And indeed, such commitments can stifle innovative thinking, but there are well-developed alternatives to logical empiricism. Contextualism, in particular, retains the epistemological empiricism of logical empiricism, but develops a much more flexible and pluralist understanding of methodology. This is an approach that is friendly to innovative thinking without abandoning the commitment to observation, experiment, and measurement that are the hallmarks of scientific thinking. I have outlined six ways to respond to diversity and change in the sciences: monist and pluralist forms of logical empiricism, holism, and contextualism. Each offers different understandings and different prescriptions. My hope is to have shown that responses to the facts of diversity and change get their support from more encompassing views about the nature of scientific knowledge, and thus that their assessment depends on the tenability of those more encompassing views.

References

Barnes, B. and Bloor, D. (1982). Relativism, rationalism and the sociology of knowledge. In M. Hollis and S. Lukes (eds.) *Rationality and Relativism*, pp. 21–47. Cambridge, MA: MIT Press.

Boyd, R. (1983). On the current status of the issue of scientific realism. In C.G. Hempel, H. Putnam, and W. Essler (eds.) *Methodology, Epistemology, and Philosophy of Science*, pp. 45–90. Dordrecht, Netherlands: Springer.

Duhem, P. (1954). *Aim and Structure of Physical Theory*. (P.P. Wiener, trans.) Princeton, NJ: Princeton University Press. (Originally published in 1906 as *La Théorie Physique: Son Objet et Sa Structure*.)

Feyerabend, P.K. (1963). Explanation, reduction, and empiricism. In H. Feigl and G. Maxwell (eds.) *Scientific Explanation, Space and Time*, pp. 28–97. Minneapolis, MN: University of Minnesota Press.

Feyerabend, P.K. (1975). *Against Method*. London: Verso.

Giere, R. (1985). Constructive realism. In P. Churchland and C. Hooker (eds.) *Images of Science*, pp. 76–99. Chicago, IL: University of Chicago Press.

Giere, R. and Richardson, A. (eds.) (1996). *Origins of Logical Empiricism*. Minneapolis, MN: University of Minnesota Press.

Hanson, N.R. (1958). *Patterns of Discovery*. Cambridge: Cambridge University Press.

Hardcastle, G. and Richardson, A. (eds.) (2003). *Logical Empiricism in North America*. Minneapolis, MN: University of Minnesota Press.

Hempel, C.G. (1945). Studies in the logic of confirmation. *Mind*, 54(213), 1–26.

Hempel, C.G. (1965). Empiricist criteria of cognitive significance: problems and changes. In *Aspects of Scientific Explanation and Other Essays in the Philosophy of Science*, 101–119. New York, NY: Free Press.

Kuhn, T. (1977). Objectivity, value judgment, and theory choice. In *The Essential Tension*, pp. 320–339. Chicago, IL: University of Chicago Press.

Kuhn, T. (1996). *The Structure of Scientific Revolutions* (3rd ed.). Chicago, IL: University of Chicago Press. (Originally published in 1962.)

Lakatos, I. and Musgrave, A. (eds.) (1970). *Criticism and the Growth of Knowledge*. Cambridge: Cambridge University Press.

Laudan, L. (1981). A confutation of convergent realism. *Philosophy of Science*, 48(1), 19–49.

Longino, H.E. (2001). *The Fate of Knowledge*. Princeton, NJ: Princeton University Press.

Longino, H.E. (2013). *Studying Human Behavior: How Scientists Investigate Aggression and Sexuality*. Chicago, IL: University of Chicago Press.

Popper, K. (1963). *Conjectures and Refutations*. London: Routledge.

Shapin, S. and Schaffer, S. (1985). *Leviathan and the Air-Pump: Hobbes, Boyle, and the Experimental Life*. Princeton, NJ: Princeton University Press.

Van Fraassen, B. (1980). *The Scientific Image*. Oxford: Oxford University Press.

Chapter 3

For objective, value-laden, contextualist pluralism

John Dupré

I am generally very sympathetic to Longino's useful survey of the various main approaches to understanding scientific change. Like Longino, I think that the most defensible approach is contextualist and pluralist, and that this is the approach that will be most useful for understanding scientific change in a field as complex and diverse as psychiatry. I shall briefly discuss in these comments some areas of probably quite minor disagreement. The main suggestion I want to make is that the taxonomy that Longino presents is in the end more complex than necessary; in particular I think the differences she describes between holism and contextualism reduce very closely to the differences between monism and pluralism, so that setting aside more minor internal debates her taxonomy can be reduced to four approaches rather than six. I shall then conclude with some very brief comments on the topics of value-ladenness and objectivity. With regard to the former, Longino doesn't say much here on this topic, but what she does say suggests a somewhat more restricted view of the entanglement of fact and value in science than I think is appropriate within the context of a pluralist empiricism. This, I think, is the site of one of the most fundamental divisions between logical empiricism on the one hand, and both holism and contextualism on the other. I'll conclude, finally, by suggesting that worries she alludes to about objectivity should not be worrying.

Longino doesn't say much about pluralist holists. She says, "A pluralist holist (of whom Feyerabend is an example) will hold that insisting on a single paradigm stifles research. For the pluralist, more 'paradigms' means more knowledge." Later she writes that "[t]he pluralist and epistemological anarchist Feyerabend, however, held that any rules (proscribing certain types of input) stifle science. Proscription of content of any kind is simply an exercise of unjustified power," and therefore rejected any way of distinguishing scientific from nonscientific inputs into the scientific process. I must confess to being rather an admirer of Feyerabend, though certainly I don't espouse unlimited epistemological anarchy. But at any rate I don't think holist pluralism needs to be associated with anarchy. Indeed, to get to my first point, I think it is very close to pluralist contextualism.

What's wrong with holism? A point that Longino stresses is that it is very hard to reconcile incommensurability of theories with their incompatibility, as Kuhn, at least, the paradigm holist, appears to want to do. As she says, "Doesn't ascertaining incompatibility require some degree of commensurability?" This is a problem, I take it, for a monist holist like Kuhn, someone who sees the progress of science as a sequence of incompatible and incommensurable theories each superseding the previous one. But surely no pluralist will want to say that different theories are always incompatible, since she is by definition someone who thinks that multiple theories should coexist?[1]

Contextualism is, moreover, in obvious respects a holistic doctrine. Kuhn argued that a theory could only be understood in relation to a paradigm, in the sense of that term that refers to the background assumptions, methods, instruments, and so on involved in the application of the theory. Similarly the Quine/Duhem thesis, which Longino sees as the starting point for contextualism, emphasizes the context—background assumptions and so on—relative to which a theory must be applied or, crucially, tested. I agree with Longino that complete incommensurability, the inability of any meanings to transfer across theoretical frameworks, is implausible; my point is just that the move to pluralism, the advocacy of concurrent theories in the same domain, already pretty much commits one to rejecting such total incommensurability. I don't mean to imply that the contextualism that Longino advances, and has done much to develop, differs from Kuhnian holism only in respect of pluralism. I do think that the moves are so closely connected that it is more helpful to think in terms of a more linear sequence of positions: logical empiricism (monist or pluralist), holism (Kuhnian, monist), and contextualism (holist, pluralist). There are of course many differences among contemporary contextualists/pluralists, but I think they are arguments within the same camp—the camp in which both Longino and myself, I think, believe that psychiatrists should pitch their tents. As for Feyerabend, I'm not sure how deep his commitment to incommensurability went, but he at least deserves credit as a pioneer of pluralism.

Longino is mainly concerned in her chapter to lay out options and she doesn't spend a lot of time defending the position that she advocates, contextualist pluralism. So let me mention what I take to be the most basic reason why this is the position that psychiatry should embrace to answer the questions posed by Kenneth Kendler. Psychiatry deals with problems of enormous complexity, the human mind and its relation to the social environment. Scientific models always and necessarily provide only partial perspectives on real phenomena and the more complex the phenomena the more necessary it will become to provide multiple such perspectives if we are to answer the full range of questions about them that we want to address. As Longino notes, scientific models address specific questions or interests. Models focus on the features of an entity that are relevant to a particular kind of concern, and ignore, as far as possible, features that are of little relevance. A model is in many respects like a map, and as Borges has reminded us, a "perfect" map is simply a recapitulation of the reality we are trying to map, and is consequently entirely useless. But given the partiality of useful maps, or models,

---

[1] A pluralist who has taken up in detail the interactions between different perspectives on complex issues is Sandra Mitchell (2003).

it seems unlikely that one such partial perspective will be sufficient to address our various interests.

Perhaps the greatest benefit for psychiatry in embracing pluralism is that it gives the right perspective, I think, on the problem that has been so central to the philosophy of the subject, nosology. There is no reason to assume that there is one uniquely best way of classifying mental illness. An obvious possibility along these lines is that classifications for purposes of social policy may be quite different from those best suited to therapeutic uses. For example (and the example is entirely hypothetical, given my lack of relevant expertise) it could be that attention deficit hyperactivity disorder is an excellent classificatory concept for addressing questions in educational policy, while being of little use for determining individual treatment. It might be, that is to say, that specific deficiencies in the education system generated a cluster of related psychiatric conditions differing substantially in their individual expression. Some of these might belong, from a therapeutic perspective, in quite different clusters.

Longino makes this point in more detail with the example of aggression. As she writes:

> Aggression is susceptible to various kinds of operationalization (that is, specification of measurable phenomena thought to be components of or signs of aggression) using tools from hospital, census, or criminal justice databases to questionnaires to self- and other-report. Different kinds of distinction (impulsive versus non-impulsive, physical versus verbal, defensive versus instinctual) are also found in the literature.

From a pluralist perspective this is just what one might expect and, crucially, there is no reason to think that there is anything fundamentally misguided about any of these operationalizations. Conversely—and this is perhaps the more important and challenging point—there is always a risk that one is using a concept of aggression that works well in one context, but does not carry over effectively into the context into which it is being transplanted.

One of the benefits that Longino claims—rightly in my opinion—for the pluralist position, is that different perspectives can be effective in detecting the biases in other, often more mainstream perspectives. This is an idea that has been influentially developed in much of Longino's earlier work. Feminist science and science studies, in particular, have been extremely successful in highlighting sexist biases in many areas of science. I would like, however, to add a slight caution. It might be concluded from what Longino says here that the aim of science is to remove biases altogether and thus recapture the logical empiricist ideal of a value-free science. But this, I suggest, is impossible.

What would be a value-free concept of aggression? The point of talking about aggression is that we think it is a bad thing, a kind of behavior that we would like to discourage.[2] It is a condition of adequacy of any operationalization of the concept that the behavior it captures is behavior of which we disapprove. The only options are value-ladenness or irrelevance. In the end, of course, this supports

---

[2] I do recall that when I first lived in the United States I was quite surprised to discover that "aggressive" was used as a fairly general term of approbation. It carried connotations, I suppose, of forcefulness, determination, and suchlike. I suppose that this kind of

Longino's main position. The values that we use in deciding what is an inappropriate level of aggression may well differ among people or groups of people, and multiple perspectives may, in the way Longino proposes, help to provide, if not a value-neutral view, at least one that reflects a wider consensus on values.[3]

Longino's paper ends with some questions that she thinks contextualism still needs to face:

> Contextualism, like its predecessors, has challenges. If pluralism is the price that must be paid for saving objectivity and rationality, are objectivity and rationality really saved? How does one place a boundary between what is context and what is contextualized? Addressing these questions lies in the future of contextualism.

I'm not persuaded that the first question is one that still needs to be addressed. I think there is a perfectly clear answer: scientific models of complex phenomena are necessarily partial and different models address different parts. I don't see why this implies any lack of objectivity or rationality. We might wonder whether at some imagined end of inquiry the sum of all possible models will equate to the complete truth about a phenomenon. I find this an extremely dubious prospect, but even if it is true I do not see why it threatens the rationality of the models we have now. As for objectivity, it is no doubt the case, for reasons that Longino herself has explored in great detail, that particular models incorporate particular value-laden assumptions and are less than fully objective. And, as again Longino is well known for insisting, the best approach to objectivity is to develop multiple perspectives that reveal the biases in contrasting approaches. I think that pluralism and contextualism offer as much rationality and objectivity as we have any reason to seek.

The second question is harder. Indeed the question of boundaries that separate an entity under investigation from its context seems to me a deep metaphysical problem posed by developing understandings throughout the life sciences. From molecular biology to sociology, I believe, what something is depends profoundly on the context on which it exists. In psychiatry, I assume, no one would suppose that an individual patient could be understood as entirely distinct from the social, familial, etc. context in which they lived and had lived. This presents problems for contextualists and everyone else, and no doubt there are other problems. Thankfully these comments are not the place to try to solve them.

References

Dupré, J. (2012). *Processes of Life: Essays in the Philosophy of Biology*. Oxford: Oxford University Press.

Mitchell, S.D. (2003). *Biological Complexity and Integrative Pluralism*. Cambridge: Cambridge University Press.

---

aggressiveness is not generally treated as calling for psychiatric treatment at least in the United States.

[3] I discuss the inextricability of science and values in much more detail in Dupré (2012, chapter 3).

Section 2
Change in psychopathology

Chapter 4

Introduction to "History and epistemology of psychopathology"

Josef Parnas

Chapter 5 by German Berrios is very dense and demanding, requiring a lot of attention and, preferably, some theoretical background as well. However, this should not scare a potential reader because the chapter is accessible even if one does not fully grasp all of its conceptual and theoretical references. The topic is "change in psychopathology," more specifically, a change in clinical manifestations over large spans of history (i.e., centuries). It is an important topic with questions such as "Has schizophrenia always existed?" and "Has the frequency or severity of schizophrenia changed over the last 100 years?" The answers to such questions have important implications, for example, on etiological considerations. Berrios makes it clear from the outset that trying to answer such questions is an extremely difficult task that depends on a host of epistemological and other philosophical assumptions. Berrios's chapter therefore presents certain preparatory steps in clarifying basic metaphysical issues and our conceptualization of the nature of mental symptoms.

First, what *is* change? It may be a quantitative or a qualitative change in properties (*metamorphosis*) or even a *replacement*, where the change is so extreme that the object changes its identity from being A to being B. The next question is *what exists* that may change, that is, what kind of entities populate our universe that may be subject to change. If we ask an ordinary man on the street the two most important metaphysical questions "What is?" and "Who are you?", he will likely answer: "There are things and I am John Smith." In fact, says Berrios, the matter is more complicated, although he refrains from addressing the second question (of the Who). We have: (1) a category of being with spatiotemporal existence, comprising *things* (e.g., tables or neurons) and *processes* (e.g., digestion, typically involving duration); (2) *events* (discontinuants), predominantly temporal (e.g., sneezes or explosions); (3) *abstract objects* (such as numbers or geometrical objects); and (4) *ideal objects* (such as beauty or justice). Consciousness and social/cultural institutions (e.g., presidential elections) are not listed as distinct categories and Berrios leaves their metaphysical status unclarified. We learn however that *mental* symptoms occupy an ambiguous metaphysical position. In the current neurobiological model of psychiatry, mental symptoms are, erroneously according to Berrios, considered as *things*, that is, *identical without any residuum* to "pathological changes in the structure or function of the brain"—a continuation of what Berrios designates as the "anatomico-clinical model of disease," introduced in France at the beginning of the nineteenth century. In other words, psychiatry, an offshoot of neurology, carelessly adopted the biomedical model of symptom formation. Yet a mental symptom cannot be equated with its putative substrate; rather it is a "hybrid," with traces of biological "signal" and with semantic components and its formation is the result of a *constructive* process of conceptualization and linguistic embodiment. The symptom is not something that arrives entirely passively but is co-constructed by the sufferer and it has often a pragmatic, *performative* significance (the patient obtains something through his symptom). Berrios' symptom model (the so-called Cambridge model) proposes—heavily relying on the analogy with external perception—that "mental symptoms result from cultural configuration of prelinguistic information that penetrates the sufferer's awareness" and "causes discomfort, bewilderment, or emotional upheaval. This information may be of biological and semantic origin."

In other words, the symptom is formed when an aberrant signal penetrates the threshold of consciousness but is unmet because it is unmatched by the repertoire of sociolinguistic "templates" available to the sufferer's mental apparatus, normally needed to configure (conceptualize) the signal in an automatic and unproblematic way. This requires therefore a novel and anomalous configuration, that is, a formation of a symptom. Unfortunately, the notions of *information* or *signal* are not well clarified in this chapter, so readers might find it difficult to understand what it is that constitutes the information *as* information or what constitutes the identity of the signal. The phenomenal nature of prereflective awareness and its relation to the linguistic level are not explored here. This is not surprising because we are approaching in these issues the "explanatory gap" or the "hard problem" of consciousness (our inability to conceive how something mental arises from the physical substrate). The Cambridge model allows for many different specific articulations, and, according to Berrios, it provides an adequate tool for analyzing historical changes in psychopathology. The Cambridge model has a predecessor and also a more contemporary, empirically oriented version. A closely similar model was proposed in 1928 by Charles Blondel, a professor of clinical psychology at the University of Strasbourg. In a fascinating analysis of seven psychotic cases, Blondel, inspired by Levy-Brühl (an anthropologist) and Bergson (a proto-phenomenological philosopher), proposed that when certain prereflective affections surpassed the subject's capacity for a socially adequate, linguistic-communicative discharge, a psychiatric symptom was formed through a sociodystonic, highly subjective conceptualization (Blondel 1928). More recently, a German research group (Gerd Huber, Gisela Gross, Joachim Klosterkötter, et al.) initiated a still ongoing research program on the so-called basic symptom model of the formation of first-rank symptoms (Klosterkötter 1988). Here, the first stage is of "basic irritation," with unspecific sensations and complaints ("signals," proximate to the physiological substrate (*"substratnahe"*)), which over time, and in interaction with the environment, become progressively (with intermediate, symptomatically more articulated stages) formed as concrete symptoms ("concretization"), infused with semantic content ("thematization"), and externalized (e.g., as voices or influence phenomena).

Berrios' analysis of basic metaphysical and epistemological issues relevant for psychiatry and his model of symptom formation is rich food for thought. This is especially important today, when psychiatry again seems to be confronting its foundational psychopathological and epistemological questions (Parnas and Bovet, Chapter 23, this volume).

References

Blondel, C. (1928). *Conscience Morbide. Essai de psychopathologie générale.* Paris: Librairie Félix Alcan.

Klosterkötter, J. (1988). *Basissymptome und Endphänomene bei Schizophrenie.* Berlin: Springer.

Chapter 5

History and epistemology of psychopathology

German E. Berrios

5.1 Introduction

It is a common clinical observation that mental symptoms do change in response to: (1) therapy or (2) the passage of time (chronicity). Treatment-related changes are mostly quantitative (e.g., reductions in frequency or severity) and may help to evaluate outcome (Berrios 2008). Time-related changes are qualitative (e.g., stereotyped, degraded, and experientially empty complaints) and are met with in the chronic stages of mental disorders (Lanteri-Laura 1972). A third form of change, affecting the phenomenological profile of symptoms or disorders may also be possible. Noticed or suspected by historians of psychiatry and theme of this chapter, this type of change: (1) occurs over centuries rather than decades (i.e., it is secular), (2) can be both qualitative and quantitative, and (3) can also preside over the disappearance of some clinical states, (e.g., acedia[1] and aural hematoma[2])

---

[1] In classical Greece the word "acedia" (*akēdia*) meant carelessness and indifference (Liddell and Scott 1994; Marinas 2004). Early in the second millennium, together with a cluster of behaviours which included tedium, sloth, and suicidal behaviour, the word acedia was made to enter into a convergence and conceptualized as a clinical cum religious "disorder." It soon became epidemic, affecting most monasteries in Europe where it led to the death or malfunctioning of novices. To deal with this serious problem abbots and heads of houses saw fit to meet on various occasions (Crislip 2005; Jehl 1984; Wenzel 1967). By the fourteenth century Acedia had almost disappeared. Efforts to diagnose it retrospectively have repeatedly failed because its unique behavioural profile can only be understood against a social and religious context which is no more (e.g., Forthomme 2000).

[2] Aural hematoma named an "effusion of blood or of bloody serum between the cartilage of the ear and its perichondrium, occurring in certain forms of insanity and sometimes among the sane". It had a prodromal period during which local turgescence and swelling appeared. Onset was sudden: "as a rule, the patient may have gone to bed with ears perfectly normal, and have a developed othematoma in the morning". The left ear was most commonly affected. The condition was worse "in those forms of insanity in which the mental excitement runs high for any length of time." Aural hematoma had a natural history, clinical correlations, pathological anatomy, genetics, etiology, and treatment. It thus became standard science and was an obligatory question in the examinations for the

and the appearance of new ones (e.g., catatonia[3], schizophrenia,[4] or anxiety disorders[5]).

Terms such as metamorphosis, becoming, modification, flow, adaptation, renewal, etc., name properties inherent in the model of "Nature" currently sponsored by both physics and biology (Coates 1998; Farago 2000).[6] Darwinian theory predicts that changes in the structure and profile of biological species (evolution) are brought about by an interplay of genetic variation, adaptation, and natural selection (Tort 1996). Social and cultural theory likewise posits that "change" is an inevitable result of human interaction (Boudon 1984; Mink 1968; Williams 1966, Wilson et al. 2013). Indeed, throughout history "change" and "flow" (and not "static" being) have been periodically considered to be the essential property of the world (Davies 1900; Graham 2006). Against this omnipresence of change, why should mental symptoms and disorders be expected to remain invariant and unchanging?

Of particular interest to the epistemologist, secular change raises important issues in regards to the nature, etiology, duration, and management of the "objects of psychiatry" (Berrios 2011). Firstly, such change would call into question the assumption that mental symptoms and disorders are ontological stable, that is, they are "natural kinds" (Campbell et al. 2011; Murphy 2006). Secondly, if they are subject to secular change then the entire body of "psychiatric knowledge" (namely, clinical descriptions and the network of correlations

---

specialization in alienism. J.F. Pieterson, its "discoverer," was a respected mental asylum superintendent and his new disease constituted a perfect example of historical convergence (word + concept + behaviour or physical change) (Berrios 1999a).

[3] Catatonia is another perfect example of convergence in the work of an alienist called Kahlbaum (1874) who in a small book brought together a neologism (Katatonie), a concept (disease of muscular tension), and a set of signs, symptoms, and behaviors (Berrios 1981). The new disease became popular and was frequently diagnosed. Kraepelin felt obliged to include it under his portmanteau dementia praecox. Clinical and statistical re-analysis of the original cases studied by Kahlbaum has shown that many were suffering from basal ganglia disorders (Berrios 1996). By the middle of the twentieth century, writers were beginning to wonder where all the patients suffering from catatonia had gone (Fink and Taylor 2006; Mahendra 1981; Ungvari et al. 2006)

[4] There is little point in rehearsing the history of the construction of "schizophrenia". It includes two successive historical convergences: one by Kraepelin that gave rise to the concept of dementia praecox; and the other, undertaken by Bleuler that, in addition to "re-naming" dementia praecox, also replaced the concept and the cluster of behaviours in question (Berrios et al. 2003).

[5] The "anxiety disorders" resulted from a series of historical convergences the first of which was proposed by Freud (Berrios 1999b). This clinical category did not exist before the 1890s (Berrios 2014).

[6] Like all the grand concepts that form part of Western culture, "Nature" has gone through various redefinitions and each in its time has governed the manner in which Nature is perceived (David 2004; Kaulbach 1984)

linking them to the brain) must be considered as temporary and in need of periodic updating (Berrios 1999c). To deal with these issues more needs to be known about the nature and constitution of the objects of psychiatry. Equally important is to have a model of symptom formation that explains how mental symptoms are inscribed in the brain. Available correlational networks bridging complaints and brain regions cannot be considered as sufficient (Berrios and Marková 2002a, 2002b).

A model of symptom formation will also clarify the issue of whether sufferers are "passive" recipients of their mental symptoms (i.e., whether they "happen" onto them as might a bolt from the sky) or whether they are active participants in the construction of their complaints. Indeed, it will be proposed in this chapter that mental symptoms are veritable "mental acts" (Proust 2010). This should not only help to understand "change" in general but also suggest new ways to manage complaints. For example, a correlation between symptom S and brain site B should no longer be considered as constituting a sufficient ethical warrant for therapeutically intervening on site B. It would also be necessary to know the level of participation of the sufferer in the construction of his complaint and his reasons for doing so.

To study change, the psychiatrist needs a metalanguage (lexicon, definitions, and concepts), a methodology (how best to map "change"), and a theory of mental symptom formation. Unavailability of these tools explains why debates on "whether schizophrenia existed before the eighteenth century" (e.g., Berrios et al. 2003; Ellard 1987; Jeste et al. 1985) or whether "catatonia has changed since the nineteenth century" (Berrios 1981; Mahendra 1981) could not reach satisfactory conclusion at the time. After a brief account of the general concepts involved, the question will be explored of whether the objects of psychiatry do suffer secular change. It will be concluded that they do, and that their change may be due both to evolution (affecting their biology) and to social shifts (affecting their construction).

5.2 Defining "change" in General

Albeit omnipresent, "change" is difficult to define and has an ambiguous meaning: "A has changed" may mean that "A" has undergone "metamorphosis" or "replacement" (Hyslop 1910; Osier 1990; Rhodes 1909). Metamorphosis refers to shifts in the properties of A; on occasions, property change may threaten the identity of A. "Replacement" means that "B" has taken the place of "A." In daily conversation, this semantic ambiguity is usually resolved by shared additional knowledge on the object under discussion, its context, and the interlocutor's intentions. Perceiving and monitoring change is easier in the case of "natural kinds," that is, concrete entities with stable baseline properties such as stones, people, dogs, or orchids (Keil 1989; Laporte 2004). It is harder for entities such as clouds, fires, and rivers, and even harder for "events" such as sneezes and explosions. One way of dealing with change affecting "events"

(Mellor 1998) may be to consider them as tokens or expressions of an "ideal type" (Rogers 1969).[7]

The obscurities surrounding the concept of "change" are deeply rooted in the past. Thus, in classical Greece concepts such as "change," "movement," and "becoming" were intertwined under the term "kinesis" (Chantraine 1968, p. 533; Liddell and Scott 1994; Weigelt 2004). Philosophical and scientific developments (particularly in mechanics) led to the separation of "movement" as an independent category (Fink 1957; Lange 1886). "Becoming" and "change" were, in due course, redefined in terms of foundational notions such as "property" and "time." This has helped to differentiate "real" change from "Cambridge change," the term that Geach introduced to refer to Russell's logical definition of change (1969, pp. 71–72).[8] Thus, when it comes to exploring "change" in relation to the objects of psychiatry, it should be important to separate their essential and accidental properties[9] and decide whether it is more appropriate for such objects the use of a "tensed" or "tenseless" definition of time (Dyke 2013).[10] To avoid becoming entangled in some of these serious philosophical issues, "change" will be defined in this chapter as both metamorphosis and exchange, and the "properties" in question will be chosen in relation to each individual mental symptom.

The world is populated by: (1) categories of being (continuants and discontinuants), (2) abstract objects (e.g., numerical sets and geometrical objects), and (3) "necessary" beings (e.g., God) (Campbell 2006). Continuants can be roughly subdivided into: things, like dogs, neurons, diamonds, tables, etc., that is, entities whose endurance in time and in space allows for a stable listing of their properties; and processes like digestion, a concert, a football match, or a revolution, whose quiddity unfolds more in time than in space. Discontinuants, also called events, occurrences, or happenings (e.g., sneezes or explosions) are entities whose essence

---

[7] For example, the statement "a change in sneezes at world level was only noticed after 2013" would only make sense if an "ideal type" for sneezes is constructed and monitored for a number of years. "Ideal type," a concept introduced by Max Weber to deal with issues in economics and sociology, can be defined as "an attempt to capture what is essential about a social phenomenon through an analytical exaggeration of some of its aspects" (Swedberg 2005, p. 115). It is not, as it is sometimes believed, an "average" of a sample of such phenomena.

[8] "Cambridge change" refers to shifts in the external properties of objects, for example, in the position of an object in relation to other objects or in its name (e.g., renaming or repositioning of a mental symptom or disorder—as it can be noticed in successive editions of DSM). This type of change does not really affect the essence or definition of the object in question and hence will not be mentioned further (Geach 1969).

[9] At its simplest, essential properties are those without which the object will cease to be what it is; accidental properties are those whose absence will not affect it.

[10] "Tensed time" refers to the view that although past, present, and future do exist, they are not equally real for future is not yet fixed or determinate. "Tenseless time" refers to the belief that all three categories are equally real and that the fact that it is known less about the future than the past is not ontological but epistemological in nature (Callender 2011).

is more related to time than space. Hence it makes sense to say that "change" affects continuants and discontinuants in a different way. How we talk about "change" in relation to the objects of psychiatry does, therefore, depend upon the type of entity the latter are considered to be (more on this later).

5.3 Change in Psychopathology

"Alienism" (now called psychiatry) was the name of a discipline and trade constructed during the nineteenth century to explain and manage madness from a medical perspective (Berrios 2012). Coined in German in 1845, the term "psychopathology" was eventually used to refer to the nascent language of alienism.[11] As a metalanguage, it was meant both to capture in words the phenomena of madness and to construct units of analysis for the objects of psychiatry (Berrios 1984). Mental disorders thus became clusters of mental symptoms (the units of analysis) held together by some notional (etiology) glue. The ensuing semiology of madness (in the image of the semiology of medicine) (Landré-Beauvais 1813)[12] presented itself as a form of "atheoretical" descriptivism,[13] that is, as a neutral narrative of what patients said and did (Berrios 1993).

In practice, the language of psychopathology operated by breaking up the categories of mental alienation in vogue at the beginning of the nineteenth century (melancholia, mania with and without delusions, dementia, and idiocy) (Pinel 1800) into fragments, some of which were to be reconstituted as "mental symptoms." This process did not carve "nature at its joints" (in the rather nonsensical manner in which Plato's metaphor has been used in psychiatry) (Campbell et al. 2011) but fractured the fluid behavior of madmen along artificial lines dictated by the psychological theory then in vogue.[14] By the 1840s, mental symptoms had become the Newtonian "atoms" of madness.[15] From this time on, papers started

---

[11] In the original German edition (Feuchtersleben 1845) the term "psycho-pathologie" appeared with a hyphen. It was transliterated in the English translation as "psychopathology" (Feuchtersleben 1947).

[12] First as *Séméiologie* and then as *Sémiologie* this term has been associated with the descriptive language of medicine since the eighteenth century. By the early nineteenth century it has been imported into alienism to refer to the description of the signs and symptoms of insanity (e.g., Landré-Beauvais 1813).

[13] The myth that it is possible to describe mental symptoms in a "neutral" manner and that descriptive psychiatry can be an "atheoretical" discipline dies hard. During the twentieth century it was wrongly associated with the "phenomenological" views of Karl Jaspers (Berrios 1992)

[14] Borrowed from the Scottish Philosophy of Common Sense, this theory conceived of the mind as a cluster of mental functions and was also important in the development of phrenology (Berrios 1988).

[15] The eighteenth century and later saw the persistent application of the analytical methods proposed by Newton (Force and Hutton 2004). "Newtonianism" not only influenced

to be published on the profile and brain associations of specific symptoms (e.g., delusions, hallucinations, obsessions, fixed ideas, etc.). The belief that mental symptoms were like atoms led to the claim that they could, without changing, participate in the formation of different mental disorders (Berrios and Marková 2009). In other words, a hallucination was a hallucination regardless of whether it was part of an acute confusional state, mania, melancholia, or dementia. This ontological fixity remains central to the current neurobiological approach to mental disorders.

5.4 Change, Evolution, and Madness in the Nineteenth Century

As philosophical categories, "change" (Adamson 1903), "becoming" (Lotze 1878), and "event" (McIntyre 1895) were well discussed during the nineteenth century. Much of this debate, however, took place in the context of the broad notion of "evolution," particularly in its pre-Darwinian meanings (Croll 1890; Richard 1903; Tort 1996). In the field of alienism, the debate on psychopathological change occurred in the context of the doctrine of degeneration (Dallemagne 1895; Genil-Perrin 1913; Larger 1917; Pick 1989). There is no space in this chapter to explore any of these issues at any great length and only two examples will be briefly mentioned.

In a section entitled "On becoming and change" of his book *Metaphysic*, Lotze (1878) discussed the ontological meaning of change, placing it in the realm of the phenomena (in the Kantian sense of this term); Lotze also believed that phenomenic change always reflected change at the level of the noumenon (essence) (Berrios 2005). Adamson (1885) attributed this view to the influenced of Herbart on Lotze. Adamson (1903) understood change as "exchange": "so in like manner simple qualities can undergo no change: change, in their regard, as in respect to notions, means simply the substitution of one for another" (p. 302).

By the end of the nineteenth century the concept of "evolution" had accumulated at least five meanings all entailing either implicitly or explicitly, the reality of change. The first meaning, which goes back to the very etymology of "evolution" ("unfolding") concerned the idea of a latent principle or form gradually emerging until fully manifest (Glare 1968). The second, also pre-nineteenth century, referred to slow, minute, almost imperceptible changes that when concatenated gave the impression of continuity (in this sense evolution became an antonym of "revolution"). The third meaning referred to progressive transformations governed by a rule or law; the fourth, to structural shifts leading from the

---

research in the natural sciences but also in those disciplines that later on were to be called "social sciences." The central principle of the Newtonian methodology was that all complex objects could be analyzed into their atoms or component parts. It has been claimed that Newtonianism was an important component of the Philosophy of the Enlightenment (Jacob 1977). The idea that diseases are made out of individual symptoms and signs is also a clear expression of this philosophy.

homogeneous to the heterogeneous (Spencer 1880, chapters xii–xviii); and the fifth to "Darwinian" evolution as such (Tort 1996).

Some of the pre-Darwinian meanings were incorporated into the notion of degeneration which some have interpreted as a real "contre-évolution" (Larger 1917). First proposed by Morel (1857), the doctrine of degeneration is still the subject of serious debate (Liégeois 1991). Its popularity in Europe well into the early twentieth century was due to the fact that it not only facilitated the description and classification of mental disorders (Genil-Perrin 1913) but also included a moral-religious perspective (Moore 2002), particularly in relation to some 'sinful' etiologies of degeneration such as alcoholism and drug abuse (Bynum 1984). Pollutants and social vice could cause in successive generations of a family the development of ever worsening forms of mental disorder culminating in dementia. Whether such a pathological chain reflected transformations of diseases remains a moot point of the doctrine.

With the advent of Darwinian theory, "evolution" (and change) began to be understood in general terms as mere biological processes and its metaphysics, as had been discussed by Lotze, Adamson, and others, ceased to be important. Because Darwinian evolution arrived late in the field of alienism, its metaphysical aspects lingered on. This explains, for example, Hughlings Jackson's idiosyncratic views on insanity (Berrios 2001) based, at least partly, on Spencer's pre-Darwinian concepts of "evolution" and "dissolution" (Laminne 1908; Spencer 1880). Interestingly enough, Jackson's ideas ended up being more influential in France (Delay 1957) and on Freud (Fullinwider 1983) than they ever were in his own country (Berrios 1977). Another effect of earlier notions of evolution and change can be found in the persistence of the Cartesian view that the soul was a unitary and intangible substance and hence madness could only be a "disease" of the body (Bynum 1976). The same view also explains difficulties found at the beginning of the nineteenth century to develop (and accept) the notion of "partial insanity" (Saussure de 1946; Tissot 1877).

5.5 Mental Symptoms as "things" or as "events"

Are mental symptoms categories of being, abstract objects, or "necessary" beings (Campbell 2006)? Given that it is most unlikely that the last two notions apply to them, the question is whether mental symptoms are substances or events. Amongst neuroscientists and affiliated philosophers it is conventional to consider them as concrete objects or natural kinds (like tables, dogs, trees, gold, etc.), i.e., as substances durably collocated in space and time (Churchland 1989). The belief that mental symptoms (and hence disorders) are natural kinds has historical and epistemological roots. During the nineteenth century the objects of psychiatry were constructed on the model of medicine and the latter's ontological assumptions were transferred over: if medical diseases were "things" invading the body then mental disorders were to be the same. The epistemological roots are to be found in etiological beliefs started in the early nineteenth century according to which all behavior (both normal and abnormal) was fully reducible to bodily structures (Berrios and Marková 2002a). For a while the brain and the stomach vied as candidate structures but in the end the brain predominated. From then on behaviors in general and madness in particular were all considered as sharing with the brain the same collocation in space and time and hence knowing the latter was sufficient to know the former (Morel 1860). This etiological reductionism has been debated ever since (Bennett and Hacker 2003; Churchland 1989).

Events are unique occurrences or happenings associated with objects which may or may not act as their agents (Hacker 1982).[16] The event "falling of an apple" is related to the objects "apple" and "tree" but neither of the latter can be considered to have acted as an agent. A "patellar reflex kick," "sneeze," "blink," "chirp," or a "speech act" are also events but in each case the objects to which they are related may be said to show degrees of agency (although the patellar reflex kick is likely to have less agency than a speech act). Events are entities primarily located in time. The debate on whether they also occur in space (like the objects to which they are related) has not been resolved. This is because, like the concept of change itself, the understanding of the structure of events depends upon the definition of time in use.

Events can be explored from common sense, philosophical, and scientific perspectives (Casati and Varzi 2008). On philosophical analysis, common-sense accounts are often found to contain paradoxes and contradictions. However, to the man in the street, philosophical accounts themselves may appear as counterintuitive. To settle these issues, others defer to accounts of events provided by "science." The latter, however, are subject to secular change and selecting a version depends upon accepting notions such as "true" and "progress." To escape this circular debate, this chapter will adopt a common-sense account of events.

Typically, events occur in time, but based on the argument that they are associated with objects, some will claim that events also occur in space (Quinton 1979). Regardless of whether their base object is or not an agent, events bring about changes classifiable along different dimensions: short or long term, routinary or novel, simple or complex, etc. For example, ordinary perceptions are concatenated events (some may want to call these "processes") related to multiple objects: percipients, stimuli, information, and so on (Zacks and Tversky 2001). Most stimuli triggering perceptual events are routinary and are dealt with automatically, that is, the percipient will match well-known stimuli to well-worn templates (i.e., interpretative accounts or "configurators"). On rare occasions, novel stimuli may alert the percipient into a conscious mode so that the adequate configurator may be found. Such novel stimuli can be external (new images or ideas) or internal (e.g., strange sensations or mental contents). It is proposed in this chapter that mental symptoms start as novel information causing alarm, distress, bewilderment, and so on, thereby inducing the percipient to communicate his inchoate experience. To do so he need to configure it into words (more on this later).

---

[16] By "agency" it is meant the voluntary undertaking of an act (Hyman and Steward 2004; Mele 1997; Morsella et al. 2009; O'Connor and Sandis 2010).

What type of ontological entities are mental symptoms? The generic term "mental symptom" names a class or collection of experiences, behaviors, and other phenomena which are dissimilar in structure and content. Hallucinations, delusions, aboulia, obsessions, irritability, sadness, anxiety, mutism, etc. have little in common and much detail would be lost if they are treated equally (Marková and Berrios 1995). The history of why they have been thrown together is beyond the confines of this chapter. Suffice it to say that it was due to the fact that they all were considered as signs, i.e., as semantic indicators of hidden pathological process (i.e., diseases) (Berrios 1996; Landré-Beauvais 1813).

Given that mental symptoms are heterogeneous entities, it would make little sense to ask whether they are, in general, things or events.[17] The question must be asked in relation to each. For example, say, "hallucinations." In a given day, a patient suffering from the first episode of an acute psychotic disorder may "experience" (and "report") various "hallucinatory episodes." Of varied duration and content, these episodes may have distinguishable end-points (i.e., the patient can indicated a beginning and an end). How can this intermittence be explained? According to the received neurobiological account, true intermittence results from oscillations in the underlying pathological process and false intermittence from shifts in attention or reporting. Crucial to this view is the fact that all hallucinatory episodes are considered as tokens (expressions, occurrences, etc.) of the same underlying pathological process. In other words, from the diagnostic point of view the study of one is enough to know them all. Hallucinatory episodes are thus reified as things (signs) standing for other things (brains or bits thereof). Hallucinatory experiences occurring early or late in the same episode of the disorder (or in different episodes thereof) or at any time of the day are no different. If differences are noticed they must be considered as clinically trivial. The hallucinating subject is considered as a mere rapporteur of intermittent or clonic expressions of a brain process, as a passive recipient of something in which he has no participation.

Given that therapeutic approaches to hallucinations based on the neurobiological model have so far had limited success (Sommer et al. 2012), it is ethically incumbent upon clinicians to search for alternative ways of understanding hallucinations. One is to explore the possibility that the replicated token account is incomplete, and that hallucinations are actually specific and particular events generated or constructed by the suffering agent (Berrios and Marková 2012). Each hallucinatory event would be a separate entity constituted by its own "tropes" (i.e., unique expressions of properties) (Keinänen 2011; Williams 1953). All that the neurobiological process would offer to the sufferer is a signal or kernel which would trigger his need to configure (Berrios and Marková 2006). On this model, all differences between hallucinatory experiences can be potentially meaningful and hence need to be recorded. A similar analysis can be undertaken in regards to delusions, obsessions, sadness, anhedonia, depersonalization, etc. This would

---

[17] To simplify matters I will only discussed here the type of symptom called "subjective" (Marková and Berrios 2009)

show that sufferers are far more active and participatory in the formation of their mental symptoms than the current neurobiological model allows.

5.6 Mental Symptoms as "passive happenings" or as "acts"

The ontological proposal that mental symptoms are events raises the question of whether they are also mental acts. A mental act has been defined as: "the process of intentionally activating a mental disposition in order to acquire a desired mental property" (Proust 2001, 2010). This capacity to exercise a mental action (e.g., configure a mental symptom) is based on the subject's intentionality, mental disposition, and agency (Geach 1957; O'Brien and Soteriou 2009). Sufferers and nonsufferers alike are able to exercise mental capacities such as perceiving, deliberating, self-reflecting, remembering, talking to themselves, etc. (Morsella et al. 2009). Given the nature of mental symptoms and the general importance of mental acts it is rather surprising that the latter are rarely discussed in relation to the former. The model of symptom formation to be discussed in later sections assumes that mental symptoms are mental acts and on this basis can explain their "change," whether short or long term.

5.7 Ascertaining Change in Psychopathology

Change can be ascertained from the historical or current perspective. In regard to the former, comparisons can be made of clinical cases retrospectively diagnosed as suffering from the "same" disorder and extracted from different historical epochs. Any consistent differences might then constitute circumstantial evidence for change. Unfortunately, retrospective diagnosis is inherently anachronistic.[18] This can be illustrated in another way. Writing on the history of any symptom or disorder requires a subject of study which is usually captured by a working definition. The presentistic assumptions of medicine and psychiatry ("latest is bestest") encourage the selection of a definition from one of the current listings (e.g., ICD-10 or DSM-5). Soon enough it is realized that this definition only allows for the study of the specific historical convergence[19] that gave rise to the category in question and nothing else. In order to link this convergence to earlier ones the historian must choose to follow the history of the word, the concept of the behaviors.

---

[18] Within the discipline of historiography, anachronism refers to the act of describing and explaining information belonging to the past in terms of concepts and ideas belonging to the present. It is also called presentism (Spoerhase 2008), the fallacy of the *nunc pro tunc*, and is closely related to linear and progressist views of history, what Herbert Butterfield (1931) called the "Whig history." There is a tendency amongst some clinical historians to interpret the history of psychiatry as a chronicle of progress from an inchoate, erroneous, and uniformed past to a scientific and truth-making present. This approach destroys the possibility of understanding the very concepts of madness or mental disorder.

[19] "Convergence" names an explanatory hypothesis for the construction of mental symptoms and disorders. According to this hypothesis the objects of alienism (now psychiatry) have been formed by the coming together (convergence) in the work of a writer (usually

Doing the first becomes an exercise in etymological history; doing the second is very difficult for concepts are parasitical upon explanatory theories and are rarely (if ever) reused in successive convergences; doing the third may certainly be possible but then the behaviors considered as abnormal in the latest convergence may not be so considered in earlier ones. In order to deal with this problem the historian must then assume that it was wrong of earlier periods not to have pathologized the said behaviors. Furthermore, there is the problem that because in earlier times such behaviors were not considered as abnormal they are not documented, and when they were, the resulting descriptions were not atheoretical and hence a bias or deformation of some sort can be expected. Given the pitfalls besetting historical comparisons, what other method is available to identify change? It will be proposed in this chapter that this can be done by means of a model of symptom formation.

5.8 Classifying Change in Psychopathology

On the basis of the analysis included earlier in this chapter, it may be possible to sketch a tentative classification of change in psychopathology. If "locus" or "subject" is used as the taxonomic criterion then change can affect either the language or the objects of psychiatry. Language changes can be arbitrary, formal, or external ("Cambridge change") (Geach 1969), or structural. Structural changes are important for they modify the very definition of the objects of psychiatry. For example, redefining properties may change the clinical profile of a mental symptom or disorder (as happened to depersonalization in DSM III) (Sierra and Berrios 2001).

The object of change can be the objects themselves; in this case, two types can be distinguished. Quantitative change affects the intensity, frequency, and duration of mental symptoms or disorders. Qualitative change may consist either in metamorphosis (which on occasions may threaten the identity of the object itself) or in exchange. Whether quantitative or qualitative changes can be immanent, that is, occurring within one individual (i.e., within a particular disease episode or along the natural history of one disease) and transcendent, that is, occurring along over large expanses of time (e.g., centuries) and effectively changing the form of a disease. As mentioned earlier, the focus of this chapter is transcendent change.

5.9 Change and the "received view" of Mental Symptoms

The possibility of change within the epistemological confines of the neurobiological model can now be examined. As it stands, it proposes that mental symptoms and

---

acting as the spokesman of a group or fashion) of a word (new or recycled), a concept (representing contemporary ways of thinking about the subject), and a set or cluster of behaviours. The success of convergences is due less to their scientific or evidential basis than to social and economic factors (Berrios 1994).

disorders can be fully naturalized, that is, reduced without residuum to pathological changes in the structure or function of the brain. This view is supported in practice by a complex and self-sustaining network of statistical correlations that maps sets of proxy variables representing the symptom or disorder under study (D) upon sets of proxy variables representing the brain (B). However, the correlations thus obtained exhibit an asymmetrical predictive capacity in the sense that only in few cases can it be claimed with confidence that "normal" subjects showing the changes in question are actually suffering from D (Berrios and Marková 2002). This model is a continuation of the so-called anatomoclinical model of disease introduced by the Paris school at the beginning of the nineteenth century (Ackerknecht 1967; Laín Entralgo 1978). The epistemological power of this model has always depended upon the quality of the representativeness of the variables entered in the correlations. During the nineteenth century, and before the development of statistical techniques, the variables in question, both for D and B, were disjunctive (i.e., "present or absent") (Georget 1820; Janet 1867; Morel 1860) but during the twentieth century, they became quantified. Disease (D) was represented by interval-type scores obtained via diagnostic scales; The brain (B) was represented by numbers obtained by means of research techniques that in historical terms have moved from the histological to the electrical, neurochemical, neuroimaging, and neurogenetic.

Can "change" be accommodated within the neurobiological model? Given that it assumes that D is an expression of disrupted or degraded B, then it should be possible to predict that changes in B will change D. Change in this sense could be short term, as in the case of shifts induced by therapeutic stabilization of B; or long term as in situations when it may be plausible to claim that B has been subject to evolutionary mutation or epigenetic modulation.

5.10 Change and the Cambridge Model of Mental Symptom Formation

The Cambridge group proposes that mental symptoms result from the cultural configuration of prelinguistic information that after penetrating the sufferer's awareness may cause discomfort, bewilderment, or emotional upheaval. This information can be of biological origin (resulting from distressed brain networks) or of semantic origin (reverberating or corollary personal or social worries) (Berrios and Marková 2006). To communicate their experience, sufferers need to configure it by means of personal, social, and cultural templates. These are no different from those used in normal perception. In this sense "mental symptoms" are not things that happen to sufferers but are genuine actions (events) undertaken by subjects in order to deal with distressful or strange experiences. On account of this configuratory act, symptoms combine biological and cultural information and hence can be considered as structurally being hybrid objects, a special type of entity different from brains (things) and from abstract objects (e.g., virtue or beauty) (Berrios 2011).

Do sufferers configure their symptoms anew every time that they experience or report them or does this process only take place during the very early, acute states of the disease (to simply quote them from memory later on)? According to the Cambridge model sufferers do, only that as they become more familiar with both the experience and the use of the configurator, the act becomes easier on each successive occasion. If this is the case, then each event (e.g., hallucination) cannot be considered as an identical replica of the others as the configuratory act may vary. For example: (1) the information in need of configuration may have changed but in spite of this the sufferer decides[20] to use the same configurators (in this case, different biological signals may give rise to the same symptom); (2) the sufferer may decide to use a different configurator for the same information (in this case, the same signal may give rise to different symptoms); (3) although no biological information has accrued the subject nonetheless decided to use a configurator for emotional or cognitive reasons external to the process itself (in this case, a symptom is produced although there is no biological signal). It goes without saying that all three options may be relevant to treatment choice.

Change, both short and long term, can be comfortably explained by the Cambridge model as due to change in: (1) brain structure and function (as per the neurobiological model), (2) type and quality of the information or material entering awareness, (3) configurators themselves, (4) sufferer's intentions and motivations, and (5) the dialogical negotiation (Gadamer 1989) between sufferer and clinical interlocutor (a mechanism so far not raised in this chapter).[21] Options (1) and (2) have been explored. Option (3) suggests that the configurators themselves are subject to cultural change thereby changing symptom profile; option (4) involves the sufferer in: (a) choice of configurator and (b) inclusion of performative function that he may wish to attach to his symptom (Austin 1962; Pennycook

---

[20] From the viewpoint of its intentionality, the mental action of configuring inputs into awareness can be variously characterized. Routine actions are likely to be automatic as this will make them speedy and mostly correct. However, novel inputs may require attention. This is the case with the information (biological or symbolic) that invades awareness during the early stages of a mental disorder. Sufferers may be bewildered and distressed and in need to communicate their experience. This encourages them to configure the information received. It has also been claimed that to do so the sufferer may "select" a configurator. Does "select" in this context refer to a deliberate, conscious decision to use a particular configurator or does it simply mean that the subject may "opt" for one? Actions are considered to have conscious or unconscious automaticity (Weathey and Wegner 2001). Given that it may be counterintuitive to believe that the sufferer will "deliberate" choose a configurator, and given that resolving this issue is not directly relevant to the question of change dealt with in this chapter, we will only want to say that the sufferer's action is automatic. Further research needs to be done to decide on whether his selecting is conscious or unconscious.

[21] As the culmination of a long history of efforts to understand the meaning of texts, Gadamer (1989) offered an interesting hermeneutic model which allows the interpreter to start with certain early beliefs ("prejudices" which have no negative connotation in Gadamer), and by iterative steps approach a stable understanding (Bilen 2000). The caveat must be entered that the complaints reported by a sufferer are likely to be more dynamic, kaleidoscopic, and changing than a text. This notwithstanding, it is clear that a model is still needed to study the manner in which clinical interlocutor and sufferer together seek a meaning for the complaints reported by the latter.

2009); lastly, option (5) refers to the contribution of the clinical interlocutor with whom the sufferer negotiates the final version of his complaint.

Configurators are cultural templates, social representations, symbols whereby sufferers give shape to information (sensations) that is inchoate, prelinguistic, and preconceptual. By choosing a way of describing, understanding and expressing it, the sufferer collocates his experience in a speech act apt for communication. Configurators can be personal (idiosyncratic renderings of experiences invading awareness), social (family and social group templates ready-made to deal with certain experiences), and cultural (general and often transparent templates built into the culture or episteme). While they last (that is, are sanctioned by culture), configurators are responsible for the stability with which humans experience their external and internal world. In the case of symptoms, configurators guarantee the stereotypical form in which they are regularly reported by sufferers. The neurobiological model attributes this invariance to the brain. In this respect, the Cambridge model is more cautious as according to symptom and situation this invariance may be attributed to either the biological signal and to the cultural configurator itself. When the latter is changed, renewed, or replaced then it is likely that the clinical profile of mental symptoms will follow suit.

Given that configurations are actions, it should be possible for sufferers to guide, albeit partially, the configuratory process. This could be done via the choice of templates or by attaching additional functions to the speech act. In this sense, whilst the content of the complaint itself could be considered as the "locutionary" act, what the sufferer wants to do with his report becomes the "perlocutionary or performative" act (Austin 1962). Very little work has been done on the pragmatic characteristics of mental symptoms; indeed, this function is invisible to the neurobiological model which would find it difficult to explain it.

Lastly, upon reporting his complaint, the sufferer enters into a dialogue with his clinical interlocutor. Less a passive amanuensis than an active participant, the interlocutor enters into the dialogical situation armed with a diagnostic hypothesis. What follows then is a dynamic, semantic negotiation during which the interlocutor may guide the sufferer in certain directions. Therefore, the final version of the mental symptom, as recorded in the casenotes, is the result of a veritable Gadamerian hermeneutic process whereby the clinical interlocutor reaches an understanding of the complaints narrated by the sufferer (Gadamer 1989). This final stage of the symptom-formation process has been little studied perhaps because according to the official view clinical history-taking is assumed to be a "theoretically neutral" operation. However, according the Cambridge model this dynamic process is of importance in regards to who should undertake the first mental state examination (i.e., a more or less directive interviewer).[22]

---

[22] Two issues need to be clarified: (1) the directiveness or otherwise of the clinical interlocutor during the mental state examination, and (2) whether the clinical interlocutor and the

5.11 Conclusions

General definitions of "change" depend on how metaphysical categories such as object, event, property, and time are themselves defined. Whether the understanding of change should be done in general or within specific metaphysical regions (e.g., physics, biology, sociology) is also a moot point. In general, both biology and sociology seem to accept the existence of change (however defined).

Psychopathology refers to the language of psychiatry. Since the nineteenth century, alienism (now psychiatry) has named a discipline and trade addressed at the understanding and management of madness. As it stands at the moment, psychiatry is considered by most as a specialism of medicine and hence as a form of applied biology. This means that medicine and psychiatry are likely to borrow the views on change entertained by the current biological sciences. Originally, the forms of mental alienation recognized by successive cultures were defined in psychological and social terms. The medicalization of madness that took place during the nineteenth century caused them to be considered as mere expressions of a diseased brain. It became the ideal of such model: (1) to identify invariant links between mental symptoms and brain regions; (2) to naturalize mental symptoms, i.e., to reduce them without residuum to their brain substratum, and (3) to diagnose mental disorders by means of changes in the brain substratum thereby bypassing the complaints themselves (this, for example, underlies the desideratum of diagnosing and treating mental disorders *before* they are behaviorally expressed). According to this model, "change" both short and long term in the nature of the complaint is to be explained as resulting from change in the neurobiological substratum.

Change in psychopathology can also be explained by means of the Cambridge model of symptom formation which considers mental symptoms are the primary objects of psychiatry. Mental disorders are considered as secondary objects, as clusters of symptoms held together by a hypothetical glue whose nature can be historical, social, biological, or statistical. Mental symptoms are considered to be events resulting from actions undertaken by sufferers to

---

sufferer share cultural configurators. In regards to the first, it is essential that the clinical interlocutor does not allow his diagnostic hypothesis to influence the sufferer's final configuration of his experience. For example, if the sufferer is not sure whether he is experiencing an idea or an image, it is important that the interviewer remains neutral even if reporting a "delusion" would fit better his diagnostic hypothesis (Berrios and Marková 2012). In regards to the second, in most cases it is expected that sufferer and clinician share the same culture and hence the same configurators (that is, templates indicating how in mental symptoms, disorders and other behaviours ought to be experienced and talked about). However, this cultural sharing was probably more likely in earlier times than now. The fact that in our time clinicians often enough work away from their continent or culture of origin should in principle create cultural and configurator dissonance. In practice, however, the globalization of medical information and common training compensate for this fact and hence it is less likely that clinicians might encourage sufferers to use culturally dissonant configurators.

make sense of distressing information invading their awareness. This information can be biological (the result of a signal released by a distressed brain network) or symbolic (meanings resulting from social interaction or personal refection).

Upon entering awareness this information is inchoate, prelinguistic and preconceptual, often emotionally effervescent, and ineffable. To talk about it sufferers must shape it by means of configurators (idiosyncratic, social, or cultural). This process creates speech acts which often have both locutionary and performative functionality. Upon being reported, the mental symptom may undergo additional changes resulting from dialogical negotiations between sufferer and clinical interlocutor. Once the negotiation has been completed the symptom crystallizes and is recorded as a fact. Within this model of symptom formation, change may be due to multiple causes, for example, changes in the information (be this biological or symbolic), in the sufferer's choice of configurators and motivation, or in the skill of the clinical interlocutor. Each will give rise to a different type of change and could potentially be recognized by a close mental state examination.

Acknowledgment

This chapter is dedicated to the late Professor Peter Geach (1916–2013) whose work on "mental acts" has been influential on my thinking.

References

Ackerknecht, E. (1967). *Medicine at the Paris Hospital 1794–1848*. Baltimore, MD: Johns Hopkins Press.

Adamson, R. (1885). Review of Lotze's "Metaphysic." *Mind*, 10, 573–788.

Adamson, R. (1903). *The Development of Modern Philosophy* (Vol. 1). Edinburgh: William Blackwood.

Austin, J.L. (1962). *How to Do Things With Words*. Oxford: Clarendon Press.

Bennett, M.R. and Hacker, P.M.S. (2003). *Philosophical Foundations of Neuroscience*. Oxford: Blackwell.

Berrios, G.E. (1977). Henri Ey, Jackson et les idées obsedantes. *L'Evolution Psychiatrique*, 42, 685–699.

Berrios, G.E. (1981). Stupor: a conceptual history. *Psychological Medicine*, 11, 677–688.

Berrios, G.E. (1984). Descriptive psychopathology: conceptual and historical aspects. *Psychological Medicine*, 14, 303–313.

Berrios, G.E. (1988). Historical background to abnormal psychology. In E. Miller and P. Cooper (eds.) *Adult Abnormal Psychology*, pp. 26–51. London: Churchill Livingstone.

Berrios, G.E. (1992). Phenomenology, psychopathology and Jaspers: a conceptual history. *History of Psychiatry*, 3, 303–327.

Berrios, G.E. (1993). Phenomenology and psychopathology: was there ever a relationship? *Comprehensive Psychiatry*, 34, 213–220.

Berrios, G.E. (1994). Historiography of mental symptoms and diseases. *History of Psychiatry*, 5, 175–190.

Berrios, G.E. (1996). *History of Mental Symptoms*. Cambridge: Cambridge University Press.

Berrios, G.E. (1999a). Anxiety disorders: a conceptual history. *Journal of Affective Disorders*, 56, 83–94.

Berrios, G.E. (1999b). Haematoma auris. *History of Psychiatry*, 10, 371–383.

Berrios, G.E. (1999c). Towards a new descriptive psychopathology: a sine qua non for neurobiological research in psychiatry. *Brain Research Bulletin*, 50, 457–458.

Berrios, G.E. (2001). Jackson and the "Factors of Insanities." *History of Psychiatry*, 12, 353–373.

Berrios, G.E. (2005). Lotze and his "Medicinische Psychologie oder Physiologie der Seele" *History of Psychiatry*, 16, 117–127.

Berrios, G.E. (2008). The history of psychiatric therapies. In P. Tyrer and R. Silk (eds.) *Cambridge Textbook of Effective Treatments in Psychiatry*, pp. 16–43. Cambridge: Cambridge University Press.

Berrios, G.E. (2011). Psychiatry and its objects. *Revista de Psiquiatría y Salud Mental*, 4, 179–182.

Berrios, G.E. (2012). The 19th-century nosology of alienism: history and epistemology. In K.S. Kendler and J. Parnas (eds.) *Philosophical Issues in Psychiatry II*, pp 101–123. Oxford: Oxford University Press.

Berrios, G.E. (2014). Robert James and Febrile Anxiety. *History of Psychiatry*, 25, 1–13.

Berrios, G.E. and Marková, I.S. (2002). Biological psychiatry: conceptual issues. In H. D'Haenen, J.A. den Boer, and P. Willner (eds.) *Biological Psychiatry*, pp. 3–24. New York: John Wiley.

Berrios, G.E. and Marková, I.S. (2002a). The concept of neuropsychiatry: a historical overview. *Journal of Psychosomatic Research*, 53, 629–638.

Berrios, G.E. and Marková, I.S. (2002b). Assessment and measure in neuropsychiatry: a conceptual history. *Seminars in Clinical Neuropsychiatry*, 7, 3–10.

Berrios, G.E., Luque, R., and Villagrán, J.M. (2003). Schizophrenia: a conceptual History. *International Journal of Psychology and Psychological Therapy*, 3, 111–140.

Berrios, G.E. and Marková, I.S. (2006). Symptoms: historical perspective and effect on diagnosis. In M. Blumenfield and J.J. Strain (eds.) *Psychosomatic Medicine*, pp. 27–38. Philadelphia, PA: Lippincott Williams and Wilkins.

Berrios, G.E. and Marková, I.S. (2012). The construction of hallucinations: history and epistemology. In J.D. Blom and I.E.C. Sommer (eds.) *Hallucinations: Research and Practice*, pp. 55–71. Berlin: Springer.

Bilen, O. (2000). *The Historicity of Understanding and the Problem of Relativism in Gadamer's Philosophical Hermeneutics*. Washington, DC: The Council for Research in Values and Philosophy.

Boudon, R. (1984). *La Place du Désordre*. Paris: Presses Universitaires de France.

Butterfield, H. (1931). *The Whig Interpretation of History*. London: G. Bell.

Bynum, W. (1976). Varieties of Cartesian experience in early 19th century neurophysiology. In S.F. Spicker and H.T. Engelhardt (eds.) *Philosophical Dimensions of the Neuro-medical Sciences*, pp. 15–33. Dordrecht: D. Reidel.

Bynum, W. (1984). Alcoholism and degeneration in 19th century European medicine and psychiatry. *British Journal of Addiction*, 79, 59–70.

Callender, C. (ed.) (2011). *The Oxford Handbook of the Philosophy of Time*. Oxford: Oxford University Press.

Campbell, K. (2006). Ontology. In D.M. Borchert (ed.) *Encyclopedia of Philosophy* (2nd ed., Vol. 7), pp. 21–27. Detroit, MI: Thompson.

Campbell, K., O'Rourke, M., and Slater, M.H. (eds.) (2011). *Carving Nature at its Joints. Natural Kinds in Metaphysics and Science*. Cambridge, MA: MIT Press.

Casati, R. and Varzi, A.C. (2008). Event concepts. In T.F. Shipley and J.M. Zacks (eds.) *Understanding Events. From Perception to Action*, pp. 31–53. Oxford: Oxford University Press.

Chantraine, P. (1968). *Dictionnaire Étymologique de la Langue Grecque. Histoire des Mots*. Paris: Éditions Klincksieck.

Churchland, P.S. (1989). *Neurophilosophy*. Cambridge, MA: MIT Press.

Coates, P. (1998). *Nature: Western Attitudes since Ancient Times*. Cambridge: Polity Press.

Crislip, A. (2005). The sin of sloth or the illness of the demons? The demon of Acedia in early Christian monasticism. *The Harvard Theological Review*, 98, 143–169.

Croll, J. (1890). *The Philosophical Basis of Evolution*. London: Stanford.

Dallemagne, J. (1895). *Dégénérés et Déséquilibrés*. Bruxelles: Lamertin.

Davies, A.E. (1900). The concept of change. *The Philosophical Review*, 9, 502–517.

David, P. (2004). Nature. In B. Cassin (ed.) *Vocabulaire Européen des Philosophies*, pp. 854–855. Paris: Seuil.

Delay, J. (1957). Jacksonism and the work of Ribot. *Archives of Neurology and Psychiatry*, 78, 505–515.

Dyke, H. (2013). Time and tense. In H. Dyke and A. Bardon (eds.) *A Companion to the Philosophy of Time*, pp. 328–344. Oxford: Wiley-Blackwell.

Ellard, J. (1987). Did schizophrenia exist before the eighteenth century? *Australian and New Zealand Journal of Psychiatry*, 21, 306–318.

Farago, F. (2000). *La Nature*. Paris: Colin.

Feuchtersleben, E. (1845). *Lehrbuch der ärztlichen Seelenkunde*. Wien: Carl Gerold.

Feuchtersleben, E. (1847). *The Principles of Medical Psychology*. (H.E. Lloyd and B.G. Babington, trans.). London: Sydenham Society.

Fink, E. (1957). *Zur ontologischen Frühgeschichte von Raum, Zeit, Bewegung*. Den Haag: Nijhoff.

Fink, M. and Taylor, M.A. (2006). *Catatonia*. Cambridge: Cambridge University Press.

Force, J.E. and Hutton, S. (eds.) (2004). *Newton and Newtonianism*. Dordrecht: Kluwer.

Forthomme, B. (2000). *De l'acédie monastique à l'anxio-dépression. Histoire Philosophique de la transformation d'un vice en pathologie*. Paris: Collection les Empêcheurs de Penser en Rond.

Fullinwider, S.P. (1983). Sigmund Freud, John Hughlings Jackson, and speech. *Journal of the History of Ideas*, 44, 151–158.

Gadamer, H.G. (1989). *Truth and Method* (2nd ed.) (J. Weinsheimer and D.G. Marshall, trans.). London: Sheed and Ward.

Geach, P. (1957). *Mental Acts. Their Content and their Objects*. London: Routledge and Kegan Paul.

Geach, P. (1969). *God and the Soul*. London: Routledge and Kegan Paul.

Genil-Perrin, G. (1913). *Histoire des Origines et de l'Évolution de l'Idée de Dégénérescence en Médicine Mentale*. Paris: A Leclerc.

Georget, E.J. (1820). *De la Folie*. Paris: Crevot.

Glare, P.G.W. (1968). *Ēuoluē*. In P.G.W. Glare (ed.) *Oxford Latin Dictionary*, pp. 627–628. Oxford: Clarendon Press.

Graham, D.W. (2006). *Explaining the Cosmos: The Ionian Tradition of Scientific Philosophy*. Princeton, NJ: Princeton University Press.

Hacker, P.M.S. (1982). Events, ontology and grammar. *Philosophy*, 57, 477–486.

Hyman, J. and Steward, H. (eds.) (2004). *Agency and Action*. Cambridge: Cambridge University Press.

Hyslop, J.H. (1910). Change. In J. Hastings (ed.) *Encyclopaedia of Religion and Ethics* (Vol. 3), pp. 357–358. Edinburgh: T. and T. Clark.

Jacob, M.C. (1977). Newtonianism and the origins of the Enlightenment: a reassessment. *Eighteenth-Century Studies*, 11, 1–25.

Janet, P. (1867). *Le Cerveau et la Pensée*. Paris: Baillière.

Jehl, R. (1984). *Melancholie und Acedia. Ein Beitrag zu Anthropologie und Ethik Bonaventuras*. München: Ferdinand Schöningh.

Jeste, D.V., Del Carmen, R., Lohr, J.B., and Wyatt, R.J. (1985). Did schizophrenia exist before the eighteenth century? *Comprehensive Psychiatry*, 26, 493–503.

Kahlbaum, K.L. (1874). *Die Katatonie, oder das Spannungsirresein*. Berlin: Kirschwald.

Kaulbach, F. (1984). Natur [Nature]. In J. Ritter and K. Gründer (eds.) *Historisches Wörterbuch der Philosophie* (Vol. 6), pp. 421–478. Darmstadt: Wissenschaftiche Buchgesellschaft.

Keil, F.C. (1989). *Concepts, Kinds, and Cognitive Development*. Cambridge, MA: MIT Press.

Keinänen, M. (2011). Tropes: the basic constituents of powerful particulars? *Dialectica*, 65, 419–450.

Laín Entralgo, P. (1978). *Historia de la Medicina*. Barcelona: Salvat.

Laminne, J. (1908). *The Théorie de l'évolution. Étude Critique sur les "Premiers Principes" de Herbert Spencer*. Bruxelles: Albert Dewit.

Landré-Beauvais, A.J. (1813). *Séméiotique ou Traité des Signes des Maladies* (2nd ed.) Paris: Brosson.

Lange, L. (1886). *Die geschichtliche Entwicklung des Bewegungsbegriffs und ihr voraussichtliches Endergebnis. Ein Beitrag zur historischen Kritik der mechanischen Prinzipien*. Leipzig: Wilhelm Engelmann.

Lanteri-Laura, G. (1972). La chronicité dans la psychiatrie moderne française. *Annales. Économies, Sociétés, Civilisations*, 27, 548–568.

Laporte, J. (2004). *Natural Kinds and Conceptual Change*. Cambridge: Cambridge University Press.

Larger, R. (1917). *Théorie de la Contre-évolution ou Dégénérescence*. Paris: Alcan.

Liddell, H.G. and Scott, R. (1994). *A Greek-English Lexicon*. Oxford: Clarendon Press.

Liégeois, A. (1991). Hidden philosophy and theology in Morel's theory of degeneration and nosology. *History of Psychiatry*, 2, 419–428.

Lotze, H. (1878). *Metaphysic* (B. Bosanquet, ed.). Oxford: Clarendon Press.

Mahendra, B. (1981). Where have all the catatonics gone? *Psychological Medicine*, 11, 669–671.

Marinas, J.M. (2004). Acedia. In B. Cassin (ed.) *Vocabulaire Européen des Philosophies*, pp. 8–9. Paris: Seuil.

Marková, I.S. and Berrios, G.E. (1995). Mental symptoms: are they similar phenomena. *Psychopathology*, 28, 147–157.

Marková, I.S. and Berrios, G.E. (2009). Epistemology of mental symptoms. *Psychopathology*, 42, 343–349.

McIntyre, J.L. (1895). Time and the succession of events. *Mind*, 4, 334–349.

Mele, A.R. (1997). Agency and mental action. *Noûs*, 31, 231–249

Mellor, D.H. (1998). Events. In E. Craig (ed.) *Routledge Encyclopedia of Philosophy*, pp. 461–463. London: Routledge.

Mink, L.O. (1968). Change and causality in the history of ideas. *Eighteenth-Century Studies*, 2, 7–25.

Moore, G. (2002). *Nietzsche, Biology and Metaphor*. Cambridge: Cambridge University Press.

Morel, B.A. (1857). *Traité des Dégénérescences Physiques Intellectuelles et Morales de l'Espèce Humaine*. Paris: Baillière.

Morel, B.A. (1860). *Traité des Maladies Mentales*. Paris: Masson.

Morsella, E., Bargh, J.A., and Gollwitzer, P.M. (eds.) (2009). *Oxford Handbook of Human Action*. Oxford: Oxford University Press.

Murphy, D. (2006). *Psychiatry in the Scientific Image*. Cambridge, MA: MIT Press.

O'Brien, L. and Soteriou, M. (eds.) (2009). *Mental Actions*. Oxford: Oxford University Press.

O'Connor, T. and Sandis, C. (eds.) (2010). *A Companion to the Philosophy of Action*. Oxford: Blackwell.

Osier, J.P. (1990). Changement. In S. Auroux (ed.) *Les Notions Philosophiques* (Vol. 2), pp. 301–303. Paris: Presses Universitaires de France.

Pennycook, A. (2009). Performativity and language studies. *Critical Inquiry in Language Studies*, 1, 1–19.

Pick, D. (1989). *Faces of Degeneration: A European Disorder, c.1848–1918*. Cambridge, Cambridge University Press.

Pinel, P. (1800). *Traité Médico-Philosophique sur l'Aliénation Mentale ou la Manie*. Paris: Richard, Caille et Ravier.

Proust, J. (2001). A plea for mental acts. *Synthese*, 129, 105–128.

Proust, J. (2010). Mental acts. In T. O'Connor and C. Sandis (eds.) *A Companion to the Philosophy of Action*, pp. 209–217. Oxford: Blackwell.

Quinton, A. (1979). Objects and events. *Mind*, 88, 197–214.

Rhodes, D.P. (1909). *The Philosophy of Change*. New York: McMillan.

Richard, G. (1903). *L'Idée d'Évolution dans la Nature et l'Histoire*. Paris: Alcan.

Rogers, R.E. (1969). *Max Weber's Ideal Type Theory*. New York: Philosophical Library.

Saussure, R. de (1946). The influence of the concept of monomania on French medico-legal psychiatry (from 1825–1840). *Journal of the History of Medicine*, 1, 365–397.

Sierra, M. and Berrios, G.E. (2001). The phenomenological stability of depersonalization: comparing the old with the new. *Journal of Nervous and Mental Disease*, 189, 629–636.

Sommer, I.E.C., Slotema, C.W., Daskalakis, Z.J., Derks, E.M., Blom, J.D., and van der Gaag, M. (2012). The treatment of hallucinations in schizophrenia spectrum disorders. *Schizophrenia Bulletin*, 38, 704–714.

Spencer, H. (1880). *First Principles* (4th ed.). London: Williams and Northgate.

Spoerhase, C. (2008). Presentism and precursorship in intellectual history. *Culture, Theory and Critique*, 49, 49–72.

Swedberg, R. (2005). *The Max Weber Dictionary*. Stanford, CA: Stanford University Press.

Tissot, J. (1877). *La Folie Considérée Surtout ses Rapports avec la Psychologie Normale*. Paris: A. Marescq Ainé.

Tort, P. (1996). Évolution. In P. Tort (ed.) *Dictionnaire du Darwinisme et de l'évolution* (Vol. 1), pp. 1422–1468. Paris: Presses Universitaires de France.

Ungvari, G.S., Caroff, S.N., and Gerevich, J. (2006). The catatonia conundrum. *Schizophrenia Bulletin*, 36, 231–238.

Weathey, T. and Wegner, D.M. (2001). Automaticity of actions. In N.J. Smelser and P.B. Baltes (eds.) *International Encyclopedia of the Social & Behavioral Sciences*, pp. 991–993. Oxford: Elsevier.

Weigelt, C. (2004). Logos as kinesis: Heidegger's interpretation of the physics in "Grundbegriffe der aristotelischen Philosophies." *Epoché*, 9, 101–116.

Wenzel, S. (1967). *The Sin of Sloth: Acedia in Medieval Thought and Literature*. Chapel Hill, NC: The University of North Carolina Press.

Williams, D.C. (1953). On the elements of being I. *The Review of Metaphysics*, 7, 3–18.

Williams, T.R. (1966). The study of change as a concept in cultural anthropology. *Theory into Practice*, 5, 13–19.

Zacks, J.M. and Tversky, B. (2001). Event structure in perception and conception. *Psychological Bulletin*, 127, 3–21.

Chapter 6

Can hybridity overcome dualism?

Helen E. Longino

Professor Berrios, in his wide-ranging and fascinating chapter (Chapter 5, this volume), is concerned with the possibility of qualitative change in psychopathological states themselves, rather than change in the representation and conceptualization of such states, which is the concern of most of the chapters in this volume. Thus, his central question is:

> "Can the basic forms of mental distress change over time (in a more than superficial way)?"

A superficial way would be changes in theory which result in reclassifying symptoms that have nevertheless remained constant, and changes in language, both language available to the sufferer of mental distress and language available to the therapeutic practitioner. And, "over time" means across centuries, thus treating forms of mental distress as transindividual entities, with characteristic patterns that are constant across individuals.

Berrios mentions various ideas about the nature of change and about the ontological status of mental symptoms. None of these offers a quick way to resolve his question. Indeed, the very fact of scientific change, that is, of change in the identification, diagnosis, or classification of forms of mental distress makes the challenge Professor Berrios has undertaken almost impossible: looking back 500, 1000, years, how do we determine whether perceived change is change in the actual symptoms or in the ways of classifying and understanding them? The development of neuroscience in the nineteenth century seemed to promise advances over previous ways of dealing with disordered mentality. Enthusiasm for a neurobiological approach has increased with increasing capacity to study the brain and brain processes, and is expressed, according to Berrios, in the locating of psychiatry as a branch of medicine. Were the neurobiological model of psychopathology correct, he suggests, the question about change would be more easily answered. We could simply study the disordered brain states/processes that generate disordered behavior to see if they exhibit some qualitative change while retaining some constant and characteristic core. While we may not be able to do so retrospectively, owing to conceptual and theoretical change and lack of adequate instrumentation, we would certainly be able to do so prospectively, at least in principle.

But, Berrios claims that the neurobiological approach has been of limited utility in alleviating mental distress. We should therefore take a different approach to the metaphysics of mental distress. He proposes that the hybrid model employed by the Cambridge group of which he is a member is both more descriptively accurate and therapeutically effective. It also permits answering the question about the possibility of qualitative change in mental symptomatology.

This hybrid model proposes that pathological states are hybrid entities with both biological and social dimensions. Berrios describes the process by which psychopathology manifests itself as follows. A brain site in distress generates a signal that initiates a cascade whose outcome is symptom formation. On the way to symptom formation, the neurological signal enters subjective consciousness as inchoate and formless experience. The discomfort thus created generates a desire to communicate what the experience is like, but its formlessness means the subject must employ the concepts and categories already in use in the subject's culture in order to represent it in communication. Because the subject is understood as representing her or his distress by means of elements from her or his cultural imaginary, Berrios thinks it appropriate to think of the subject as actively involved in the construction of her or his symptoms. The psychopathological episode is not a passively experienced mental event, but a mental act. Thus, the hermeneutic act of a therapist is preceded by a prior hermeneutic act of the sufferer who interprets her or his experienced, but inchoate, inner states.

This multidimensional, hybrid, character of psychopathological states makes them, according to Berrios, susceptible to change. This reflects the view that qualitative change that preserves the continuity of the changing entity requires compositional heterogeneity. There can be changes in symptom clusters produced by changes in structure and processes of neural networks, in the inchoate material that presents itself to consciousness, in the choices and motives of the subject, in available cultural configurations (including salient imagery, and the looping effects described by Ian Hacking that make symptoms themselves part of the available cultural imaginary), and by changes in the dialogical interactions of subjects with clinical interlocutors (for example, by means of changes in interview protocols or typical clinical interactions). As long as there is continuity in one dimension of a persistent entity, there can be change in another.

I would like to raise some questions about the line of thought Professor Berrios has developed in his chapter: two about the tenability of some of the specific proposals and one more general concern about the overall approach taken.

First, Professor Berrios's chapter emphasizes two points that, taken together, stand in some tension with the aim of identifying change. One is that the qualitative experience of the sufferer is integral to the phenomena of psychopathology. The other is that each psychopathological episode is unique, made so by the very centrality of the qualitative dimension to the nature of the episode. Presumably this means that what might be identified as the same or similar neurobiological disturbance could, through the individual's different choices at different times, have different manifestations. Similarly, what might be identified as different neurobiological disturbances could, through the individual's different choices, have similar manifestations. This would seem to suggest that it is just not possible to group or classify disordered states, thus undermining the possibility of answering the question whether a condition presently classified as a kind of mental disorder/distress has changed over time.

This leads me to wonder whether some relevant progress is not being made in some related fronts. Oliver Sacks (2012) offers a veritable zoo of hallucinatory kinds, some of which are apparently closely related to brain states. For instance, Sacks reports that frontal lobe epileptic seizures are associated with distinctive hallucinatory patterns. Visually impaired elderly people experience two patterns of a kind of second sight, some simple geometric images, and some complex images. The forms of hallucination Sacks concerned himself with were recognized as such by the individuals having them, unlike the delusions and hallucinations we associate with conditions such as schizophrenia or "acute psychotic episodes" and that command the affected individual's assent. Does the apparent success in identifying distinctive patterns associated with distinctive physiological states or conditions such as epilepsy or migraine challenge the uniqueness claim and offer hope that a more systematic understanding can be developed for the distress of schizophrenia or bipolarity? Or does it suggest that schizophrenia and acute psychosis belong to a totally different ontological category?

Secondly, Professor Berrios is at pains to stress that he is interested in the possibility of interindividual, diachronically identified change, as he puts it, "transcendental" change. The heart of the matter for Berrios seems to be, can there be change in something more substantial than the cultural materials available for the representation of distress, which vary from individual to individual and even within individuals? I take this to be asking whether there could be changes to the process leading to the expression of mental distress. If so, what kind of change would this be? And, in light of the uniqueness claim, how would we ever know? In the end (literally, in the final paragraph), Berrios does give us a picture of change, but this is really change within an individual. What he calls "transcendent" change, or we might call transindividual change, remains elusive.

More generally, in his quest for a comprehensive hybrid model, Professor Berrios seems to be treading a fine line between several contesting forms of thought hoping to incorporate what is true or valuable from each. The effort at hybridity rather than autonomy, that is, the effort to incorporate insights from each of these forms of thought, may, however, be less fruitful that at first seems. Professor Berrios seems to want to say that only a dogmatic commitment to a strictly biological model of psychopathology would say there cannot be change in the kinds of disorder in the functional systems that generate the cascade into disordered behavior and states of consciousness. Do we really know enough about the neurobiological processes themselves to claim that forms of biological disorder remain stable over generations? In spite of the miracle of neuroimaging, not enough is known about the biology of the brain and nervous system to give a settled and comprehensive account of either the functions, the forms of neurological disruption, or the nature of the cascades from neural distress to psychopathological symptoms.

Speaking as a philosopher, I suspect that the Cambridge model, as well as the models it seeks to displace, is still too caught up in the old Cartesian dichotomization of mind and body. To try to link independently defined physical (neurophysiological) phenomena with independently defined psychological (mental, subjectively experienced) phenomena through causality is a losing proposition. Professor Berrios's alternative effort to see this as quasi-voluntary, intentional, interpretation does not, in the end, provide a model adequate to answer the question he set himself. It might be more fruitful to think of constitution instead of either causation or interpretation—to think of brain states as (partially) constitutive of mental/psychological states rather than as their causes. On this view, psychological distress will always have a biological component, but that doesn't mean that the biological causes the psychological or that the biological is independent and the psychological dependent or that the biological is real and the psychological eliminable. Constitution enables us to think not of the biological causing the psychological, but of biologically constituted psychological/mental states (that is, brain states or processes experienced as states of consciousness whether choate or inchoate) causing other biologically constituted psychological/mental states. I wish I could point to a well-worked out model of this constitutive way of thinking. I can't. I think the hybrid model is an effort at producing one, but it is still too conceptually dependent on a separation of mind and body. In this, it is a victim of the very thought processes from which Professor Berrios seeks to free us.

Reference

Sacks, O. (2012). *Hallucinations*. New York: Knopf.

Section 3
Scientific disagreement in the medical context

Chapter 7

Introduction to "Expert disagreement and medical authority"

Kenneth S. Kendler

One of the important antecedents to this meeting was my reading of Solomon's stimulating book, *Social Empiricism* (Solomon 2001). Reading over the historical examples contained therein (in chapters 5 and 7), I could see the clear applicability of her approach to a number of episodes in the history of psychiatry. Indeed, I would argue that psychiatry is a quite fertile discipline for the kind of analyses she undertakes.

Solomon begins this chapter by introducing the reader to her conceptual framework of empirical and nonempirical decision vectors. Let me here do a "pre-introduction." The question she tries to address is how to classify the kinds of things that impact on the evaluation of scientific theories. This can be asked with a wide historical perspective: Why did theory A win out over theory B over some historical time period? Or, it can be asked at the individual level: What caused scientist X to prefer theory A over theory B at time C? She suggests two broad categories of "kinds of things." She wants to arrange them into what she calls "decision vectors." She calls the first category "empirical decision vectors" that she ties tightly to the concept of "empirical success." Roughly, these are reasons (or causes) for preference of theories that "do real work in the world." Such theories predict new things. They explain why things are the particular way they are. These vectors are especially strong when they produce empirical success, which is particularly salient to the community or individual scientist. Salience is not typically regarded as "internal to the field of science" (it is traditionally viewed as a "biasing factor"). However, empirical decision vectors all require that the theory be empirically successful. Traditionally, empirical success is viewed as an "internal" (or "rational") reason for preferring scientific reasons. She calls her other major category "nonempirical decision vectors" and it is defined largely negatively as "causes of preference for aspects of theories other than their empirical success." This includes a wide variety of kinds of processes that would have generally been called "external" to the scientific process, and some factors that have traditionally been called "internal." It includes economic forces (funding priorities), social processes or preferences by scientists that are unrelated to empirical success such as beauty, simplicity, and elegance of theories.

Solomon suggests that science would work fairly well when the nonempirical vectors are roughly balanced. Empirical decision vectors should not be balanced (they reflect the differing empirical success of each theory), and only those theories with no unique empirical decision vectors should be dropped. A bad outcome might arise if there is a strong asymmetry in the nonempirical vectors that might then keep a theory with poor empirical support around (or dominant) longer than it should. Indeed, in Chapter 32 of this book, I ponder whether just this sort of process contributed to the extraordinary longevity of the dopamine hypothesis of schizophrenia.

To capture Solomon's concept it is important to realize that in her view each working scientist is at any one time under the influence of a range of decision vectors, some of which act in the same direction and some of which act in different directions. The same process is occurring at the higher level of the scientific community, which might be reflected in consensus conferences, funding decisions, or the outcome of paper or grant reviews.

Readers who keep going in this book will see the impact of Solomon's framework in later chapters, especially on the dopamine hypothesis of schizophrenia and on premenstrual dysphoric disorder.

The focus of this chapter is scientific disagreement. She begins by noting that, contrary to what might be a first impression, a number of weighty philosophers of science have sung the praises of disagreement. It is, they argue, not to be shied away from. Indeed, in general, it is a good thing for the field. In her section 8.4, she gives a list of eight negative views of scientific disagreement and rejects all of them. Centrally, she argues that consensus for a field of inquiry is not, generally, a desirable outcome.

In section 8.5, she turns away from this laudatory view of disagreement in basic science to argue for quite a different conclusion in applied research, as in medicine more generally or psychiatry specifically. Two trenchant examples that show negative outcomes from the public display of disagreement in medicine would be: (1) the substantial negative public health effects of spurious evidence of the possible causative relationship between certain childhood vaccinations and autism; and (2) the one Solomon explores at length, the controversy about screening mammography. She emphasizes the problem of trust between the "general public" on the one hand and the "medical establishment" on the other. Eroding that—as controversies often do—can have aggregate adverse consequences on public health.

I had raised with her my concern that her brush was a bit too broad here. Many aspects of medical research, although meeting a broad definition of "applied," are actually closer to basic science in practice. They are so far from the public eye that the adverse effects of disagreements are very unlikely to have any impact on public trust. She responds in her footnote 3, which the reader may wish to consult.

Before concluding, she provides her take on the story of premenstrual dysphoric disorder (PMDD) and the DSM (see Chapter 41, this volume). She suggests that scientific dissent was closed off prematurely in this disorder in large part because of the US Food and Drug Administration (FDA) approval of an antidepressant for treatment of PMDD. This would, I think, be an example of an adverse effect of an unbalanced set of nonempirical vectors. To show the subtleties of these issues, nearly all of the experts on the DSM-5 subcommittee on PMDD would disagree with this conclusion. They would have said that a scientific consensus that PMDD belonged in the DSM manual (and had better scientific support that most other diagnoses contained therein) was inappropriately delayed by strong and ill-informed nonempirical decision vectors. Such historical examples are open to varying interpretations.

This chapter and the conceptual framework it introduces merit study by the interested reader given the utility the approach and its ready applicability to the analysis of historical change in psychiatry.

Reference

Solomon, M. (2001). *Social Empiricism*. Cambridge, MA: MIT Press.

Chapter 8
Expert disagreement and medical authority

Miriam Solomon

8.1 Introduction

Scientific disagreement is, on the whole, good for science. Three reasons for this are regularly given. The first, from John Stuart Mill (Mill et al. 2003), Karl Popper (1963), Paul Feyerabend (1975), Helen Longino (1990), and others is that disagreements stimulate criticisms, and responding to criticism often improves theories. The second is that disagreements can produce an efficient division of cognitive labor, when scientists choose to work on those theories or approaches that they find the most promising, while disagreeing about which theories or approaches are the most promising. David Hull (1988), Alvin Goldman (1991), Philip Kitcher (1993), and I (Solomon 2001) have all written about this benefit of disagreement. The third benefit of disagreement is that it can produce a useful social distribution of knowledge. Consensus often leads to loss of information, skills, data, and modes of engagement. Donna Haraway (1991), Helen Longino (1990), Cass Sunstein (2003), and I argue this.

At the same time, there is a general tendency to see disagreement in science as a situation in need of resolution in order to produce stable knowledge. Consensus is often regarded as the *telos* of a period of scientific investigation, by both philosophers and historians of science. When I wrote *Social Empiricism* (Solomon 2001) I argued that this view is mistaken, and that consensus is not necessary for scientific progress or scientific knowledge. I think that consensus is overrated and often unfortunate. Dissent,[1] on the other hand, is often—although not always—fruitful.

While writing *Social Empiricism* I was thinking primarily about research science in the research community. I was not thinking about science in the public sphere. And I was not thinking about *applications* of science. Medicine is a quintessential applied science in that the contexts of application require consideration of ethical, political, professional, social, economic, ideological, national, and other factors. Many of the applications are controversial and require discussion, even when the science is uncontroversial. When the science is controversial and

---

[1] For my purposes, it is not necessary to distinguish "disagreement" and "dissent" and I use the two interchangeably.

scientific experts disagree, the authority of these experts in the wider deliberative context is, in practice, diminished. (Maybe it shouldn't be—but it is.) This diminished authority can be undesirable in situations where other interests—such as the interests of medical insurance companies—are only too happy to exploit any rhetorical weaknesses of the scientific experts. In this chapter I consider how I would modify my previous claims about dissent for the context of medicine, including psychiatry (the topic of this conference). To give away the punch line in the interests of clarity: I will argue that scientific disagreement is, on the whole, good for science and bad for medicine.

8.2 Causes of Scientific Disagreement: The Decision Vectors Framework

This section and the next will summarize the descriptive and normative frameworks of *Social Empiricism* (Solomon 2001) and use them to describe the causes of disagreement and state some epistemic norms for disagreement. (For detailed arguments, please see *Social Empiricism*.) I developed the vocabulary of "decision vectors" in order to give neutral descriptions of the factors that, in more judgmental language, "bias" researchers in one direction or another. A decision vector is a cause, or a reason, for preference of one theory over another. Scientific disagreement results when scientists have different decision vectors. Typically, each scientist is affected by more than one decision vector, and members of scientific communities (when the community is sufficiently diverse) are affected by different decision vectors. The decision vectors act together, and their strength and direction determine the scientists' commitments. For normative reasons that come later, I distinguish two types of decision vector: empirical decision vectors and nonempirical decision vectors. The distinction is subtle and does not quite correspond to traditional bifurcations such as "rational" versus "biased," or "cognitive" versus "social."

Empirical decision vectors are causes of preference for theories with empirical success (which can be predictive success, manipulative success, or explanatory success). For example, cognitively salient supporting data can be a cause of preference for the theory with those supporting data. Data become salient because of immediacy (direct experience), sensory vividness, or emotional resonance. For example, geologists who directly observed the folded structure of the Alps (salient field observations) were more likely to be sympathetic to the idea that the Earth's crust can move laterally to produce continental drift than geologists who did not make these observations, but knew about them from reading (Solomon 2001). Thus, empirical decision vectors are not the same as the traditional "evidence": they include weighing some data more heavily, and without justification for this partiality.

Nonempirical decision vectors are causes of preference for aspects of theories other than their empirical success. They include traditionally described "external" or "social" factors such as cohesion with ideologies and interests but also include traditionally described "rational" or "cognitive" factors such as simplicity (a structural feature of theories) and conservatism (the smallest distance between accepted knowledge and a new theory).

8.3 Norms of Scientific Disagreement

According to *Social Empiricism*, there are just two epistemic norms for scientific disagreement:

1. *Presence* of empirical decision vectors for each theory.
2. *Balance* of nonempirical decision vectors.

The first requirement is quite weak—weaker than in most normative accounts—but not vacuous. Each theory should have some empirical decision vectors specifically in its favor. This requirement excludes theories with no unique evidential support. Thus not all dissent is appropriate or useful. Dissent on theories with no empirical successes or with empirical successes that other theories also have is not useful dissent. (Intelligent design theory and climate change denial theories are, in my assessment, in the category of scientifically inappropriate dissent.) Secondly, the nonempirical decision vectors should be balanced as well as possible. The idea is that they should not be excluding theories from consideration or even giving them short shrift or excess attention. In practice, since we have no way of measuring the magnitude of decision vectors, I make an improper linear model[2] for the nonempirical decision vectors and sum them up on both sides (or on each side, if there are more than two options of theories to pursue). The smaller the gap between the totals, the better distributed the nonempirical decision vectors. Even though numbers are involved, this is a crude calculation. It is, however, better than forgoing assessment altogether (Solomon 2008). I encourage others to try to improve methods for calculation of the balance of decision vectors. (In this volume, Kenneth Kendler attempts to do so by estimating magnitudes as well as the direction of decision vectors.)

Many, perhaps most, epistemologists of science (e.g., Kitcher, Lakatos, and Laudan) argue that it is appropriate to pursue the theory with the most (or the "best") evidence. I do not offer the same advice—indeed, I advise against it—because more than one theory can contain important knowledge. A theory should be given up only when it has no evidence of its own. From a scientific point of view, pluralism is welcome, and insofar as scientific disagreement contributes to pluralism, scientific disagreement is also welcome.

8.4 What does Scientific Disagreement Mean?

Scientific disagreement is commonly thought to mean any or all of the following:
1. We do not know anything in the area of disagreement.
2. At least one person is wrong about something.

---

[2] An improper linear model counts each decision vector as one unit in a particular direction and does not estimate the size or strength or pervasiveness of that decision vector. Improper linear models do better than "seat of the pants" judgments (see Solomon 2008).

3. We have an embarrassing situation.
4. There is some failure to follow scientific method (because if we all followed scientific method, we would agree with each other).
5. We have a crisis.
6. We are "going through a stage" on the way to consensus.
7. There is incommensurability.
8. We can't work together (consensus is necessary for joint action).

I do not think that scientific disagreement, properly understood, means *any* of these. There can be knowledge in more than one theory—even when the theories are inconsistent with one another. Of course, we may not be able to pinpoint which features of our theories are responsible for their successes. (We cannot identify the "truth in the theory," except perhaps in hindsight.) It is true that at least one person is wrong about something, but that is typically the case when scientists agree as well as when they disagree: it is not the import of dissent. So long as the importance and meaning of dissent are understood, it should not be thought of as an embarrassing situation, a scientific failure, or a crisis when scientists disagree. Consensus is not the *telos* of inquiry, so the situation should not be framed as "going through a stage" on the way to consensus. And disagreement does not mean that scientists disagree about everything: there are still large areas of overlap. In particular, scientists may wish to standardize some measures, such as temperature measurement, in order to make clearer their areas of agreement and disagreement (Chang 2004).

If scientific disagreement does not mean any of these things, what does it mean? I suggest that it means "science as usual," with imprecise methodology and fallible results. It also means that there is a social structure in which mutual criticism will take place (as Mill, Longino, and Sunstein recommend) and that research effort as well as knowledge may be distributed and thereby increase the range of inquiry, avoiding narrowness and excess duplication of efforts.

8.5 Applied Research (Including Medicine and Psychiatry)

Scientific disagreement is often useful when doing basic research. In applied contexts, however, especially those involving public policy, it is difficult to plan collective action without some agreement on the impact of that action. When making environmental policy, for example, there needs to be some agreement about the influence of changing carbon emissions on global warming. Moreover, it is difficult to garner public support for an action when the acknowledged experts are in disagreement. The authority of experts depends on their unanimity. When they disagree, other interests are more likely to take over. (This is a remark about rhetoric, not about logic.) For example, if the medical community is in disagreement about the benefits of long-term psychiatric hospitalization, insurance companies and governmental agencies are more likely to go with their own interests, and to deny funding for this intervention. The slogan "Doubt is our product," began in cigarette companies, where it was quickly realized that the best way to reduce scientific authority is to produce an apparent expert who disagrees with the experts (Oreskes and Conway 2010; Proctor 2008).

Sociologists and historians of medicine have remarked that professionalization depends on having shared standards (see, e.g., Freidson 2001; Marks 1997; Timmermans and Berg 2003). Professionalization, of course, contributes to the perceived authority of an expert group. Members of a professional group do not have to completely agree about everything—Freidson in particular writes about the importance of some individual autonomy in making professional judgments—but they have their greatest authority in those areas in which they agree, and they need to have large areas of agreement in order to have authority at all.

In fact, the institution of medical consensus conferences (started at the National Institutes of Health (NIH) in 1977) was intended to produce more consensus on clinical care than was occurring by the usual means of research dissemination. The idea is that a formal consensus of neutral experts can make an authoritative statement about standards of care. The medical consensus conference movement quickly spread, both nationally and internationally. What happened with consensus conferences is a long story that I can't tell here (see Solomon 2007, 2011, forthcoming). The bottom line, though, is that medical consensus conferences were, and indeed still are (although to a lesser degree) institutions that are charged with delivering authoritative statements about medical care. When the experts disagree, they can easily lose their authority. When such conferences fail to reach consensus, or when different groups reach different conclusions on the same topics, authoritative statements cannot be made.[3]

8.6 Illustrative Case Study: Screening Mammography for Women Aged 40–49

Here is an example in which medical experts disagree about clinical (i.e., practical) recommendations. I have not (yet) worked out a detailed example for psychiatry, but Peter Zachar and Kenneth Kendler have, in Chapter 41 in this volume. In section 8.9 of this chapter I use their case study to suggest how my discussion of dissent and its management extends to psychiatry.

Recommendations for screening mammography have been controversial ever since the technology was developed in the late 1960s. Despite the fact that mammography has been more extensively evaluated by randomized trials than any

---

[3] Ken Kendler suggested to me that consensus is important only for part of medicine: the part that is involved in clinical recommendations. He thinks that basic science in medicine can tolerate disagreement to the same extent as the pure (nonapplied) sciences. This is a fair point. Much of the time, however, differences in clinical recommendations occur at least partly *because of* differences in basic research, and consensus on clinical recommendations cannot occur without substantial consensus on the basic science.

other screening method (Wells 1998), it continues to be controversial, especially for routine use in women aged 40–49. The length and persistence of controversy—over 40 years, with the same issues frequently rehashed—is extraordinary. The Canadian Preventative Services Task Force, re-established in 2010, selected screening mammography as its first topic for discussion, indicating the continuing importance of making authoritative statements about it. Currently, in the United States,[4] the American Cancer Society, the National Cancer Institute, the Society for Breast Imaging, and the American College of Radiologists all recommend annual screening starting at age 40, while the United States Preventative Services Task Force (USPSTF) and the American College of Physicians recommend against routine mammography for women aged 40–49. These recommendations are made by groups of experts—physicians, researchers, and statisticians—who typically construct a consensus statement after examination and discussion of the evidence.

Judgments on the topic differ sharply. Michael Baum, a breast surgeon from the United Kingdom, has said that screening mammography is "one of the greatest deceptions perpetrated on the women of the Western World" (quoted in Ehrenreich 2001), while the American College of Radiology has a statement on its website about the "ill advised and dangerous USPSTF mammography recommendations" which claims that "The [USPSTF] recommendations make unconscionable decisions about the value of human life" and predicts that the recommendations will lead to more women dying of breast cancer.[5] In response to such comments, Jane Wells, a British public health physician, asserts "The debate over the necessity of screening for breast cancer among women in their 40s has assumed an importance out of proportion to its potential impact on public health" (Wells 1998, p. 1228).

Let's take a look at how the decision vectors framework describes the causes of the mammography controversy. First, what are the empirical decision vectors? Nine randomized trials have shown zero, small positive, or small negative effects for screening mammography for women aged 40–49. The results of meta-analyses depend on the evidence hierarchy selected (Goodman 2002), also indicating a small effect, if any. Clinicians often present evidence from individual cases, arguing that they have seen patients' lives saved by the detection and treatment of early-stage breast cancer. These cases are salient, but the evidence is not robust because it is subject to a number of biases such as mistaken attribution of causation. One estimate suggests that only about one in eight of women diagnosed by mammography and treated for early-stage breast cancer have their lives saved by early diagnosis (Welch and Frankel 2011). And those who are harmed rather than helped by mammography and unnecessary

---

[4] There is similar controversy in other developed countries, but I am most knowledgeable about the United States.

[5] See <http://www.acr.org/About-Us/Media-Center/Position-Statements/Position-Statements-Folder/Detailed-ACR-Statement-on-Ill-Advised-and-Dangerous-USPSTF-Mammography-Recommendations>.

treatment are not salient. In summary, empirical decision vectors are present for both sides of the mammography controversy—different trials have different results—and there is some salient (although not robust) evidence for the effectiveness of mammography in women aged 40–49. According to social empiricism, all that is needed of the empirical decision vectors is that they are present for both sides of the mammography controversy, and they are (although not robustly). The empirical decision vectors do *not* need to be balanced with approximately the same on both sides.

Nonempirical decision vectors are well known. They include the self-interest of radiologists, who stand to gain from a broad and frequent screening policy (see, e.g., (Quanstrum and Hayward 2010) and the widespread view—reinforced by organizations such as the American Cancer Society—that we can control cancer through responsible individual efforts such as annual screening examinations. Furthermore, the established practice, from early days when it was expected that screening mammography would work, is to screen women aged 40–49, so conservatism favors broad screening. That is three nonempirical decision vectors on the side of screening. There may be one nonempirical decision vector on the side of not screening: the desire to cut costs by not doing unnecessary screening. But this nonempirical decision vector does not have much force in the United States, where the politics of breast cancer has led to policy decisions not to restrict reimbursement for mammography. (In some European countries, cost-saving incentives probably function as nonempirical decision vectors against screening mammography for women aged 40–49.) Thus in the United States, there are three nonempirical decision vectors favoring screening, and none on the other side. (In some European countries, there are three nonempirical decision vectors favoring screening, and one disfavoring it.) This is an imbalance of nonempirical decision vectors, particularly in the United States. Nonempirical decision vectors do not need to be exactly balanced—the improper linear model of balancing decision vectors is not all that precise—but gross imbalance is notable. According to the framework of *Social Empiricism*, there is more attention paid to positive recommendations for screening than there should be from a scientific point of view.

From the point of view of the standardization and authority of the practice of medicine, however, scientific dissent is troubling, whether or not nonempirical decision vectors are balanced. Not surprisingly, there have been continued efforts on the part of the medical profession to end the dissent about mammography screening. Some consensus conferences have failed to produce consensus—most notably, the 1997 NIH Consensus Development Conference on Screening Mammography. Others have achieved consensus only to be disputed by other groups' consensus conferences (as when the USPSTF disputed the consensuses of the American Cancer Society and the American College of Radiologists). Other efforts to end the disagreement are worth taking a look at. I'm going to continue this chapter by mentioning four of these ways. They are not unique to breast cancer screening, although breast cancer screening makes particularly good use of them.

8.7 "Managing" Disagreement

Four ways of managing disagreement in medicine are: (1) guideline syntheses, (2) reframing areas of uncertainty as opportunities for autonomy for both physicians and patients, (3) use of methodological hierarchies, and (4) promoting trust. Since disagreement in medicine tends to damage medical authority, it is not surprising to find efforts to manage and contain it.

8.7.1 Guideline Syntheses

The National Guidelines Clearinghouse (NGC), managed by the Agency for Healthcare Research and Quality (AHRQ), lists up-to-date clinical guidelines, provided that they are produced by a recognized organization and include an examination of relevant scientific evidence. Sometimes, this results in listing guidelines that conflict with one another; in these cases NGC often publishes a "Guideline Synthesis" that addresses the areas of dispute. In late 2010, I took a look at the guidelines on screening mammography that were listed by the NGC. The included the American College of Physicians 2007 guideline, the US Preventative Services Task Force Guideline from 2009, the American Cancer Society 2007 guidelines, and the American College of Obstetricians and Gynecologists 2006 guideline. The first two guidelines are in agreement that routine screening mammography should *not* be offered to women aged 40–49 and the second two guidelines are in agreement that it *should* be offered. However, the "Guideline Synthesis" statement includes only the first two guidelines, and thus presents more consensus than exists. I sent an inquiry to the NGC, asking why the other guidelines were listed by NGC (and therefore presumably of high enough quality) and yet not included in the synthesis. Their response was that the other guidelines are not up to date with the evidence. I sent another query, asking why guidelines can be listed (which requires that they be up to date with the evidence) and yet not used for the guideline synthesis. This inquiry did not receive a response.[6] Obviously, if selected guidelines are dropped from syntheses, it can look as though there is less dissent than there actually is.[7]

8.7.2 Reframing

It is common to reappropriate areas of disagreement as a locus for the "individualized" judgments that support either physician autonomy (framing them as "clinical judgment"), patient self-determination, or both. Hence we find a common recommendation that each woman discuss with her physician whether or not to have screening mammography in her 40s. This turns the area

---

[6] My contact was Vivian Coates at the ECRI Institute, which manages the NGC for AHRQ. Our communications were by e-mail in Fall 2010.

[7] Recently the NGC updated its material on guidelines for screening mammography. Interestingly, it still lists guidelines that are not used in the guideline synthesis. I discuss this update in detail in Solomon (forthcoming)

of epistemic uncertainty into an area of professional judgment and preference, making a virtue out of the uncertainty by using it as an area in which to extol physician autonomy and patient-centered medicine. It also, subtly, encourages confining the area in which personal judgments and preferences make a difference to women in their 40s. But personal judgments and preferences *could* be used for women in their 50s and beyond, to weigh benefits and risks for each woman. For example, for some women the anxiety associated with false positive results may be severe, and for them the potential harms of mammography will be greater. *The magnitude of benefits and risks is not the same as the magnitude of uncertainty in the data.* However, such expansion of patient and physician discretion is not encouraged by any party to the debate. In my view, there is a compromise here between the desire to be guided by the evidence and the desire to acknowledge both clinical judgment and patient self-determination. A "gray area" is defined where guidelines are not governing. Quanstrum and Hayward are a particularly clear example of endorsement of this strategy when they write of "a gray area of indeterminate net benefit, in which clinicians should defer to an individual patient's preferences" (Quanstrum and Hayward 2010). The strategy is not limited to the case of mammography; similar recommendations have been made recently for prostate cancer screening with the prostate-specific antigen test.

8.7.3 Methodological Hierarchies

Disagreements can sometimes be avoided if some methods or approaches are regarded as having privilege over others. For example, since 2000 the NIH Consensus Development Conference Program has required a systematic evidence review to take place *before* the panelists meet. This review is done by the AHRQ according to the standards of evidence-based medicine, and the result is a published evidence report. Then consensus conference discussions start off anchored in the evidence report. It is likely that this has reduced disagreement for some medical controversies. The practice may or may not be justified, depending on the reliability of the evidence report. It has not helped to reduce disagreement over screening mammography, in part because there is not unanimity in the evidence syntheses; different meta-analyses of the same data have reached different conclusions (Goodman 2002). Moreover, positions in the mammography debate were staked out before the development and widespread use of evidence-based medicine techniques.

8.7.4 Promoting Trust

It is common for guidelines that do not recommend routine screening mammography for women aged 40–49 to insist, at the same time, that such mammography continue to be covered by health insurance or government reimbursement programs. For example, the 1997 NIH Consensus Development Conference statement says, "For women in their forties who choose to have mammography performed, the costs of the mammograms should be reimbursed by third-party payers or covered by health maintenance organizations so that financial impediments will not influence a woman's decision."[8] Such a statement is designed to prevent dissent from being amplified by distrust.

8.8 Disagreement and Agnotology

Disagreements can be distracting. Barbara Brenner, the former Executive Director of Breast Cancer Action, said this eloquently in 1997:

> If there is any reason for outrage, it is this: as long as we are spending our time, energy and money on the mammogram debate, we are distracted from finding a nonradiation-based detection method that works, discovering effective treatments and offering primary prevention. Just as Nero fiddled while Rome burned, we are spending enormous resources on an aspect of breast cancer that ultimately does very little, if anything, to save lives. (Brenner 1997)

Likewise, the oncologist and epidemiologist Steven Goodman writes:

> even under the most optimistic assumptions, mammography still cannot prevent the vast majority of breast cancer deaths. Improving methods of risk prediction, communication, disease detection and treatment will probably yield more public health benefit than continued debate about mammography. (Goodman 2002, p. 364)

Brenner and Goodman are arguing that continued debate over mammographic screening is actually harmful (not only fruitless) because it diverts attention and research resources that would be better spent on other forms of diagnosis or on prevention and treatment. Their warnings have not been generally heeded and the debate over mammographic screening is still live (witness the choice of the newly reconstituted Canadian Preventative Services Task Force to do screening mammography for its first topic in 2010). Live controversies can have the unintended (or sometimes intended, in cases of intentionally manufactured dissent) effect of keeping us ignorant in other (not so live) areas.

Agreement can have an epistemological downside, also. After we reach or negotiate an agreement, we tend to forget the terms of that agreement. We no longer remember exactly what was at stake. When knowledge or practices change, this forgetting can make it difficult to revisit and revise earlier negotiations. "Agnotology" is a term coined by Robert Proctor (2008) to describe the ways in which we are, or we become, ignorant. Agreement has agnotological consequences.

8.9 Application to Psychiatry

I have used the case of medical disagreement about mammographic screening because it is a case I know particularly well. But I should also say something about how psychiatry, as a branch of medicine, produces and manages disagreement. The case of premenstrual dysphoric disorder (PMDD), explored by Peter Zachar and Kenneth Kendler in Chapter 41 in this volume, is a good example

---

[8] See <http://consensus.nih.gov/1997/1997BreastCancerScreening103html.htm>.

to discuss. Zachar and Kendler show that disagreement about the existence of this disorder was produced by a range of empirical and nonempirical decision vectors. The disagreement was not left alone to run its scientific course; perhaps it might have generated a number of different lines of research. Instead, efforts were made starting in the 1980s to settle the matter in the pages of the *Diagnostic and Statistical Manual of Mental Disorders* (DSM). The DSM is a lengthy consensus statement of the US psychiatric community on the classification of mental disorders. It is intended for use by clinicians, who often need to make a diagnosis before selecting an appropriate treatment.[9] (It is also used by clinicians for billing purposes.)

What is the purpose of the DSM? If psychiatrists completely agreed about disease classifications, there would be no need for it. Indeed, the rest of medicine has much more agreement about disease classification and rarely introduces diagnostic categories that are as complex and difficult to apply as those in the DSM.[10] The DSM uses the authority of expert consensus to reduce dissent in the psychiatric community. As all consensus statements, the DSM needs to avoid going too far by trying to force consensus when there is clear dissent; if it is seen as making premature judgments that will only decrease its authority. But it can use its authority to nudge along the consensus a little.

The first time PMDD was added to the DSM was in 1987. The details are interesting: late luteal phase dysphoric disorder (a category close to PMDD) was added to "Appendix A" of the DSM-III-R as a proposed disorder in need of further study. As Zachar and Kendler write, "In fact, this DSM appendix was created largely to contain PMDD" (Chapter 41, this volume). Why create Appendix A? I think that if PMDD had been included in the main body of the volume, the dissent around it might have undermined the authority of the DSM as a whole. The appendix is a compromise between including PMD and not including it.

The most recent DSM-5 moves PMDD to the main body of the text, classified with mood disorders. Zachar and Kendler (Chapter 41, this volume) point out that the 1999 Food and Drug Administration (FDA) approval of the drug Sarafem® specifically for PMDD paved the way for DSM-5 to unhesitatingly add PMDD to the mood disorders. The FDA approval was strongly influenced by pharmaceutical interests and is scientifically controversial. This is a case in which scientific dissent was prematurely ended by a combination of pharmaceutical interests and the need for clinical authority.

---

[9] As Robert Michels has argued (Chapter 20, this volume), the DSM also serves constituencies other than clinicians. It is used by educators, in order to train clinicians. And it is used by researchers, who need clinical trial inclusion and exclusion criteria.

[10] There is no equivalent to the DSM for physical diseases as a whole. The World Health Organization's ICD classification system is important for epidemiological and billing purposes, but it is a much thinner volume. There are complex and disputed classifications for some areas, such as rheumatology (I am grateful to Ken Kendler for pointing this out).

8.10 Conclusions

Medical disagreement, like scientific disagreement, can produce a beneficial division of intellectual labor. A "decision vectors" analysis can go some way toward assessing whether or not the division of intellectual labor is appropriate for research in a particular domain. The downside, however, is that medical disagreement tends to reduce the authority of medical experts. In order to maintain unanimity (and thus authority), the medical community has (consciously or unconsciously) developed strategies for reducing and containing scientific disagreements. It is important to remember that such strategies can obscure issues and lead to loss of knowledge.

Acknowledgments

The material on the mammography case in this chapter is taken from Solomon (2012). Work on this chapter was supported by NSF grant SES-1152050 and a Temple University Research and Study Leave during 2012–2013. I am most grateful to Kenneth Kendler and to the participants in the conference "Philosophical Issues in Psychology III" for their feedback on this chapter.

References

Brenner, B.A. (1997). Fiddling while Rome burns: the latest mammogram controversy. *Breast Cancer Action Source*, 41.

Chang, H. (2004). *Inventing Temperature: Measurement and Scientific Progress*. New York: Oxford University Press.

Ehrenreich, B. (2001). Welcome to cancerland. *Harper's Magazine*, November, 43–53.

Feyerabend, P. (1975). *Against Method: Outline of an Anarchistic Theory of Knowledge*. London: Newleft Books.

Freidson, E. (2001). *Professionalism: The Third Logic*. Chicago, IL: University of Chicago Press.

Goldman, A.I. and Shaked, M. (1991). An economic model of scientific activity and truth acquisition. *Philosophical Studies*, 63(1), 31–55.

Goodman, S.N. (2002). The mammography dilemma: a crisis for evidence-based medicine? *Annals of Internal Medicine*, 137(5), 363–365.

Haraway, D.J. (1991). *Simians, Cyborgs, and Women: The Reinvention of Nature*. New York: Routledge.

Hull, D.L. (1988). *Science as a Process: An Evolutionary Account of the Social and Conceptual Development of Science*. Chicago, IL: University of Chicago Press.

Kitcher, P. (1993). *The Advancement of Science: Science Without Legend, Objectivity Without Illusions*. New York: Oxford University Press.

Longino, H.E. (1990). *Science as Social Knowledge: Values and Objectivity in Scientific Inquiry*. Princeton, NJ: Princeton University Press.

Marks, H.M. (1997). *The Progress of Experiment: Science and Therapeutic Reform in the United States, 1900–1990*. New York: Cambridge University Press.

Mill, J.S., Bentham, J., Austin, J., and Warnock, M. (2003). *Utilitarianism; and, On Liberty: Including Mill's 'Essay on Bentham', and Selections from the Writings of Jeremy Bentham and John Austin* (2nd ed.). Malden, MA: Blackwell Pub.

Oreskes, N. and Conway, E.M. (2010). *Merchants of Doubt: How a Handful of Scientists Obscured the Truth on Issues from Tobacco Smoke to Global Warming.* New York: Bloomsbury Press.

Popper, K.R. (1963). *Conjectures and Refutations: The Growth of Scientific Knowledge.* London: Routledge & Kegan Paul Limited.

Proctor, R.N. (2008). Agnotology: a missing term to describe the cultural production of ignorance (and its study). In R.N. Proctor and L. Shiebinger (eds.) *Agnotology: The Making and Unmaking of Ignorance*, pp. 1–33. Stanford, CA: Stanford University Press.

Quanstrum, K.H. and Hayward, R.A. (2010). Lessons from the mammography wars. *The New England Journal of Medicine*, 363(11), 1076–1079.

Solomon, M. (2001). *Social Empiricism.* Cambridge, MA: MIT Press.

Solomon, M. (2007). The social epistemology of NIH consensus conferences. In H. Kincaid and J. McKitrick (eds.) *Establishing Medical Reality: Methodological and Metaphysical Issues in Philosophy of Medicine*, pp. 167–177. Dordrecht: Springer.

Solomon, M. (2008). *Norms of Dissent.* Contingency and Dissent in Science Project Discussion Paper Series. London: London School of Economics CPNSS.

Solomon, M. (2011). Group judgment and the medical consensus conference. In F. Gifford (ed.) *Philosophy of Medicine*, pp. 239–254. New York: Elsevier.

Solomon, M. (2012). "A troubled area." Understanding the controversy over screening mammography for women aged 40–49. In C. Jager and W. Loffler (eds.) *Epistemology: Contexts, Values, Disagreement. Proceedings of the 34th International Ludwig Wittgenstein Symposium*, pp. 271–284. Heusenstamm: Ontos Verlag.

Solomon, M. (forthcoming). *Making Medical Knowledge.* Oxford: Oxford University Press.

Sunstein, C.R. (2003). *Why Societies Need Dissent.* Cambridge, MA: Harvard University Press.

Timmermans, S. and Berg, M. (2003). *The Gold Standard: The Challenge of Evidence-Based Medicine and Standardization in Health Care.* Philadelphia, PA: Temple University Press.

Welch, H.G. and Frankel, B.A. (2011). Likelihood that a woman with screen-detected breast cancer has had her "life saved" by that screening. *Archives of Internal Medicine*, 171(22), 2043–2046.

Wells, J. (1998). Mammography and the politics of randomised controlled trials. *BMJ (Clinical research ed.)*, 317(7167), 1224–1229.

Chapter 9

Trust, dissent, and decision vectors

Ian Hacking

9.1 Solomon on Dissent

Miriam Solomon's *Social Empiricism* (2001) sketched a very useful framework in which to portray the forces that act on people making up their minds, individually or as a group, about which scientific theories to take seriously, work on, or simply accept and use. The forces are of different types and come from different directions, so she names them "decision vectors." Since a vector is a quantity that has both magnitude and direction, this is a metaphor—we seem to have no ready-made noun for forces with direction but indeterminate magnitude. Her framework is a "social" one, in which there are two types of vector, empirical and nonempirical; the nonempirical vectors are, to speak coarsely, social rather than data based. "Scientific disagreement results when scientists have different decision vectors."

This all seems very plausible to me, but I am not an apt commentator, for I have never thought seriously about the questions that have interested so many philosophers of the sciences, namely questions about the acceptance of scientific theories and norms for so doing. To tell the truth, the idea of deciding to work on a theory, to join a lab, to decide among possible places at which to do a postdoc—all that makes excellent sense. I decide which expert to consult or to hire. But I have never well understood the idea of a person or a community "deciding to accept" a theory. Hence, I shall not venture into such questions, and so far as is possible, take Solomon's lucid framework for granted.

In the chapter under discussion, Solomon coins an aphorism: "scientific disagreement is, on the whole, good for science and bad for medicine," and indeed for applied science in general. When she wrote about science in previous work, she "was thinking primarily about research science in the research community." There, disagreement is on the whole valuable to the enterprise. But she "was not thinking about *applications* of science," or "science in the public sphere" (quotes from Chapter 8). There, she maintains, dissent can do a good deal of harm.

Compare the aphorism: "Dissent is good for science, bad for application," with Francis Bacon's "Knowledge is power." Bacon said something important and illuminating, although you have to see what he means, and also acknowledge that it is not literally true. We are well aware that to know is all too often not to have power. There are men in jail, for example, who know they are innocent, but are powerless to convince their jailers. Solomon's aphorism is not quite as snappy as Bacon's. But as with Bacon, we do have to know what it means, and when it is not literally true. Innumerable applications of science have had disastrous consequences, and disagreement would have been good for the applications, for those who apply the science, and for those to whom the science was applied. One wishes, for example, that there had been more disagreement about the probabilities of earthquakes, which might have led to different designs and prevented the Fukushima Daiichi nuclear disaster. I don't think Solomon's qualification "on the whole" quite evades the difficulty.

I should also register caution about the distinction between "research science in the research community" and "applications." The noun popularized by Bruno Latour might be a good corrective: "technoscience." Much research is mission oriented, conducted and funded with uses in mind; some scientific research really is done solely to find out about the nature of things, with no application in view. But there is such a continuum between the two that I hesitate to follow Solomon's distinction; I very much doubt that she would strongly disagree with this caution.

Moreover, unless the idea of medical research is very severely constrained, there is a lot of "research science in the research community" that is funded by the US National Institutes of Health (NIH), French Institut National de la Santé et de la Recherche Médicale (INSERM), or the UK Medical Research Council (MRC), and so on. I am told that if you are applying for a grant for research on voltage-gated potassium channels that are involved in interaction between neurons, it is prudent to add a paragraph about how this might bear on Alzheimer's disease—all those old geezers on the panel will perk up and welcome your proposal. But that is window dressing: potassium channels are, at present, pretty much "research science in the research community"—in the United States, mostly funded by the NIH. Is it not "medicine?" A really whopping discovery in that field would likely qualify for a Nobel Prize in Physiology or Medicine. For example, the 1962 prize in medicine for Perutz and Kendrew, doing research science on hemoglobin, was less sensational but almost as important as the 1962 prize in chemistry given to Watson and Crick.

9.2 Screening Mammography of Breast Cancer

Solomon proceeds in exactly the way I always favor: careful examination of a particular case, that of "screening mammography for breast cancer, for women aged 40–49." She tends, perhaps, to run together this specific question, with the slightly more general issue of screening mammography for women, period. Many of her more virulent quotations seem not to be age specific, for example, Michael Baum's "one of the greatest deceptions perpetrated on women of the Western World." He and others whom Solomon cites are against mammography screening overall, which is a quite distinct issue from screening women aged 40–49, under the tacit assumption that screening 50–69-year-old women is worthwhile. Baum rejects that tacit assumption, while the debates considered by Solomon accept it.

You might think Solomon has provided ample information in presenting her example, but I propose to go one more layer down. Solomon twice mentions the Canadian Preventative Services Task Force. That is actually the nomenclature of the similar US body. The correct designation is the Canadian Task Force on Preventative Health Care established under the aegis of the Public Health Agency of Canada. Everything that I shall say about the Task Force is taken from well-indexed parts of their website (Canadian Task Force on Preventative Health Care (n.d.). The Task Force is a panel of 14 acknowledged experts, mostly physicians, with adequate staff, intended to give clear and explicit advice to the medical community of the current judgment about, among other things, screening.

I should preface by saying that every province in Canada has Universal Health Insurance which pays all costs of mammography recommended by a physician. In contrast, prostate-specific antigen (PSA) screening for prostate cancer is not covered in my province (Ontario), but is routinely available at cost ($25 per test). I may also mention that a PSA test is totally painless—a pinprick to take a dab of blood, while many women find mammography demeaning and/or painful. (Disclosure: every year I pay the $25 because I have immediate (free) access to a first-class urologist who says the PSA count is always one tidbit of evidence that helps diagnosis. Without that access, I would not take the test. I cite this as an instance of what Solomon calls "management" of disagreement.)

Solomon writes that the Task Force was re-established in 2010, and that it "selected screening mammography as its first topic for discussion, indicating the continuing importance of making authoritative statements about it." I would modify this a bit. "Re-established" suggests there was an issue, which would support Solomon's inference. In fact it was re-established because the mandate of its predecessor was for 25 years, which had simply expired. In 2010 it was renewed.

The Canadian Guide to Clinical Preventive Health Care (Canadian Task Force on Preventive Health Care 1994) is an enormous document covering screening for a great many conditions, running from (1) "Routine Prenatal Ultrasound Screening" to (81) "Screening for Asymptomatic Bacteriuria in the Elderly." "Breast Cancer" is 65th, occupying pages 786–795. It includes an excellent run-through of the then-available evidence, and recommends screening from age 50 to 74, but says the evidence for women aged 40–49 is equivocal, and the *Guide* does not recommend screening. The recommendations rely heavily on seven studies, four from Sweden, and mention a great many studies then underway. Thus the 2010 Task Force put mammography up front because the previous guidelines radically needed updating, not because of "the continuing importance of making authoritative statements about it," but because massively more information was obtained from 1994 to 2009. Solomon mentions many of those very studies.

At its first meeting, April 26-27, 2010, the Task Force established working groups for its future methodology, focusing on (in its own order): diabetes, breast cancer, hypertension, depression, and cervical cancer, for each of which there was substantial new data after 1994. At its next meeting, June 28, 2010, it set up a priority ranking for topics to consider, as follows: screening for breast cancer, hypertension, depression, diabetes, cervical cancer, obesity, moderately elevated multiple cardiovascular and metabolic risk factors, colorectal cancer, prostate cancer, and five other conditions, ending with cognitive impairment and dementia in the elderly.

In 2011, the Task Force produced, in the case of breast cancer screening, one of the most easily understood authoritative documents I have ever read, so I reproduce it here in full (Canadian Task Force on Preventive Health Care n.d.):

- For women aged 40–49 we recommend *not routinely screening* with mammography. (Weak recommendation; moderate quality evidence)
- For women aged 50–69 years we recommend *routinely screening* with mammography every 2 to 3 years. (Weak recommendation; moderate quality evidence)
- For women aged 70–74 we recommend *routinely screening* with mammography every 2 to 3 years. (Weak recommendation; low quality evidence)

Note that the recommendation is *never* for annual screening at any age. Note that all three recommendations are qualified as weak (in comparison, for example, to screening for hypertension where there are strong recommendations). The evidence in two cases is qualified as moderate and in one as of low quality.

After the recommendations, there is a succinct summary with full references of the studies on which these recommendations are based. The recommendations are effectively the same as in 1994, but are based on massively more evidence.

We might modestly call this the official Canadian consensus. Solomon mentions that in the United States there is still no consensus, with the American Cancer Society, the National Cancer Institute, and the American College of Radiologists recommending annual screening after age 40. I am not clear from her paper whether the US Preventive Services Task Force or American College of Physicians, both of which reject routine screening in the age range 40–49, favor *annual* routine mammography for older women, or not.

Canadian consensus? The advice given by the Canadian Cancer Society (n.d.) is totally different from that given by its American opposite number:

- If you are 40–49: talk to your doctor about your risk of breast cancer, along with the benefits and risks of mammography.
- If you are 50–69: have a mammogram every 2 years.
- If you are 70 or older: talk to your doctor about how often you should have a mammogram.

Of course there are cancer advocacy groups in Canada who favor more mammography, usually drawing on US activists. A respected Canadian health science journalist with whom I discussed these matters unkindly calls them lobbyists, and says they have to be reported in the media out of "fairness." She holds that this is the skewed notion of fairness that insists that climate change deniers get equal time with the vast majority of climate scientists, but her bosses insist that if she does not give them equal TV time, the "lobbyists" will counterattack.

Why this substantial difference between Canada and the United States? One wants almost to invoke stereotypes. Canadians are just more respectful of authority in general, and many of us lament that fact. There have been horrendous errors because of excessive trust; the most notable is the "tainted blood scandal." For most of the twentieth century, blood collection and distribution was administered by the Canadian Red Cross—almost all the blood collected by voluntary donation. All college campuses have intensely competitive blood drives, which helps. But then in the late 1970s there was an incredible incidence of HIV and hepatitis B among hemophiliacs. Yet all the Red Cross experts said this could not possibly have come from tainted blood, so rigorous was the testing. And who would doubt the Red Cross? We were desperately in need of more scientific dissent.

But there is something more specific than trust in authority. Every indicator shows that the broad mass of Canadians, despite complaints about excessive waiting times for nonurgent surgery and other problems, are solidly behind universal health care. We trust the system to look after us.

9.3 Social Empiricism

I mentioned earlier my hesitation over the very language of "deciding to accept scientific theories." Happily there is no need to speak that way anywhere in this story. The Canadian Task Force and the Canadian Cancer Society had to decide which recommendations to make, on the basis of an increasingly large number of somewhat conflicting studies. Theory acceptance does not arise. Hence, I am content with Solomon's framework of decision vectors.

How well does my local story fit into that framework? Solomon mentions that European health systems might have a strong bias toward cost-cutting, not present in the United States. So that would be a nonempirical decision vector relevant in Europe but not in the United States. Is it relevant in Canada, with an even more universal system than anywhere in Europe? (In Canada a two-tier system is forbidden by Act of Parliament.) Perhaps cost was considered by the Canadian Task Force; only real social research and interviews would determine the extent of that. But let us suppose that cost has been and is an active nonempirical decision factor in Canada.

Solomon mentions three American nonempirical decision factors favoring screening (in the age group 40–49). (1) Conservative: in the early days it was thought, lacking evidence, that screening would apply over all mature ages. (2) Enterprise individualism: we can control cancer by individual efforts including screening. (3) Special interest: the radiologists have a financial stake—different from in the United States, but still, the more screening, the more jobs. We would expect all three vectors to be present in Canada as well. Are we to explain the Canadian phenomenon by saying that they must have been weaker in Canada than in the United States, while they were countered by a nonempirical vector of cost-cutting? Frankly, that is too easy a fit with the framework to provide a rich and satisfying explanation. The "social" context is just so much richer than that, and I confess I would prefer more science studies/sociology of science than the rationalist model of decision vectors.

Yes, I suggest that when we get down to details, Solomon's framework is all too "rationalistic." Unlike most traditional "rationalists" (e.g. Popper or Lakatos) she allows nonempirical factors into the equation. But the social reality seems to me to be somewhat more complex than can be described within the framework. Should I put "readiness to trust authority" in as a nonempirical decision vector? Should we put "the existence of well-financed lobbyists" as a nonempirical decision factor that bears on the American Task Force, but not to the same extent as on the Canadian one? That would at least lead us a little closer to social reality.

If we are considering medicine, there is a social element that it is very important to recognize. In the past 50 years, advocacy groups—what my journalist unkindly calls lobbyists—have come to the fore in connection with almost every medical condition. In Chapter 38 in this volume, I have urged that the lobbyists for autism have been vastly more important than the medical people who are not personally connected to an autistic person. *And that has unequivocally been a good thing.* "Lobbying" is not necessarily a bad thing. It is actually a useful way of bringing dissent to the fore in medical affairs.

I suggest advocacy as a fundamental feature of twenty-first-century medicine as opposed to "research science." It might be at the heart of the difference Solomon finds between research science and medicine. Advocates, who are personally involved, directly or indirectly, in any particular disorder, now have an immense effect on decisions reached, research pursued, and data analyzed. I am not sure that this is all to be classified as nonempirical. The existence of advocacy groups is nonempirical (with respect to the disorder), but they participate in the generation and use of empirical factors. Solomon regretted that she had not had the time to choose a psychiatric example, in which dissent was bad for medicine. I believe (anecdotally) that advocacy is far more effective in mental health than in physical health—with good reason! We understand so little about mental ill health, and antagonistic advocates have, in my opinion, been essential to questioning overconfident psychiatry of all persuasions.

I conclude with a major doubt. Solomon's aphorism says that disagreement is bad for medicine. I have already suggested cases where medicine desperately needed dissent. Indeed, *disagreement is bad for medical authority.* But is it bad for medicine? We need dissent: because medical authority is sometimes wrong. I do not see a strong difference between application, in this case, and scientific research in the research community. I do see a real difference in the role of activists in connection with schizophrenia, and research into carbon nanotubes, for example.

References

Canadian Cancer Society (n.d.). *Screening for Breast Cancer.* [Online] Available at: <http://www.cancer.ca/en/prevention-and-screening/early-detection-and-screening/screening/screening-for-breast-cancer/?region=bc>.

Canadian Task Force on Preventive Health Care (1994). *The Canadian Guide to Clinical Preventive Health Care.* Ottawa: Health Canada.

Canadian Task Force on Preventive Health Care (2011). *Screening for Breast Cancer: Summary of Recommendations for Clinicians and Policy-Makers*. [Online] Available at: <http://canadiantaskforce.ca/guidelines/2011-breast-cancer/>.

Canadian Task Force on Preventative Health Care (n.d.). *Canadian Task Force on Preventative Health Care*. [Online] Available at: <http://canadiantaskforce.ca/>.

Solomon, M. (2001). *Social Empiricism*. Cambridge, MA: MIT Press.

Section 4
The social, the cultural, and psychiatric kinds

Chapter 10
Introduction to "Varieties of social constructionism and the problem of progress in psychiatry"

Kenneth S. Kendler

In this tightly reasoned yet challenging chapter, Schaffner and Tabb (S&T) explore the knotty and controversial issue of how and in what form "social construction" might apply to psychiatric illness. Their answers are nuanced and well grounded in both the philosophical and psychiatric literatures. They interweave their observations and reflections about psychiatric illness—particularly schizophrenia—with parallel aspects of the history of the HIV/AIDS story. The similarities and contrasts are illuminating.

They develop a typology of social construction defined by two dichotomies. The first they term *inclusionary* and *exclusionary*. Inclusionary social construction makes the rather uncontroversial claim that "any psychiatric description that excludes the social is incomplete." Examples of such social processes might be as obvious as competition between scientific groups for students and funding, the impact on research programs of alterations in insurance coverage and hospitalization patterns, changes in federal funding due to influential politicians or National Institutes of Health leaders, and the rewards versus detractions for collaborative research programs. Exclusionary social construction is quite a bit more radical and would basically claim that psychiatric illness is "nothing but" the social.

The second dichotomy they propose is *token* and *type* social construction. Is it the overall category (= type) of a disorder or the specific manifestation such as the affected individual (= token) that is socially constructed? I will leave it to the interested reader to work through the four possible combinations of these two dichotomies.

What this approach does is to provide a more subtle and graded view of the possible ways in which psychiatry might be "social constructed" or may be more accurately "socially influenced." In the minds of many in the field of mental health, the phrase "social construction" constitutes "fighting words." They raise the specter of fervent antipsychiatrists parading outside meeting halls yelling curses (e.g., "Nazi Doctor") at those who breach their picket line. It is as if any questioning of the hegemony of the biomedical model of psychiatry could only lead to the adoption of the principles of scientology that deny any legitimacy to the field of mental health or to any of its key diagnostic and treatment approaches. But this is simply not the case.

In a reasoned voice, S&T "deconstruct" this position. They lay out the space of possibilities in the (rather tired) debate over social construction, and offer a taxonomy of the widely varying stances that have been articulated over the last 30 years. They end up advocating a role for inclusionary social construction. One of their strongest arguments shows how the inclusionary constructivist approach was central to the reduction of the disease burden of HIV. While biomedical progress in the development of retroviral therapies was important, a sole focus on the biology of HIV was counterproductive. Social programs to reduce the spread of the virus were also crucial. In the many shades of gray S&T illustrate, particularly informative are the various "subtypes" of dissenters both to HIV/AIDS and schizophrenia.

S&T also make the useful distinction between what they term "the social construction of a concept (an epistemological claim) and the social construction of an entity (a metaphysical claim)." That is, it is perfectly possible that the concept of schizophrenia has been strongly influenced by a range of historical and social processes, and poorly reflects any reality out there in the world; yet the current concept does encompass patients who are really suffering from severe mind/brain dysfunctions. That is, questioning the legitimacy of DSM diagnoses is not the same as questioning the validity of mental illness with all the suffering thereby entailed. Indeed, I have argued elsewhere that while anyone with extensive clinical or personal experience with mental illness can see the superficiality of the exclusionary social constructivist position (e.g., "just an alternative lifestyle"), a skeptical position toward any current instantiation of psychiatric diagnostic criteria (i.e., DSM-5) is quite defensible and reasonable.

The broader theme of this chapter is how the social and biomedical perspectives have and should interrelate in our consideration of psychiatric illness. Their view is broader than simply explanatory pluralism whereby social and biological factors are seen to act and interact in etiologic pathways to psychiatric illness. They also consider social forces that impact on the historical development, nosologic structure, and treatment delivery in mental health. Understanding the important role of social factors in the field of psychiatry does not thereby imply that the field cannot be making progress in biological understanding, treatment, or even nosology. The dichotomy between the rigorous biomedical perspective and a sober consideration of the importance of social factors in psychiatry is a false one. We should not have to choose.

S&T provide early in their chapter what I might take to be their overall conclusion that the "deserved prejudice among psychiatrists against exclusionary construction should not give way to prejudice about inclusionary construction, which is beneficial, even necessary, for progress in medicine—especially psychiatric medicine."

Chapter 11

Varieties of social constructionism and the problem of progress in psychiatry

Kenneth F. Schaffner and Kathryn Tabb

11.1 Introduction

There is a growing consensus among psychiatrists and philosophers of psychiatry that the failures of the discipline to establish etiological explanations of mental disorder are due to the enormous diversity of causal pathways leading to the syndromes characterized in the *Diagnostic and Statistical Manual of Mental Disorders* (DSM). Particularly problematic for accounts based on neurological mechanisms is the interplay of genes and environment affecting that biological pathway diversity (Sullivan et al. 2012). Despite early optimism that behavioral genetics would ultimately validate psychiatrists' taxonomies, recent findings from genome-wide association studies indicate that even the very signs and symptoms of mental disorder may have thousands of different genes affecting them (Goldstein 2009). Furthermore, even when there is evidence of the implication of certain genes in psychopathology, the character the disorder takes in each individual case is likely the result of personal experience. It is time to take seriously the role of environmental factors in the etiology of mental disorder, but there is no consensus on how to do so.

Even worse, there is an *anxiety* about doing so on the part of many psychiatrists and philosophers of psychiatry, thanks to the sting of historical challenges to the legitimacy of the biomedical paradigm by advocates of social constructionism. Such critics have suggested that categories of psychiatric disorder do not correspond to real kinds of disease, and that individuals diagnosed with mental disorder have merely a social label, rather than an organic condition. The present discussion attempts to clear the way for a philosophical treatment of psychiatric classification that can take seriously how environmental factors—specifically *social* factors—contribute to thinking about mental illness. Rather than avoiding the convoluted history of social constructionism about psychiatry we hope to address the vagueness of the term head-on by offering a taxonomy of our own, classifying the various ways in which mental disorder has been said to be socially constructed.

We argue for the value of some of these diverse positions, which can offer correctives for the reductionistically biomedical characterization of psychiatric progress in vogue in the United States since the advent of psychopharmacology and genetic approaches in the second half of the twentieth century. At the same time the history of psychiatry reveals the dangers of certain critiques that have flown the social-constructionist banner, which have rejected any physiological account of mental disorder and encouraged a dangerous form of taxonomic nihilism as well as mind–body dualism. By revisiting the fraught literature on social construction in psychiatry, we aim to argue for the place of the social without excluding the grounds on which psychiatry can be said to be—even theoretically—progressive.

In some ways the question of progress in medicine is an easier one than that of progress in science, which has been hugely divisive within the philosophical literature (Niiniluoto 2011). Elsewhere one of us has suggested the best approach to progress in psychiatry is a coherentist one, in which new theoretical developments are considered progressive when they fall into alignment with basic phenomenological facts about mental disturbance *and* when they contribute to the maximization of psychiatric values (Schaffner 2012). There is little dispute that the goal of psychiatry is to prevent, treat, and ideally cure human mental disorder, though the definition of "disorder" is also a complex challenge for philosophers. Accordingly here we define progress in psychiatry as the increase in the ability to prevent, treat, or cure mental disorder. Scientific progress can contribute to psychiatric progress insofar as knowledge of etiology and epidemiology, pharmacological interventions, and physiology contribute to these aims.

We believe that progress in medicine includes, but is not fully constituted by, scientific progress, and suggest that, due to the nature of psychiatric objects, the role of supra-biological features may be more prominent in psychiatry than in other branches of medicine. Thus the importance of paying attention to the way we talk about and theorize the social in psychiatry. However, we do not claim that psychiatry is unscientific, or that its progress is reducible to the construction of a set of social norms or practices. Rather, we aim to elucidate the integration of diverse progressive forces that can best assure the success of psychiatric theory and practice.

In order to tease apart the role of the social in medical explanation, we start by distinguishing between two views on how social factors can contribute to psychiatry. The first, which we call *inclusionary social constructionism*, maintains that psychiatric classifications are, in some part, either caused by or constituted by (more on this distinction later) social factors. Inclusionary social construction is generally seen as innocuous, and recognizes the social dimensions of science and medicine, including standard peer review, collaboration, role of research funding, education, health insurance, patient support networks, and financial support (disability payments), as well as social factors such as stigma and folk-psychiatric theories about, and treatment of, the mentally ill. On the level of the individual, recognized inclusionary-constructive factors include the importance of self–other relationships in the experience of the mentally ill (Parnas 2008) and what have been called the "looping effects" of psychiatric kinds (Hacking 1995). Generally this aspect of social construction is mainstream in terms of paradigm acceptances—in a sense it captures the social aspects of Kuhnian normal science.

Exclusionary social constructionism is more contentious, akin to the view that psychiatric objects are entirely the result of processes described by Dupré (2012, pp. viii, 308) as "making things up" and by Mallon as both "antiscientific" and often "covert." Essentially, exclusionary social constructionists hold that (idiosyncratic) personal values, radically different views of science, and contentious political or religious views significantly affect psychiatric beliefs, up to the point of generating distinctly different ontologies inconsistent with standard science of the time (see Dupré 2012; Mallon 2008) or with what some psychiatric professionals and philosophers view as "the real." Though characterized as a form of *social* constructionism, the theses urged by such constructionists may involve physical or biological claims, albeit embedded in their exclusionary social context. In psychiatry, *exclusionary* social constructionists sometimes argue that psychiatric classifications do not correspond to medical conditions and are merely "problems of living," though in some cases more extreme versions of such problems.

We explore these two views on social constructionism, and introduce some further divisions, using two partial analogies between the current state of schizophrenia research and the history of HIV/AIDS in its first two decades. Our analogue in somatic medicine was selected on the grounds of the resonances between the urgent need for medical advancement and the frustrating lack of scientific knowledge that characterized the HIV/AIDS situation in the 1980s and 1990s and the state of contemporary theories and treatment of schizophrenia. HIV/AIDS was also appealing to us as a case study because while it is now widely accepted as a paradigmatic monocausal disease, we shall see later that the "reality" of the etiopathogenetic relationship between HIV and AIDS was the source of great dissention (and still is, in some quarters). However, we do *not* mean to offer a prediction about the future of schizophrenia research; we recognize there are nearly countless *disanalogies*, and our aim is not to elide these, but to draw some of them out as well through our analysis.

Our first comparison between the two cases looks at the similarities and differences in disorder characterization and etiology, as well as at what most would call "rational" treatments based on etiology. Our second comparison contrasts the kinds of social-constructionist dissenters that have appeared both in the psychiatric area and the HIV/AIDS domain. This second comparison will allow us to explore what we think are positive and negative aspects of the two forms of social construction we have proposed above. We conclude that deserved prejudice among psychiatrists against exclusionary construction should not give way to prejudice about inclusionary construction, which is beneficial, even necessary, for progress in medicine—especially psychiatric medicine.

11.2 Another Look at Social Construction in Psychiatry

The term "social construction" has a complicated history in psychiatry, which has led to uncertainty about what is actually being claimed when it is said that schizophrenia, for example, is a construct.[1] One source of confusion is about the nature of the "construction"—is it a metaphor, and if so, of what sort? One may distinguish between claims of *causal construction,* the original generation of an object via a social or cultural process (an American flag, or the pattern created by dancers in a Virginia reel) and *constitutive construction,* the formation of an object by reference to social relations (a husband, or income tax) (Haslanger 1995; Mallon 2007). In the case of schizophrenia, a causal constructionist claim would be that the signs and symptoms which lead individuals to be so classified are caused by, say, cultural stressors, whether the ultimate result is a neurobiological pathology or not. An exclusionary constitutive constructionist might argue that schizophrenia *only is* the product of certain incompatibilities between the sufferer and their social milieu, such that it would evaporate if those incompatibilities were alleviated, whereas an inclusionary constitutive social constructionist would make the more modest argument that schizophrenics would be other than they are in the absence of social factors.

Hacking (1999) has pointed out another source of confusion in the ambiguity of the referent, or the *what* that is being constructed. The common referents seem to be claims either about the social construction of a kind concept or the social construction of a fact about an entity: what we will call either "category" construction or "case" construction. These two sorts of claims are not exclusive—many critics who employ the term "social construction" mean to suggest that both the concept and the instances to which it are applied are in some sense constructed. As we discuss later, in the 1970s R.D. Laing, Thomas Szasz, and others who spearheaded the antipsychiatry movement argued that the collection of signs and symptoms known as schizophrenia was in fact socially constituted by the conflicts between the patient and society. They denied that patients diagnosed as schizophrenics in fact have a "brain disease," and considered claims about schizophrenia's ontology that use medical language in a nonmetaphorical manner deeply problematic (Szasz 1987). We call social constructionists of the sort who target the nature of manifestations of purported schizophrenia in patients *case social constructionists. Category social constructionists* present their argument in terms of the concept itself, arguing that "schizophrenia" does not refer to anything in reality and fails to describe a natural kind of entity.

Such critics may acknowledge the mental suffering of patients diagnosed with schizophrenia and may locate it in the brain but believe that the diagnosis itself does not, to use a well-worn phrase, "cut nature at its joints." Instead, these critics argue, the idea of schizophrenia is a contingent product of historical and social forces—the development of the term out of the Kraepelinian "dementia praecox" is often rehearsed and shown to exhibit multiple vagaries (Berrios and Hauser 1988; Berrios et al. 2003). Some psychiatrists have suggested that it may be as fruitless to attempt to map "schizophrenia" onto real types in the world as it is

---

[1] Indeed the ambiguity of the term "social construction" in general has been well remarked upon for decades—cf. Latour and Wolgar (1979, p. 281)

"phlogiston" or "the luminiferous ether" (Bentall 1993, p. 227). Most writers in this camp acknowledge the seriousness of the symptoms of schizophrenia for those experiencing them—they may see them as tokens of another type, produced by social pressures (if they are exclusionary social constructionists) or by a combination of environmental and biological processes (if they are inclusionary social constructionists). Or they may not be constructionists about individual cases at all, but may explain them using a completely different typology under which they are a natural entity of a different sort. As we shall see later, it is possible to be an exclusionary social constructionist about a category while thinking its instances can be explained naturalistically as cases of another (nonsocially constructed) category entirely.

As Hacking has noted, the claim that the concept x is socially constructed is usually made in the service of raising awareness of its contingency in order to argue against the inevitability of the category and make way for suggestions about how it might be reformed. An example of exactly this motivation in the contemporary literature is the recent work of Steven Hyman, who has argued that the unjustified reification of the category of schizophrenia has been deeply problematic for the discovery of psychiatric research and treatment practices that could benefit those so diagnosed. Hyman writes of realizing, during his time as director of the National Institute of Mental Health (NIMH), that the constructed categories of the DSM had created "an unintended epistemic prison that was palpably impeding scientific progress" (Hyman 2010, p. 157). The NIMH's Research Domain Criteria initiative was created specifically to avoid the constriction of research by socially, rather than scientifically, constructed kinds.

These two sorts of social constructionist approaches, category and case, are cross-cut by the dichotomy introduced earlier that will be the main focus of the discussion here—between inclusionary social construction and exclusionary social construction. They can also be characterized as constitutive or causal. We do not mean to suggest that any self-identified social constructionist can be mapped onto these dichotomies, but rather that they can serve heuristically to characterize the sorts of claims that have been and are being made.

Social constructionism is often viewed as antithetical to any grounded belief in scientific progress because it can conflict with a naturalistic approach, and is often taken to refute claims that science has successfully attained knowledge about the real world. Considering the possible stances resulting from the three dichotomies discussed earlier, however, it is clear that there are a variety of ways that social constructionist critiques can engage with ontological and explanatory claims about scientific objects, concepts, and theories about entities. The analogy with HIV/AIDS will demonstrate how, retrospectively, different types of social factors have been described as having aided or impeded the understanding and treatment of AIDS. Even in the case of this prototypical medical disorder, whose etiology is well established, social factors feature importantly in the changing characterization of the disease in ways that, in retrospect, can be normatively evaluated. This historical case demonstrates how describing a disease as socially constructed can mean any number of different things, and we show that the term is no easier to apply to judgments about progress in schizophrenia.

11.3 The First Comparison: Disorder Characterization using Etiology and "Rational" Treatments

The first general lesson to be drawn from the history of HIV/AIDS is that medical progress includes, but does not consist exclusively in, scientific progress. We suggested earlier that while scientific progress can be defined as the advancement of knowledge, medicine is successful when it is able to prevent, treat, and cure disease. While the discovery of the HIV virus transformed research and treatment of AIDS, it was insufficient to resolve the huge number of challenges on both fronts. Debates over whether there was sufficient evidence of HIV's role as the necessary and sufficient pathogen behind the syndrome raged through the 1990s, and the discovery of the role of a RNA-based retrovirus in the etiology of AIDS stalled, but did not halt, the growing epidemic. Only through the integration of the theoretical advance with new technologies, social practices, public policies, and education were real advances made in the prevention and treatment of the disorder.

At first HIV/AIDS, much like schizophrenia in most current views, was identified as a syndrome with no known etiology. When the syndrome first became recognized in the early 1980s the use of amyl nitrate, popular at some gay clubs, was suspected as a cause, and one small study seemed to support that view. Others thought multiple infections due to a promiscuous lifestyle in the gay community was a contributor to a loss of infection-fighting capability, leading to the appearance of a rare cancer (Kaposi's sarcoma) or a rare pneumonia (*Pneumocystis jirovecii* pneumonia). Another early research program theorized that a viral pathogen (cytomegalovirus, which almost everyone carries) had gone awry. Yet another group at the National Institutes of Health thought AIDS symptoms were caused by a fungus that produced a fatal toxin.[2]

The Centers for Disease Control formulated several "surveillance definitions" as they tried to track the appearance of this putatively new disease in the absence of any etiological tests or clear pathophysiology (subsets of T cells were not known or used initially). These surveillance definitions attempted to codify the disparate signs and symptoms associated with the mysterious syndrome. Scientific progress over the following decades was achieved by identifying an etiological agent (HIV), understanding its life cycle, and using that knowledge to develop drugs that intervene at key points in the life cycle. For example, the first drug, AZT (zidovudine/

---

[2] There are several good histories of AIDS/HIV we have been able to draw on, including Harden (2012) and Shilts (1987). Especially sensitive to social construction issues is Epstein (1996). Gerald Stine's yearly publication *AIDS Update* has much useful information, including successive surveillance definitions.

azidothymidine), is an inhibitor of reverse transcriptase that the HIV virus needs to transform itself from RNA to DNA, prior to its insertion into the host cell's machinery.

Schizophrenia is also a surveillance definition, insofar as its etiology and pathophysiology have yet to be established. Attempts in biological psychiatry over the past 50 years have not revealed any simple etiological pathway for schizophrenia, or any mental disorder, for that matter, that could act as an analogue for the HIV virus. One of us, writing with Kenneth S. Kendler, has described how the dopamine hypothesis, which speculated that a single neurotransmitter accounted for the substantial effects of what is observed in schizophrenia, turned out to be a will-o'-the-wisp (see Kendler, Chapter 32, this volume; Kendler and Schaffner 2011) And a 2010 article by Sun and colleagues, including Kendler as a coauthor, identified a minimum of 24 possible pathways to the disease (Sun et al. 2010).

In a review of the implications for simple or complex (messy) etiological pathways of very recent GWAS and CNV advances in psychiatry, including schizophrenia, Kendler writes:

> What should we expect to see? The most pessimistic prediction that we will observe only a mess is unlikely. But discovering a highly coherent single pathway to illness also seems improbable. We can hope that the heterogeneity is not too great and the real level of illness not too hidden in the upper reaches of the mind-brain system. If this is true, important insights into the nature of psychiatric illness are likely to await our efforts. (Kendler 2013, p. 1065)

Our view is that if a primarily biological explanation for schizophrenia is obtained, it will likely be constituted by many pathways involving multiple and distinct sets of INUS conditions.[3] These INUS conditions will likely include genes as well as interacting environmental factors, and will not be analogous with the simpler pathway displayed by HIV infection.

The hope remains among many that what still amounts to a surveillance syndromic definition of schizophrenia will, as occurred with AIDS, function as a guide to an etiological pathway that will in turn help direct the development of effective therapies. However, the search for a simple biomedical cause and the possibility of exploiting that knowledge as was done in the case of HIV may mislead. It may well be that there is not any necessary and sufficient biological property or set of properties

---

[3] The notion of an INUS condition was developed by John Mackie on the basis of his reflections on John Stuart Mill's discussion of the plurality of causes problem. Mill recognized the complication of a plurality of causes by which several different assemblages of factors, say ABC as well as DGH and JKL, might each be sufficient to bring about an effect P. If (ABC *or* DGH *or* JKL) is both necessary and sufficient for P, how do we describe, for example, the A in such a generalization? Such an element, A (or any of the B … L factors, taken individually) is for Mackie an *i*nsufficient but *n*on-redundant [alternatively 'necessary'] part of an *u*nnecessary but *s*ufficient condition—a complex expression for which Mackie uses the acronym "INUS condition". Using this terminology, then, what is usually termed a cause is an INUS condition (Mackie 1974).

that all cases of schizophrenia share. If this is the case, critics who take an exclusionary constructionist approach to the category of schizophrenia may be correct that the diagnostic construct does not map on to a natural kind in the world, and that the seeming homogeneity of schizophrenia cases is in fact in part due to extrascientific factors rather than a shared etiopathogenesis. Nonetheless, though we anticipate some additional complexity in the concept of schizophrenia, we still oppose the critical accounts of schizophrenia that verge on, or clearly fall into, our sense of exclusionary social construction. We discuss that issue in the following section.

The waste of time and resources that overzealous optimism about a monocausal account of schizophrenia can induce is well demonstrated by the case of the disappointing dopamine hypothesis (Kendler, Chapter 32, this volume; Kendler and Schaffner 2011). An analogy could be drawn between the HIV hypothesis and the dopamine hypothesis to rationally reconstruct the factors that led one to contribute to medical progress more than the other. Our purpose here, however, is to examine the role of *social* factors in psychiatric progress, and to that end it is worth noting that the HIV hypothesis and the pharmacological interventions that followed from it were not alone enough to halt the AIDS epidemic.[4]

Though these drugs individually have greater or lesser effects depending on the circumstances of the particular patient, it is their effect working in concert, typically involving agents that affect each phase of the HIV cycle, that has had the major results in AIDS treatment. This multiple antiviral drug therapy goes by the name of HAART, standing for highly active antiretroviral therapy. It was the advent of HAART that produced what has sometimes been termed the "Lazarus effect" in AIDS patients and the following comment:

> Dr. Steven Deeks of the San Francisco General Hospital said in 1996 "everybody hailed the three-drug cocktail or highly active antiretroviral therapy (HAART) as the major breakthrough at that time." People who were lying on their deathbeds in the hospital got up and walked out. (Stine 2013, p. 83)

Unfortunately, Dr. Deeks added that it was then "realized that the tremendous benefit of HAART was only happening in half of our patients." Such a variable response to powerful drugs is, unhappily, quite common both in HIV/AIDS and in schizophrenia and other mental disorders. Though drugs that work to a better or worse degree in psychiatry have been discovered in the absence of etiological and pathophysiological information of the type detailed above, it remains to be seen what lessons can be inferred from that story in contrast to the more rational way anti-HIV drugs are positioned in the HIV life cycle.

Even in cases where the drugs do work, distribution and patient compliance are huge obstacles to their efficacy in practice.[5] Success stories in the AIDS epidemic

---

[4] See <http://media.hhmi.org/biointeractive/posters/2007%20aids.jpg> for a poster graphic of the life cycle of HIV and the drugs that interfere with various steps in the life cycle.

[5] For an accessible introduction and references to the HIV/AIDS literature on this and the next few points see Stine (2013).

often include advances in social programming that give patients the support they need to obtain and successfully complete their drug regimens. Additionally, given the failure of the drugs in many cases, efforts aimed at prevention—clean needle programs, safe sex campaigns, and so on—have been hugely important in curbing rates of fatality from AIDS. We expect the same is true in the case of schizophrenia, namely that independently of current or future advances in psychopharmacology, local social support systems as well as government programs and policies could help people with schizophrenia live and even flourish with their disorder. However, without the financial motivations that cause the pharmaceutical industry to thrive or the benefit of powerful lobbyists, such social interventions are currently woefully neglected. Nonetheless, a cursory look at the history of the HIV/AIDS crisis or other epidemics underscores their value.

11.4 The Second Comparison: Dissenters and the Flourishing of Exclusionary Social Construction

Our second comparison between HIV/AIDS and mental disorders, including schizophrenia, notes that in the first half-dozen years of HIV/AIDS characterization a position of "AIDS dissention" developed that still has advocates today. Some HIV/AIDS dissenters do not believe there is any natural kind "AIDS" that explains the death of purported AIDS victims—in our language, they believe the category is socially constructed, or they may put it in terms of the cases (purported AIDS deaths) belonging to a different category entirely, such as what mainstream medical professionals would consider the "secondary cause"—the viruses, cancers, and infections that fatally impact the compromised immune system. AIDS deniers frequently maintain that HIV is an innocuous infection that is universally found in the severely immune-compromised, and use this correlation to explain away evidence for the etiogenic role of HIV in AIDS.

Some AIDS dissenters are similar to exclusionary social constructionists about cases of schizophrenia insofar as they deny that schizophrenics in fact have a disease at all, or can be classified as cases of any sort of non-socially-constructed category. These individuals deny that an epidemic is underway, and counter claims about death rates in countries like Zimbabwe, in which 15% of people between 15 and 49 have AIDS, by attributing these fatalities to impoverishment and poor sanitation instead of to a specific disease (Stine 2013). Such critics believe that the diagnosis of such individuals is a social, rather than a biological, fact about them. A poignant and disturbing case of such "AIDS denialism" is that of Christine Maggiore, an HIV-positive woman who, 3 years after the death of her daughter, herself died of disorders believed to be opportunistic infections (Stine 2013). Maggiore had refused to take the medications that would lower the risk of transmission of HIV to her daughter based on her belief that the virus was benign.

Others, exclusionary social constructionists who direct their criticism at the category rather than the cases of the disease, believe that there is an epidemic of deaths referred to as "AIDS" but deny that there is any shared medical condition causing the deaths that meets the definition of "AIDS." Historically influential advocates of this position include prominent scientists such as Peter Duesberg, who still denies any causal role to HIV, and also politicians such as South African President Thabo Mbeki, who initially rejected HIV as the cause of AIDS. Duesberg has asserted that AZT, the first anti-AIDS drug that became available in 1987, was in fact a contributing cause of AIDS, rather than a defense against it. Dissenters also reject the use of standard drugs and preventive measures based on the HIV causation thesis. Duesberg's explanations of the evidence of an AIDS epidemic are variegated and complex, and display a variety of social constructionist strategies. It is worth considering his perspective in more detail.

The theses of Duesberg's early work were that: (1) HIV (in either its HIV-1 or HIV-2 form) is neither necessary nor sufficient for AIDS, though HIV is a good "marker" for American AIDS; and (2) AIDS is actually an autoimmune disease caused by as yet unknown pathogens, probably acting in concert with a variety of environmental insults, including hard psychoactive as well as medical drugs (AZT) and blood transfusion (particularly in the case of hemophiliacs) (Duesberg 1988, 1991, 1992). One of Duesberg's major arguments is that HIV fails to satisfy Koch's postulates.[6] Though he admits that various viral elements (and, by definition of the disease, antibody to HIV) can be found in most AIDS patients, he contends that HIV is not present in ways that can account for the loss of T cells or for the clinical course of the disease, which lags years behind infection. Further, with respect to Koch's second postulate, Duesberg contends that there is an "often over 20% failure rate in isolation of HIV from AIDS patients" (Duesberg 1989). Finally, citing Koch's third postulate, Duesberg notes that HIV does not produce AIDS in any animal model (chimpanzees have not been inoculated successfully), and the data from accidental inoculations of humans (through donor semen, laboratory accidents involving HIV researchers, and blood transfusions) are not consistent with the role of HIV as the sole cause of AIDS.

The response to Duesberg's arguments has been threefold. First, a number of commentators have pointed out that Koch's postulates fail to be satisfied in a number of other diseases, primarily of the viral and immunological type encountered in AIDS, and that the postulates need to be taken as "guidelines" and supplemented by broader epidemiological evidence. Second, when a broader, more epidemiological conception of causation is implemented using epidemiological data, the evidence for HIV as the cause of AIDS is overwhelming. Finally,

---

[6] Koch's postulates can be summarized as follows: (1) the infectious agent occurs in every case of the disease in question and under circumstances which can account for the pathological changes and clinical course of the disease. (2) It must be possible to isolate the agent from all cases of the disease and to grow the agent in pure culture. (3) After being fully isolated from the diseased animals (or humans) and repeatedly grown in pure culture, it can induce the disease anew by inoculation into a suitable host. For a discussion of Koch's postulates and Duesberg's responses, with citations, see Schaffner (2000).

molecular investigations of HIV pathophysiology have deepened in recent years. New co-receptors for the virus have been identified that explain some resistance to HIV and may also help explain its oddly delayed pathogenesis. These receptors have also permitted better animal models of HIV/AIDS to be created. Duesberg has rejoined to this criticism, arguing that appeals to epidemiological considerations do not make the case that the proponents of HIV think they do, and continues to aggressively defend his own theory.

It took some years for the scientific questions about HIV that Duesberg initially raised, such as where the missing free virus might be sequestered, to be satisfactorily answered. In 1996, however, the advent of a powerful drug cocktail—the highly active antiretroviral therapy (HAART) mentioned previously—provided the sort of convincing evidence, according to one historian of AIDS, that no buttressing of Koch's postulates' types of evidence could accomplish, and changed the minds of some AIDS dissenters (Harden 2012). Nonetheless AIDS dissenters continue to be active, especially via the Internet (see <http://www.virusmyth.com/aids/>).

Thus one lesson that seems extractable from the AIDS comparison is that even strong etiological and pathophysiological evidence may not suffice to convince "psychiatric dissenters," though proof of the efficacy of drugs *built on* that etiopathogenic evidence might do so. This suggests that even exclusionary social constructionism has its limits among its initial defenders, though exactly what they may be and how to characterize them is a longer-term project. We suspect that it will likely be analogous to what is known as Kuhnian resistance to paradigm change, a phenomenon that we believe was illuminated by the physicist-philosopher Pierre Duhem a half-century before Kuhn's *Structure of Scientific Revolutions* appeared. Duhem wrote, citing the great French physiologist Claude Bernard, that:

> Since logic does not determine with strict precision the time when an inadequate hypothesis should give way to a more fruitful assumption, and since recognizing this moment belongs to good sense, physicists [and we might add biologists and psychiatrists] may hasten this judgment and increase the rapidity of scientific progress by trying consciously to make good sense within themselves more lucid and more vigilant.
>
> [...] [and as] so clearly expressed by Claude Bernard: The sound experimental criticism of a hypothesis is subordinated to certain moral conditions; in order to estimate correctly the agreement of a physical theory with the facts, it is not enough to be a good mathematician and skillful experimenter; one must also be an impartial and faithful judge. (Duhem 1914/1954, p. 218)

Duesberg's views amount to exclusionary social constructionism about the category "AIDS"—he thinks the term refers to a class of things that do not share any sort of natural essence, but are only grouped together as the result of social practices. When it comes to case constructionism, however, his position is more complicated. He is an exclusionary social constructionist about AIDS victims in Africa, denying that there is an epidemic of any unique class of cases that corresponds to the label "AIDS." Rather than arguing that AIDS cases have been mischaracterized, Duesberg argues that there simply are no such instances: "the presumably new AIDS epidemic can be neither distinguished epidemiologically nor clinically from conventional African diseases and mortality."[7] In the case of the United States, however, he does not deny that individuals diagnosed with AIDS would continue to be sick if social practices changed; he attributes their deaths to the exhaustion of the immune system. In the American context the condition is *caused* by social factors (the gay lifestyle, pill-taking) but has a physiological manifestation in the body that persists even if those factors are removed. Duesberg should not be considered an exclusionary social constructionist about cases of AIDS in the United States, since he does not think they are members of a socially constructed category, but rather tokens of another disease type entirely: severe autoimmune deficiency.

Duesberg's position can be contrasted with not only advocates of a hard biomedical conception of HIV/AIDS but also with those who take an *inclusionary* social constructionist approach to the category. An example of this sort of position is that of Eric Sawyer, an American activist and founder of ACT UP (an organization of profound importance to the history of HIV/AIDS awareness in the United States) who has been actively involved in the Health Global Access Program and the United Nation's HIV/AIDS Initiative. In the early stages of the epidemic, ACT UP sought to force a government response to the epidemic that would extend prevention and treatment efforts to then-stigmatized populations such as homosexuals and needle users. While Sawyer is entirely committed to the biomedical claim that AIDS is caused by HIV, he nonetheless emphasizes that social factors have caused the epidemic to take the form it has, noting at the opening ceremony for the International Conference on AIDS in 1996 that "[t]he fact that the protease-combination drug treatments are showing a lot of promise in the blood tests of the very few people who can get them, does not mean that the cure is here. Yes the preliminary results from these hugely expensive combination treatments look great. But we are a long way from a cure, even for the rich who can afford the treatments." In his remarks Sawyer emphasizes that scientific innovation is only a part of the solution to the epidemic: "Governments are killing poor people in developing countries because they are providing only a tiny amount of AIDS funding which is limited to prevention efforts and does not pay for AIDS care."[8]

Sawyer can be viewed as believing that social factors contribute in both a constitutive and a causal way to the concept of AIDS. As his powerful quote makes clear, he believes that governments have blood on their hands due to their inaction, which caused the growing threat of AIDS to be downplayed for

---

[7] <http://www.duesberg.com/subject/africa2.html>. Duesberg has offered other explanations for the reported death rates in Africa, including problematic sampling procedures and general nutritional and hygienic challenges (Duesberg et al. 2011).

[8] From Sawyer's Remarks at the Opening Ceremony of the XI International Conference on AIDS, Vancouver, Canada, July 7, 1996. Available at <http://www.actupny.org/Vancouver/sawyerspeech.html>.

nearly a decade and the disease to be mischaracterized. On the other hand, Sawyer also believes that social factors have continued to shape both the idea of AIDS and the experience of having it due to the negative impact of stigma and misunderstanding prevalent since the discovery of the first cases. While these factors do not explain the presence of the disorder in individual cases—the contraction of the virus HIV explains that—Sawyer believes that they help constitute the experience of having AIDS, such that if the social environment changed, the experience of having the disorder would change as well. Thus we may call him an inclusionary social constructionist about both the category and the cases, that is, the individual disease states of people suffering from AIDS.

The kind of strong exclusionary social construction (or *deconstruction*) of a disease undertaken by AIDS dissenters is mirrored in psychiatry by the antipsychiatrists and their kindred doubters about mental disorders. For example, in the 1960s, Laing and Esterson argued in *Sanity, Madness, and the Family* that schizophrenia was a normal reaction to a nonnormal social environment, and thus not a disorder. Szasz argued up until his recent death in 2012 that the concept of mental disease is an oxymoron, since diseases are by definition physical. In his view, all mental illness is a myth, and symptoms are actually constituted by the tensions between the individual and societal norms. "The contention that mental illness is brain disease," Szasz writes, "is as old as psychiatry itself: it is an integral part of the grand lie that psychiatry is a branch of medicine and healing, when in fact it is a branch of the law and social control" (Szasz 2006). Szasz can provide us with the archetype of an exclusionary social constructionist, who believes that the categories of mental illness as well as facts about their manifestation in individuals are all constituted by social practices.

Other critics of psychiatry consider categories like schizophrenia to be constructions while maintaining that they describe cases of disease—here we will consider Richard Bentall—or even blame the very existence of diagnostic categories on drug marketing.[9] How far does the dissenter analogy go in such cases, and where do the differences in AIDS and psychiatry diverge to reveal interesting differences in the ontologies of disorders and criteria for progress?

In the 1990s, Bentall wrote the following, which formally resembles some of Duesberg's claims about AIDS:

> [W]e are inevitably drawn to an important conclusion: "schizophrenia" appears to be a disease which has no particular symptoms, which has no particular course and which responds to no particular treatment. It is therefore not surprising that aetiological research has revealed that it has no particular cause (Bentall et al., 1988). One obvious implication of this account is that, if we wish to make progress in the understanding of serious psychiatric disorder, the concept of 'schizophrenia' will have to be abandoned. In this regard the concept of 'schizophrenia' is similar to a number

---

[9] See, for example, the work of Peter R. Breggin (<http://www.breggin.com>).

of other concepts; for example 'phlogiston' and 'the luminiferous ether', which were widely employed by scientists for a time but which turned out to be scientifically misleading in the long term. (Bentall 1993, p. 227)

Like Duesberg in the case of AIDS in the United States, Bentall is not an exclusionary social constructionist about cases of schizophrenia—he believes them to be pathological states requiring medical attention. He may view them as tokens of diverse types, or as instances of a family-resemblance kind. Unlike Duesberg, however, he is intensely concerned with the social factors that feed into mental disorder, and is not interested in providing an alternative physiological account (Bentall 2009).

Bentall is certainly an exclusionary constructionist about the category "schizophrenia." While as noted above there is a good deal of evidence for the heterogeneity of patients classified as schizophrenic, some support also goes against Bentall's dramatic dismissal of the classical concept as the psychiatric equivalent of phlogiston and the luminiferous ether.[10] Several studies examine both the genetic and the reasonably coherent syndromic features of schizophrenia. These studies include one by McGrath et al. (2004), and Kendler et al.'s bottom-up latent class analysis (Kendler et al. 1998). That study utilized some "twenty-one items, chosen to represent a broad range of symptoms and signs," and concluded that "latent class analysis defined a class of probands—characterized by positive psychotic symptoms, prominent negative symptoms, chronicity, and a poor outcome with deterioration—which closely resembles the classic descriptions of Kraepelin and Bleuler" (Kendler et al. 1998, p. 496). Even more recent are the stronger results from an LCA analysis that support the idea that "Kraepelin was right" (Derks et al. 2012).

Whether or not Bentall has good reason to insist on the incoherence and uselessness of the concept of schizophrenia, our point here is that at this stage in the development of theories of schizophrenia there is as much uncertainty about the disorder as there was about AIDS in the early 1980s. While the dopamine hypothesis *might* have served as a profoundly influential biomedical model of schizophrenia akin to the HIV virus, it has failed to do so, and no other single etiological candidate is, at this point, promising. Thus we cannot fault Bentall's insistence that while cases diagnosed as schizophrenia should be acknowledged to integrate social and biological factors both in their constitution and causal pathways, it is doubtful that our concept of schizophrenia has been constituted by exclusively scientific factors. We also value Bentall's stance because it demonstrates the possibility, and occasional necessity, for being an exclusionary social constructionist about a category while being more moderate about its cases. To say that schizophrenia is a construct need not be to say that those diagnosed with schizophrenia are not suffering from a disorder.

---

[10] As an aside, and in the interests of full disclosure, one of us admits that in an earlier life he was the author of an extensive study of the latter nonexistent entity—see Schaffner (1972).

11.5 Some Further Analogies and Disanalogies between HIV/AIDS and Psychiatric Disorders

Above we discussed how a medical disease, HIV/AIDS, progressed from a syndromic surveillance definition to an etiological characterization with strongly beneficial effects on prognosis and therapy. We noted the similarity of a surveillance definition in schizophrenia, but also indicated that to date no such real progress has occurred analogous to the etiological simplicity found in the HIV/AIDS example. In point of fact, it appears that schizophrenia pathways will be manifold, and likely require diverse treatment interventions. We also noted the existence of dissenters about both AIDS and schizophrenia that represent heretical exclusionary accounts of disorders in those areas, and speculated, albeit only provisionally in connection with the significance of HAART therapy, on what kinds of evidence, both etiological and therapeutic, might convince such dissenters that they should alter their beliefs.

Our analysis would be incomplete however, if we did not also indicate some important differences between medical disorders such as our AIDS example and mental disorders including schizophrenia. Most obviously, schizophrenics are vulnerable to the sort of looping effects discussed in Hacking (1995). Relatedly, our conception of schizophrenia is dependent on the *subjective experience* of those so classified in a way that AIDS is not. As suggested above, progress in psychiatry is movement towards the treatment of the symptoms of mental illness, which are, for the most part, subjective and partially behavioral—that is, subjectively perceived and then orally reported. Psychological evidence plays an important role in the diagnosis, prognosis, and treatment of the patient. While an engagement with the lived experience of every *medical* patient is essential toward providing holistic support (such as assuring compliance with pharmacological regimens and taking into account comorbidities), in psychiatry the category as well as the diversity of the cases of mental disorder are dependent on personal and interpersonal factors. In HIV/AIDS, such subjective symptoms as forms of pain and angst are largely irrelevant to T-cell counts, viral load measures, and the effects of HAART. But they still constitute the primitive elements of a coherentist theory of mental illness.

As Parnas, Sass, and Zahavi have written, "The psychiatric object (symptoms, signs, behaviors, suffering, and altered existential patterns) always plays itself out in the phenomenal-experiential realm" (Parnas et al. 2013, p. 274). We agree with this, though we would extend the "playing field," as it were, to also include the biological and the molecular aspects of psychiatric disorders. We stress the word "include" here, since our approach is pluralistic and multi-level, and does not reduce the phenomenal realm to the biological. It is precisely with regard to the integration of such extrabiological factors that an inclusionary constructionist approach is appealing.

One of us has previously published the graphic in Figure 11.1 to indicate how, as psychiatry progresses, the phenomenal (subjective/behavioral/cognitive) realm

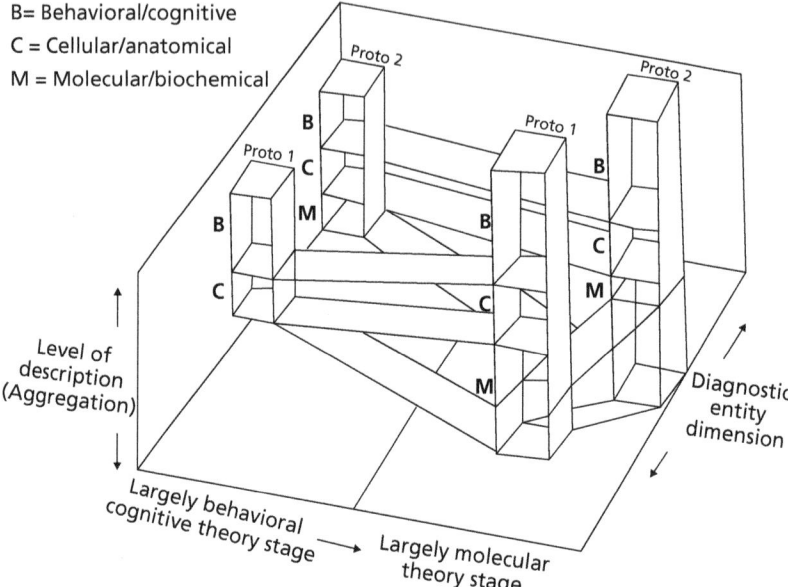

Fig. 11.1 Evolving and converging disorders with subjective and neuroscientific developments show the importance of retaining the behavioral/phenomenological.
The two towers show molecular (as well as neurocircuit) progress over time, but a retention of higher levels as well. In addition, a unification of sorts at the molecular level is depicted for these two disorders, as seems to be happening for bipolar disorder and schizophrenia.[11]

B is not only retained, but can also be further refined and utilized in improved diagnostic and potentially interventionist ways.

Phenomenological research indicates that disturbance of the basic sense of self and the self's relationship to others may be a core phenotypic marker of schizophrenia spectrum disorders. An example of this inclusion of the phenomenological is illustrated by the recent use of the Examination of Anomalous Self-Experience (EASE) instrument to detect subtle early signs of psychosis, as well as to predict the onset of conversion to psychosis (Parnas et al. 2005). In a preliminary study by McGorry group (Nelson et al. 2012), self-disorder scores predicted transition to psychosis in a small sample of ultra-high risk (UHR) subjects, and appeared to be selectively associated with a schizophrenia spectrum diagnosis (schizophrenia and schizotypal disorder), a finding previously reported in clinical (Nordgaard

---

[11] At the suggestion of Dr. Berrios, we have investigated the possibility of adding a "fourth floor," as it were, to our tower diagram. That additional floor might be labeled S for a generalized "social" aspect, and could include significant aspects of the complex analysis of psychiatric symptoms described in Dr. Berrios' comments on this chapter. Such an analysis would require, however, another article.

and Parnas 2014) and genetic population samples. These results are preliminary, but do suggest in a concrete way that a deeper understanding of the phenomenological subjective features of a psychiatric disorder in the schizophrenic spectrum area can be improved.

It is possible that these experiential aspects of the disorder will provide the sort of shared "particular" symptom that Bentall sees as lacking in the contemporary diagnostic concept (Bentall 1993; Reininghaus et al. 2013). While the emphasis on self-experience suggests that certain aspects of schizophrenia are constituted by social interaction between the patient and their environment, these aspects could be integrated with a biological account, perhaps with the help of our prospective social (S) addition to our towers model, allowing for progress even in the absence of a convincing etiogenic theory.

There is another interesting issue that the inclusion of the phenomenological subjective dimension in the psychiatric realm generates. The intrinsic (at least for the present) subjectivity of the phenomenal realm also allows exclusionary constructionist dissenters about cases to argue for alternatives that maintain that such experienced disorders are "just experiences," rather than being patterns that meet the criteria of standard scientific evaluation. The inclusion of the subjective, as necessary and useful as it is for psychiatry, thus amount to a "double-edged sword." On the one hand, this sword assists in cutting through the opaqueness of prodromal characterizations in a felicitous inclusionary constructionist way, and avoiding the exclusion of patients who fail to meet behavioral diagnostic criteria but are nonetheless suffering from mental illness. On the other hand, it provides material for the exclusionary constructionist claim that such disorders are just "made up." Differentiating between inclusionary and exclusionary social construction should help clarify what such approaches entail on both the epistemic and ontological levels.

We may broaden the point to note that the characterization of a disease as socially constructed can have both positive and negative effects on medical progress. In the HIV/AIDS case, inclusionary treatments have been more conducive to progress. For example, advances in understanding and containing the spread of the disease was significantly impeded in the years 1981–1983 by political and cultural factors, including the conservatism of established institutions such as blood banks that worried about costs and liability and the stance of the Reagan administration, which was in denial about the scope of the epidemic. Such resistance was due in part to the perception that AIDS was primarily a social problem facing a marginalized population rather than a medical problem. Details of this medico-political story are presented in the award-winning book by Shilts (1987). However, a purely medical approach to the problem was also damaging—as described by Sawyer in the earlier quote, the development of drug therapies alone was insufficient (and continues to be insufficient).

An inclusionary approach was taken to the concept of the disease when the global epidemic was widely recognized to have both social aspects and medical ones, and when social changes were discovered that could contribute to medical progress. From the 1980s onwards, social and political activists began to emphasize the importance of other sorts of interventions such as clean needle programs, condom distribution, and public health awareness campaigns. These efforts suggest that, despite the scientific advances in AIDS research, social advances are crucial too and AIDS should not be thought of as "just" HIV. We can see that the important role played by both positive and negative social factors make inclusionary social constructionism the right attitude to take when attempting to reconstruct the past, characterize the present, or envision the future of HIV/AIDS.

This is not to deny that inclusionary social constructionist hypotheses can also potentially be dangerous and degenerating. In the case of AIDS, the early widespread belief by medical researchers that factors of the "gay lifestyle" caused AIDS led to discrimination and prejudice against alternative lines of investigation and theorizing, as well as horrific stigma against homosexuals. "Outlier" cases, like hemophiliacs and needle users, were at first excluded from consideration, due to the power of a causal social-constructionist hypothesis about the importance of lifestyle factors over biological ones in cases of AIDS. A similar phenomenon in the history of schizophrenia is the theory of "the refrigerator mother," an etiological account that also posited a causal construction of the disease by experiential factors. In our concluding section we argue that nonetheless, inclusionary social constructionism is the best perspective to take in regards to schizophrenia because it is in philosophical alignment with pluralist philosophies of psychiatry that best cope with "the dappled world" (Kendler 2012).

11.6 **Conclusion**

Favoring inclusionary social constructionism over exclusionary is, of course, begging the question if there are not independent reasons to believe that biological factors as well as social ones play a role in the constructed object. We have suggested that schizophrenia fundamentally relies on the self-experience of the patient and their ability to communicate this experience to others, and if space allowed, we would further argue that social factors such as government-funded medical services, social stigma against the mentally ill, and key environmental stressors such as poverty are profoundly important causes behind the high rates of schizophrenia today. Yet our best theories of schizophrenia suggest that even this deeply subjective condition has equally key biological features that may someday shape a new diagnostic category, set of categories, or spectrum (Lewis et al. 2012).

Without retreating to ontology, however, the rewards of an inclusionary constructionism can be defended on a coherentist approach to progress in medicine, where medicine is understood as a practice which depends on both social and biological factors in order to achieve its goals of curing and preventing disease. In the case of psychiatry, social constructionist critics have argued that to ignore the "self" as well as social factors such as medical and personal norms is to allow crucial aspects of mental illness to go unaddressed. Furthermore, the role of social policy in not only treating disorder but also our conceptions of it have been undertreated in the literature. However, in light of the recently published DSM-5, there has been a renewed attention to the risk stigma and classification pose to patients, an issue that has been wrestled with extensively in the AIDS area.

Despite controversy, early testing for AIDS is becoming a consensus position. Recent mass shootings in the United States have raised in public awareness the need to adopt some mental health surveillance and help approaches in psychiatry, though there is no equivalent to the HAART treatment to offer as a "reward" for such early testing, and the risk of stigma is enormous. Further, social support networks for AIDS-infected individuals are extensive, and comparatively well funded. Schizophrenia is also a serious disease with major morbidity and significant mortality in the United States due to suicides (which far outnumber the victims of shootings by putative schizophrenics, though these figures often get more press). In order for the treatment and prevention of schizophrenia to progress, an inclusionary social constructionism should be adopted. One possible direction forward for philosophers of psychiatry is to extend the Perspectives model of McHugh and Slavney (1998) to capture the unique ways social factors construct psychiatric categories and cases, in contrast to a more limited biomedical model of scientific progress. Significantly, the Perspectives model does not include social (and global) dimensions, though an extension of the model to those areas would not be inconsistent with it.

The rhetoric of social construction is often invoked to raise awareness of the potential for the revolution of an idea or entity that has long been taken as inevitable—to remind us of what is, ultimately, under our control (Hacking 1999). While exclusionary constructionist critiques of psychiatry encourage the abandonment of lines of inquiry that may be crucial to scientific progress, inclusionary ones can do the opposite by encouraging fruitful avenues of research and treatment that fall outside of the biomedical paradigm. As seen in the case of HIV/AIDS, how we define the problem can determine the solution. Throughout the twentieth century, psychiatry has been fearful of failing to meet the standards of validity and reliability of somatic medicine, and as a result has been overzealous in its *ex*clusion of the social. In response, inclusionary constructionist critics can challenge the depressing determinism that accompanies doggedly biomedical characterizations of mental disorder. And they need not be antipsychiatric in order to do so: as Ron Mallon has written, "constructionist accounts of human kinds often involve a quite general denial of biological accounts of those same kinds, but this need not be necessary" (Mallon 2008, p. 11). Along the lines of Bentall's vision, rather than being damned by their genetic predispositions or neurochemistry, schizophrenics can be seen as complex social as well as organic beings, whose self-experience, in fundamental ways, constitutes their disease. Ironically, inclusionary social constructionism may be necessary for psychiatry to become truly medical.

Acknowledgments

We want to thank Drs. Berrios, Kendler, and Parnas for comments on earlier drafts of this material, as well as participants of the 2013 IASPM's satellite workshop on philosophy of psychiatry. We are also indebted to Elizabeth O'Neill and Aleta Quinn for useful criticisms and feedback.

References

Bentall, R. (1993). Deconstructing the concept of 'schizophrenia'. *Journal of Mental Health*, 2, 223–238.

Bentall, R. (2009). *Doctoring the Mind: Is Our Current Treatment of Mental Illness Really Any Good?* New York: New York University Press.

Berrios, G.E. and Hauser R. (1988). The early development of Kraepelin's ideas on classification: a conceptual history. *Psychological Medicine*, 18(4), 813–821.

Berrios, G.E., Luque, R., and Villagrán, J.M. (2003). Schizophrenia: a conceptual history. *International Journal of Psychology and Psychological Therapy*, 3(2), 111–140.

Colpe, L.J., Strine, T.W., Dhingra, S., McGuire, L.C., Elam-Evans, L.D., and Perry, G.S. (2010). Public health surveillance for mental health. *Preventing Chronic Disease*, 7(1), A17.

Derks, E.M., Allardyce, J., Boks, M.P., Vermunt, J.K., Hijman, R., and Ophoff, R.A. (2012). Kraepelin was right: a latent class analysis of symptom dimensions in patients and controls. *Schizophrenia Bulletin*, 38(3), 495–505.

Derks, E.M., Allardyce, J., Boks, M.P., Vermunt, J.K., Hijman, R., and Ophoff, R.A. (2012). Kraepelin was right: a latent class analysis of symptom dimensions in patients and controls. *Schizophrenia Bulletin*, 38(3), 495–505.

Duhem, P. (1954). *Aim and Structure of Physical Theory*. Princeton, NJ: Princeton University Press. (Work originally published in 1914.)

Duesberg, P.H. (1988). HIV is not the cause of AIDS. *Science*, 241, 514–516.

Duesberg, P.H. (1989). Human immunodeficiency virus and acquired immunodeficiency syndrome: Correlation but not causation. *Proceedings of the National Academy of Sciences of the United States of America*, 86, 755–764.

Duesberg, P.H. (1991). AIDS epidemiology: inconsistencies with human immunodeficiency virus and with infectious disease. *Proceedings of the National Academy of Sciences of the United States of America*, 88, 1575–1579.

Duesberg, P.H. (1992). The role of drugs in the origin of AIDS. *Biomedicine & Pharmacotherapy*, 46, 3–15.

Duesberg P.H., Mandrioli, D., McCormack, A., Nicholson, J.M., Rasnick, D., Fiala, C., et al. (2011). AIDS since 1984: no evidence for a new, viral epidemic—not even in Africa. *Italian Journal of Anatomy and Embryology*, 116(2), 73–92.

Dupré, J. (2012). *Processes of Life*. Oxford: Oxford University Press.

Epstein, S. (1996). *Impure Science: AIDS, Activism, and the Politics of Knowledge*. Berkeley, CA: University of California Press.

Goldstein, D.B. (2009). Common genetic variation and human traits. *New England Journal of Medicine*, 360(17), 1696–1698.

Hacking, I. (1995). *Rewriting the Soul: Multiple Personality and the Sciences of Memory*. Princeton, NJ: Princeton University Press.

Hacking, I. (1999). *The Social Construction of What?* Cambridge, MA: Harvard University Press.

Harden, V.A. (2012). *AIDS at 30: A History*. Washington, DC: Potomac Books.

Hyman, S.E. (2010). The diagnosis of mental disorders: the problem of reification. *Annual Review of Clinical Psychology*, 6, 155–179.

Kendler, K.S. (2012). The dappled nature of causes of psychiatric illness: replacing the organic-functional/hardware-software dichotomy with empirically based pluralism. *Molecular Psychiatry*, 17, 377–388.

Kendler, K. S. (2013). What psychiatric genetics has taught us about the nature of psychiatric illness and what is left to learn, *Molecular Psychiatry*, 18(10), 1058–1066.

Kendler, K.S., Karkowski, L.M., and Walsh, D. (1998). The structure of psychosis: latent class analysis of probands from the Roscommon Family Study. *Archives of General Psychiatry*, 55(6), 492–499.

Kendler, K.S. and Schaffner, K.F. (2011). The dopamine hypothesis of schizophrenia: an historical and philosophical analysis. *Philosophy, Psychiatry, & Psychology*, 18(1), 41–63.

Laing, R.D. and Esterson, A. (1964). *Sanity, Madness, and the Family*. London: Penguin Books.

Latour, B. and Woolgar, S. (eds.) (1979). *Laboratory Life: the Social Construction of Scientific Facts*. Beverly Hills, CA: Sage.

Lewis, D.A., Curley, A.A., Glausier, J.R., and Volk, D.W. (2012). Cortical parvalbumin interneurons and cognitive dysfunction in schizophrenia. *Trends in Neurosciences*, 35(1), 57–67.

Mackie, J.L. (1974). *The Cement of the Universe: A Study of Causation*. Oxford: Clarendon Press.

Mallon, R. (2008). Naturalistic approaches to social construction. In E.N. Zalta (ed.) *The Stanford Encyclopedia of Philosophy* (Winter 2008 ed.). [Online] Available at: <http://plato.stanford.edu/archives/win2008/entries/social-construction-naturalistic/>.

McGrath, J.A., Nestadt, G., Liang, K.Y., Lasseter, V.K., Wolyniec, P.S., Fallin, M.D., et al. (2004). Five latent factors underlying schizophrenia: analysis and relationship to illnesses in relatives. *Schizophrenia Bulletin*, 30(4), 855–873.

McHugh, P.R. and Slavney, P.R. (1998). *The Perspectives of Psychiatry* (2nd ed.). Baltimore, MD: Johns Hopkins University Press.

Nelson, B., Thompson, A., and Yung, A.R. (2012). Basic self-disturbance predicts psychosis onset in the ultra high risk for psychosis "prodromal" population. *Schizophrenia Bulletin*, (38)6, 1277–1287.

Niiniluoto, I. (2011). Scientific progress. In E.N. Zalta (ed.) *Stanford Encyclopedia of Philosophy*. [Online] Available at: <http://plato.stanford.edu/entries/scientific-progress/>.

Nordgaard, J. and Parnas, J. (2014). Self-disorders and the schizophrenia spectrum: a study of 100 first hospital admissions. *Schizophrenia Bulletin*. First published online: January 29, 2014.

Parnas, J. (2008). Varieties of "phenomenology": on description, understanding, and explanation in psychiatry. In K.S. Kendler, and Parnas J. (eds.) *Philosophical Issues in Psychiatry*, pp. 239–278. Baltimore, MD: Johns Hopkins University Press.

Parnas, J., Møller, P., Kircher, T., Thalbitzer, J., Jansson, L., Handest, P., and Zahavi, D. (2005). EASE: Examination of Anomalous Self-Experience. *Psychopathology*, 38, 236–258.

Parnas, J., Sass, L. A. and Zahavi, D. (2013). Rediscovering psychopathology: the epistemology and phenomenology of the psychiatric object. *Schizophrenia Bulletin*, 39(2), 270–277.

Reininghaus, U., Priebe, S., and Bentall, R.P. (2013). Testing the psychopathology of psychosis: evidence for a general psychosis dimension. *Schizophrenia Bulletin*, 39(4), 884–895.

Schaffner, K.F. (1972). *Nineteenth Century Aether Theories*. Oxford: Pergamon Press.

Schaffner, K.F. (2000). Philosophy of method. In J. Lederberg (ed.) *Encyclopedia of Microbiology*, pp. 227–239. San Diego, CA: Academic Press.

Schaffner, K.F. (2012). A philosophical overview of the problems of validity for psychiatric disorders. In K.S. Kendler and J. Parnas (eds.) *Philosophical Issues in Psychiatry II: Nosology*, pp. 167–89. New York, NY: Oxford University Press.

Shilts, R. (1987). *And the Band Played On: Politics, People, and the AIDS Epidemic.* New York: St. Martin's Press.

Stine, G. (2013). *AIDS Update 2013*. New York: McGraw-Hill.

Sullivan, P.F., Daly, M.J., and O'Donovan, M. (2012). Genetic architectures of psychiatric disorders: the emerging picture and its implications. *Nature Reviews Genetics*, 13(8), 537–551.

Sun J., Jia P., Fanous, A.H., van den Oord, E., Chen, X., Riley, B.P., *et al.* (2010). Schizophrenia gene networks and pathways and their applications for novel candidate gene selection. *PLoS One*, 5(6), e11351.

Szasz, T. (1987). *Insanity: The Idea and Its Consequences.* Syracuse, NY: Syracuse University Press.

Szasz, T. (2006). Mental illness as brain disease: a brief history lesson. *Ideas on Liberty*, 56, 24–25.

Chapter 12

The role of cultural configurators in the formation of mental symptoms

German E. Berrios

12.1 Introduction

Chapter 11 explores the role that "social factors" may play in the workings (or progress) of psychiatry as a science. The authors conclude that such a role is ambivalent: on the one hand, social factors make etiological sense and counteract the reductionistic excesses of neurobiology; on the other, they may act as confounders when not properly dovetailed into the explanatory frame of psychiatry. With the help of some philosophical categories and historical comment, the authors then proceed to illustrate the way in which social factors may be accommodated into the explanatory framework of both schizophrenia and HIV/AIDS.

In keeping with Otto Neurath's advice,[1] the authors have not attempted to change more than one deck plank at a time. Given that it is the hull rather than the deck of psychiatry that is in need of repair, some may deem their choice timorous. Indeed, in relation to the question of whether there is "progress" in psychiatry I feel that their effort might have been more effective had they instead explored: (1) the epistemological structure of both the discipline itself and its objects (mental symptom and disorder), (2) what "social factors" mean in relation to the structure of psychiatry and what their role may be in the actual formation of psychiatric objects, and (3) which of the available definitions of "progress" can actually be predicated of psychiatry. The comments that follow expand upon these three points and are meant to complement the views expressed in this interesting chapter.

12.2 The Epistemological Structure of Psychiatry and its Objects

12.2.1 The Historical Construction of Psychiatry

There was no "psychiatry" (as there may have been a "surgery" or a "gynecology") before the nineteenth century. Constructed after the 1810s, "alienism" was the

---

[1] I am referring here to his well-known analogy: "There is no way to establish fully secured, neat protocol statements as starting points of the sciences. There is no tabula rasa. We are

European solution to the social problems posed by individuals called mad, insane, manic, or lunatic. It was Enlightenment philanthropy rather than "scientific progress" that engendered the belief that the medical solution was the more efficient and palatable. This is not to say that medics in the West have not been interested in madness, indeed, their views have been well known since Classical times. Until the nineteenth century, however, their narratives were not exclusive or predominant or underwritten by legislation.

The officialization of an alliance between madness and medicine meant that the entire epistemological apparatus of the latter could be applied to the former. Part of this process was the importation of the (recently constructed) anatomoclinical view of "disease" (Ackerknecht 1967). This was based on the: (1) construction of a "semiology" (later called descriptive psychopathology) and a "pathology" of madness, and (2) the search for methodologies (e.g., postmortem studies) that might allow for the matching of complaint and brain sites. *Ab initio*, the links in question were treated as categorical but as statistics penetrated medicine they became probabilistic.

However, from the start it became clear that the standard analytical approaches of medicine did not work when applied to madness. For example, whilst in medicine "somatic" correlates were soon converted into "diagnostic markers," this rarely if ever happened in psychiatry. Alienists explained this away (and still do) by claiming that exploration of the brain is much harder than that of kidneys, heart, or stomach. To keep their hopes going, alienists also resorted to quoting "organic" conditions of the brain (e.g., general paralysis of the insane, tumors, Parkinson's disease, epilepsy, Lewy body disease) which were often enough accompanied by "mental symptoms" redolent of those seen in conventional psychiatric conditions. To strengthen their case they argued (they still do) that the mental symptoms seen in neurological and psychiatric diseases were in fact the same phenomenon.

As current diagnostic listings show, for example, the ICD-10 (World Health Organization 1993), the fact of the matter is that madness remains a descriptive concept and that the hundreds of correlations generated by neuroimaging, genetics, or other research techniques are not usable as diagnostic tools, *simpliciter*. Given their professional and emotional investment, it is understandable that the neuroscientists are not worried about the strange resistance that madness offers to the conventional medical approach. Far less understandable is a similar untroubled attitude on the part of historians and philosophers of psychiatry who by now should be exploring alternative epistemological approaches to madness (on this more later).

It remains unclear what were all the nineteenth century forces that led to the alliance between medicine and madness. The view that such an alliance simply resulted from "progress" in the brain sciences is historically untenable and epistemologically counterproductive for it may generate a false sense of security and

---

like sailors who have to rebuild their ship on the open sea, without ever being able to dismantle it in dry-dock and reconstruct it from the best components" (Neurath 1932/1983, p. 92).

the wrong belief that the alliance is irreversible. Even those who firmly believe that medicine is the only solution to the problem of madness should continue asking what has kept the alliance going so far. Given that even the most conventional amongst the historians of science would be happy to countenance the view that social and economic factors are relevant to the functioning of the sciences, should not historians of psychiatry be watching over the possibility that the "medical" approach to madness may become superfluous to requirements if new ways are found of managing madness that are considered as cheaper and ethically acceptable? Reconceptualizing madness as an object or event that is not a "disease" would not, of course, negate the existence of personal or social suffering nor the dire need to develop means to alleviate it. Against this new historical backdrop, should the philosopher of psychiatry explore "progress" as only meaning change within the medical view of madness or perhaps should he broaden its compass to consider change in the general manner in which the suffering of madness could be alleviated?

12.2.2 The Concept of Mental Symptom and Disorder

According to the nineteenth-century Parisian anatomoclinical model, "disease" consisted of a cluster of signs and symptoms glued together by structural lesions affecting the relevant bodily organ (Ackerknecht 1967). Alienists applied this view to madness *tout court*. Up to the 1830s, the most popular candidate organs for madness were the stomach and the brain; in the event the latter won the day. To make sense of all postmortem findings linking complaints to brain sites, a neuropsychological map was required and this was soon provided by phrenology, successfully developed on the classification of mental powers proposed by the Scottish Philosophy of Common Sense (Berrios 1988). As in general medicine, "symptoms and signs" were also to become the units of analysis of madness which, in various combinations, were thought to give rise to its different forms. The glue that kept mental symptoms together was considered to be "neurobiological" and this has remained an article of faith to this day. From time to time, however, and to the credit of some psychiatric thinkers, glues other than biological (e.g., social, historical, and statistical) have been proposed. The cluster model of mental disorders conceives of symptoms as primary and of disorders as secondary objects. In other words, the ontology of the latter is parasitical upon that of the former.

During the first half of the nineteenth century, the development of a working concept of biological "function" (and of physiology as the science of functions) added to the explanatory power of the anatomoclinical model of disease.[2] Structural lesions affecting bodily organs were now believed to distort "function" and formed the basis of symptoms and signs in medicine. Symptoms were

---

[2] Although writers like Foster (1901) talk about a 'physiological' approach during the sixteenth century, it seems clear that the current notion of function and its direct application to practical medical thinking only appeared during the early nineteenth century (Hall 1969).

redefined as degraded expressions of specific functions and hence became indicators of what organ might be compromised. In keeping with this model, mental symptoms also started to be considered as expressions of disrupted "mental functions," themselves the result of putative lesions in brain sites (or regions, networks, modules, pathways, etc.).

The problem with this approach is that a structural analysis of mental symptoms shows that they are far more than the expression of a disturbance in a "specific" brain function. Indeed, very rarely, a function can be found that matches their complex form and content (Marková and Berrios 2009). Given this problem, the Cambridge group has developed a model of symptom formation to explain how the original inchoate experience (caused by the disruption of a putative "mental function") is caught into the vortex of a configurative process (Marková and Berrios 2011). According to this model, the configurators that format the inchoate experience are cultural ("supra-biological" to use one of the authors' terms) factors intervening: (1) at a level which is deeper than what is usually allowed for social factors, and (2) playing a role which is more than "causal" (in the conventional or INUS sense of this term). According to the Cambridge model, social factors "are" part and parcel of the symptom itself and hence effect and cause (more on the role of social factors in the following section).

12.3 Social Factors in the History of Psychiatry

The concept of "social factor" needs unpacking before it can be of any use; and doubly so in relation to madness. If used in a broad sense, it can be claimed that social factors have been well recognized since the time alienism was first constructed. For example, in the 1830s, Esquirol (1838, p. 62) listed life events (social factors) that "caused" madness. Twenty years later, Bucknill and Tuke (1858, chapter III) asked whether civilization (social factor) was relevant to the increase in the rates of madness in the nineteenth century. They argued that it was, and their view was accepted in other European countries. By the end of the century a number of books had been published on the specific issue of the role of social factors in madness (Duprat 1900; Lunier 1874).

It could of course be objected that Esquirol, Tuke, and the others were entertaining a view of "social factor" far less "exact" than what we have nowadays. A look at the 1970s debate on the role of "life events" in the etiology of mental disorder should deal with this objection (Brown and Harris 1989). In fact, that debate was the last important effort to factor "social factors" into the causal equation before the neurobiological approach took over completely. Indeed, I know of no serious current effort to make "social factor" operational and meaningful. Although those practicing transcultural psychiatry have also been interested in the role of "cultural factors" in the formation of mental disorder, the level of their conceptualization is no different from that informing the older debate on "life events."

If thus, then, what does it mean for the authors of the chapter under comment to ask for "social factors" to be given a role in the formation of mental disorders? We are told: "due to the nature of psychiatric objects, the role of supra-biological features may be more prominent in psychiatry than in other branches of medicine." This is an interesting claim for three reasons: (1) there are specialisms in medicine other than psychiatry (e.g., epidemiology, dermatology, and gastroenterology) to which social factors seem absolutely fundamental. Indeed, there will be those who might claim that medicine is a social enterprise, *simpliciter*. (2) "Supra-biological features" (the nearest the authors actually get to defining "social factor") comes across as an apophatic (negative) definition. Given that some have argued that the boundary between the biological and the social needs to be trespassed in favor of the biological (Barkow et al. 1992), this definition may not be very helpful. (3) The general point by the authors that as a discipline psychiatry may be more dependent upon "social factors" than other medical specialisms is interesting and well taken. It does need, however, additional unpacking.

What are "social factors"? Given that since Durkheim (1895) there has been a debate on the ontology and epistemology of social facts (Gilbert 1989; Greenwood 2003; Little 2007) and that the use of the metaphor factor adds to such social facts a dimension of agency or causality, the need to develop an operational definition of "social factor" that may mean something in the context of mental symptoms and disorders seems rather obvious. A number of options are available in this regard. Recourse could be had to common sense to state that everyone is able to recognize how certain life events (say, the loss of a child) and about of anxiety or depression are related. Others may feel that whilst this is so, it remains essential for therapeutic purposes to know more about the way in which the life event and the person interact. Such an analysis seems to require that more is known about the structure and affordances of the life event, the context, and the personal characteristics of the individual concerned. For example, one may want to know whether the impact of the life event is nonspecific (i.e., it causes just blunt stress) and the manner in which the person responds depends upon intrinsic, personal features or whether the life event already carries shaping or molding configurators that determine the reaction of the individual concerned, or whether the reaction in question is in fact molded by the context (environment, social mores, culture, etc.) in which the individual is embedded.

In this latter sense, the role of "social factors" becomes particularly difficult to conceptualize. For example, it is not clear whether it can be simply considered to be a "cause" of the mental disorder (and hence mappable by a causal model such as Mackie's INUS) or whether the "social" actually becomes the material out of which the mental disorder is "made." It is an interesting observation that the conceptualization and classification of "causes" have been an early preoccupation of medicine. There is no space here to talk about the history of the role played by the concept of etiology in medicine and psychiatry (Berrios 2000) but it could be claimed that a large part of the debate on the very concept of cause in the Western world has been carried out within medicine and medical models and problems have been the origin of certain philosophical ideas about causality. For example, dichotomous categories such as primary versus secondary, one versus many causes, causes versus risk factors, distant versus proximate causes, modifying versus predisposing factors, causes versus enabling conditions, and so on were all first discussed in the context of medicine and carry a hidden medical dimension (Pariset 1813). It goes without saying that during the nineteenth century alienism followed medicine in its conceptualization of "cause." So, in what way might utilizing Mackie's INUS concept help to integrate social factors in the etiological fabric of mental disorder? After all, all that INUS offers is a way of logically mapping plural causes and of allocating to each an etiological valence according to their loci in a given etiological system.

12.3.1 Social Factors and the Formation of Mental Symptoms

For "social factors" to be of use in psychiatry they must be more than a putative presence in an etiological map. So far, their participation has been limited to triggering or giving content to mental symptoms and disorders. The former was the conventional role that "life events" were attributed during the 1970s. It was claimed that, mediated by stress (another complex concept), social factors brought about mental disorders. The latter has been used for decades by transcultural psychiatrists to explain why Chinese people might hallucinate dragons and Bolivian people llamas. It is clear that this is not sufficient. Part of this insufficiency relates to the fact that far more is required from social factors in psychiatry than in sociology itself. In the latter discipline, social facts are attributed sufficient activity and agency as is required to act upon other social facts. In psychiatry, what is required is that social facts intervene, effectively changing the course or behavior of neurobiological systems.

This demands ontological and epistemological furniture of a different nature and models to account for such intervention that have not yet been developed by philosophers of psychiatry. This can clearly be seen in the new discipline of cultural neuroscience where interesting empirical work seems to be showing that "culture" (whatever that means) seems to influence not only the manner in which the perceptual systems function but the actual information they seem to obtain. This intervention is far deeper than the mere providing of different perceptual "contents." A similar mechanism has been proposed by the Cambridge model of mental symptom formation. Inchoate experiences (signals from distressed brain sites) would be culturally configured upon entering consciousness giving rise to mental symptoms with a moderate level of invariance. The latter, however, would be due not to the fact that the signal comes from a particular brain site but from the fact that it is configured by the same cultural configurator (see Berrios, Chapter 5, this volume). Were this to be the case, then social factors would be found to have a real role in mental symptom and disorder formation.

12.4 The Concept of Progress in Relation to Psychiatry

It is unclear whether the editorial brief for this chapter was to explore psychiatry in relation to "progress in general" (Bury 1920; Delvaille 1910; Nisbet 1980) or "scientific progress" in particular (Dilworth 1994; Laudan 1977; Losee 2004). This is important to know for these two concepts apply differently to psychiatry. The former concerns the broader question of whether successive narratives about madness can be listed in a hierarchical, evaluative order; the latter focuses on the narrower issue of whether successive versions of the current medical narrative are approaching some intrinsic psychiatric truth but capturing the noumenon of madness.

For the effects of this comment, progress can be simply defined as evaluated change, in other words it relates to the belief that the later modifications of a system or process are better, superior, more efficient, etc., than the earlier ones. The issue here is why it should be hoped or believed that change must lead to improvement. Clearly, such expectation only can occur against complex assumptions about nature and the world in general. Interestingly enough such a notion of progress was absent in Classical thinking and only begins to develop with the philosophy of Christianity and takes off during the Enlightenment (Delvaille 1910). Particularly useful to the sociology of science, it flourished during the nineteenth century in philosophies such as positivism and Darwinian evolution and it has remained a selling point of the natural sciences (Losee 2004). Much as the philosophy of science may have since then shown that the concept of progress is burdened by epistemological complexities, the fact of the matter is that at a popular level science continues appearing as the only human activity that is getting closer to the truth of the world and hence deserves the most respect and financial support.

How should the concept of progress be applied to psychiatry? It seems clear that change does affect: (1) psychiatric narratives, (2) the objects that they construct, and (3) the opaque biological and social reality that they intent to capture (see Berrios, Chapter 5, this volume). The issue is whether the newer versions of the narratives or the objects they construct are in any way better or superior (at this stage the evaluative yardstick does not need to be specified) than the older ones. In historical terms, it cannot be denied that since Classical times there have been successive narratives about madness. Each was linked to its specific episteme and until the historical staging offered by Comte during the nineteenth century no one had seriously tried to compare them according to some value judgment and list them accordingly. Indeed, it is difficult to know how such a comparison could be justified. However, the construction of nineteenth-century alienism occurred precisely during the period when European history and philosophy of science was starting to pay notice to Comte, Whewell, Mill, and Spencer. After the 1850s, it is clear that progress from a "dark past to an enlightened present" also became an important selling point of the medical view of madness.

Progress can also be explored not across all psychiatric narratives but within the ongoing one, started, as has been show, during the nineteenth century. Now that we "know" that mental symptoms and disorders are diseases of the brain, has there been progress since the light-microscope studies of the nineteenth century? The answer should depend upon the evaluative yardstick: if is to be technical advance the answer has to be yes; if it is to be statistical reduction of people affected, the answer is unclear; if it is to be understanding of madness, the answer is probably no.

Lastly, the issue of whether the notion of progress should be applied to the narratives of madness at all must be briefly discussed. The answer is that it all depends upon whether a useful evaluative yardstick is made available. If madness is as much about meaning as it is about brain changes then such a yardstick is not going to be found in some abstract concept of truth, or in statistical significance, or in a putative primacy of the natural sciences. Surely, the only yardstick is the sufferer's satisfaction. Whatever narrative is capable of alleviating the suffering caused by madness, and is acceptable to those in need, then it should be considered as fit for purpose and defined (if one so wishes) as "progress" when compared to narratives that are imposed upon the sufferer simply because some considered them as the "truth."

12.5 Conclusions

From time immemorial, the ancient forms of behavior that fall under the generic compass of madness have elicited many (more or less successful) descriptive and explanatory narratives, and each of these has in its time contributed to social organization and order and to sufferer's satisfaction. Although very early medical narratives were part of this general effort, it is only during the nineteenth century that they were to achieve predominance, becoming legitimized by the social construction of a new profession called alienism.

Whether or not the current medical narratives should be considered as superior in relation to all others remains a moot point and requires far more informed debate than what has gone on so far. This means that those interested to create new narratives about the meaning and amelioration of madness should be encouraged to continue. What seems clear, however, is that the current alliance between madness and medicine must be considered as historical and hence temporal. This means that it is up to those who fervently believe that medicine should forever be the discipline in charge of madness to make sure that what medicine offers has an edge over all other narratives.

It should not be the job of the historian and philosopher of psychiatry to construct cosmetic justifications of what clinicians and researchers state is the case but instead to insist in the essential historicity of all narratives about madness and open up protected conceptual spaces within which new narratives may be safely constructed.

References

Ackerknecht, E. (1967). *Medicine at the Paris Hospital 1794–1848*. Baltimore, MD: Johns Hopkins Press.

Barkow, J., Cosmides, L., and Tooby, J. (eds.) (1992). *The Adapted Mind: Evolutionary Psychology and the Generation of Culture*. New York: Oxford University Press.

Berrios, G.E. (1988). Historical background to abnormal psychology. In E. Miller and P. Cooper (eds.) *Adult Abnormal Psychology*, pp. 26–51. London: Churchill Livingstone.

Berrios G.E. (2000). Historical development of ideas about psychiatric aetiology. In M. Gelder, N. Andreasen, J. Lopez-Ibor, and J. Geddes (eds.) *New Oxford Textbook of Psychiatry* (Vol. 1), pp. 147–153. Oxford: Oxford University Press.

Brown, G.W. and Harris, T.O. (eds.) (1989). *Life Events and Illness*. New York: Guilford Press.

Bucknill, J. and Tuke, D.H. (1858). *A Manual of Psychological Medicine*. London: Churchill.

Bury, J.B. (1920). *The Idea of Progress*. London: Macmillan and Co.

Delvaille, J. (1910). *Essai sur L'Histoire de L'Idée de Progrés. Jusqu'a la fin de XVIII Siècle*. Paris: Alcan.

Dilworth, C. (1994). *Scientific Progress*. Dordrecht: Springer.

Duprat, G.L. (1900). *Les Causes Sociales de la Folie*. Paris: Alcan.

Durkheim, E. (1895). *Les Règles de la Méthode Sociologique*. Paris: Alcan.

Esquirol, E. (1838). *Des Maladies Mentales* (Vol. 1). Paris: Baillière.

Foster, M. (1901). *Lectures on the History of Physiology. The Sixteenth, Seventeenth and Eighteenth Centuries*. Cambridge: Cambridge University Press.

Gilbert, M. (1989). *On Social Facts*. Princeton, NJ: Princeton University Press.

Greenwood, J.D. (2003). Social facts, social groups and social explanation. *Noûs*, 37, 93–112.

Hall, T.S. (1969). *Ideas of Life and Matter*. Chicago, IL: University of Chicago Press.

Laudan, L. (1977). *Progress and its Problems: Towards a Theory of Scientific Growth*. Berkeley, CA: University of California Press.

Little, D. (2007). Levels of the social. In S.P. Turner and M.W. Risjord (eds.) *Handbook of the Philosophy of Science: Philosophy of Anthropology and Sociology*, pp. 343–372. Amsterdam: Elsevier.

Losee, J. (2004). *Theories of Scientific Progress*. London: Routledge.

Lunier, L. (1874). *De L'influence des Grandes Commotions Politiques et Sociales sur le développement des maladies mentales*. Paris: Savy.

Marková, I.S. and Berrios, G.E. (2009). Epistemology of mental symptoms. *Psychopathology*, 42, 343–349.

Marková, I.S. and Berrios, G.E. (2011). Epistemology of psychiatry. *Psychopathology*, 45, 220–227.

Neurath, O. (1983). *Philosophical Papers*. Dordrecht: Reidel. (Work originally published in 1932.)

Nisbet, R. (1980). *History of the Idea of Progress*. New York: Basic Books.

Pariset, E. (1813). Cause. In Adelon, Alard, Alibert, *et al*. (eds.) *Dictionnaire des Sciences Médicales*, pp. 356–375. Paris: Panckoucke.

World Health Organization (1993). *International Statistical Classification of Diseases and Related Health Problems: Tenth Revision*. Geneva: WHO.

Part II

History of broad movements/structures within psychiatry

Section 5
The psychiatric history of the diencephalon

Chapter 13

Introduction to "Biography of a brain structure: studying the diencephalon as an epistemic object"

Josef Parnas

This fascinating, historico-sociological chapter attempts to illustrate the nature of scientific developments in psychiatry by examining the evolution of the role of the diencephalon (which some readers may better recognize as the thalamus and hypothalamus). The scientific development is examined here through the vicissitudes of an "epistemic object" or *epistemic thing* (e.g., an organ, enzymatic system, etc.) rather than through the evolution of concepts, topics, problems, disciplines, or institutions. In our context, the study of the diencephalon as an epistemic object of the first half of the twentieth century (until the early 1950s) provides an example of a "territory of convergence" (see also Berrios, Chapter 5, this volume), a research field targeted and invested by different, interacting, pragmatic, and theoretical scientific interests (e.g., physiology, neurology, neurosurgery, endocrinology, and psychiatry) and mutually influencing their respective developments.

There are several issues in this chapter, which a reader unfamiliar with the mechanisms of the scientific development, may extract and retain as useful insights. First, for many readers it will be a novelty to learn that the diencephalon was implicated in the pathogenesis of a quite broad range of psychosomatic and mental illnesses (from autonomic dysfunctions to schizophrenia). The significance of this role was reflected in considering the so-called "diencephalic hypothesis" as a "doctrine," "big current issue," or "the most successful current explanation for mental disorders," considering the diencephalic pathology as a "common substrate of the emergence of psychosis" (see also Kendler, Chapter 32, this volume, on the third version of the dopamine hypothesis of schizophrenia). We are of course more familiar with the subsequent "grand theories," for example, concerning the limbic system and neurotransmitters, specifically, the dopamine hypothesis of schizophrenia (see Kendler, Chapter 32). Second, this chapter portrays the evolution of science as a mainly continuous series of interpenetrating steps, where certain ideas, explicitly articulated only recently, were already vaguely anticipated much earlier. This should counteract the contemporary tendency of *presentism*, an intellectual attitude, which in a nutshell claims that the world, as we know it, has only emerged quite recently, at the latest since our own birth (e.g., that the *science of psychiatry* only began with the publication of the DSM-III in 1980 or later). Finally, the chapter illustrates a historical recurrence of ideas, retaining their substance and only changing their clothes. The most persistent and ineliminable idea seems to be a desire for and a belief in the possibility of a straightforward reduction of the mental to a well-circumscribed neural substrate (see, e.g., Cuthbert 2014).

Reference

Cuthbert, B.N. (2014). The RDoC framework: facilitating transition from ICD/DSM to dimensional approaches that integrate neuroscience and psychopathology (followed by 13 peer commentaries). *World Psychiatry*, 13, 28–55.

Chapter 14

Biography of a brain structure: studying the diencephalon as an epistemic object

Emilie Bovet

14.1 Why Study the Cerebral Hypotheses of Mental Pathologies in the History of Psychiatry?

This chapter will deal with the history of the diencephalon, written mainly from a sociological perspective. The diencephalon, located in the center of the brain, principally comprises the hypothalamus, the thalamus, and the pituitary and the pineal glands. Its spatial location between the cortex and the brainstem, and the close connections of the diencephalon to the endocrine system make it an important player in the functioning of the brain. From this chapter's perspective, which is an exploration of the interactions between the empirical and the extra-scientific influences on the evolution of psychiatry as a clinical neuroscience, the diencephalon presents itself as an ideal candidate theme to examine. This is so for several reasons.

The diencephalon, being a shared focus of interest of several different scientific approaches, is an interesting tool for the history of psychiatry. Psychiatry, as a practical science and a branch of medicine, is characterized by an intertwinement of multiple theoretical, therapeutic, and institutional interests, constantly interacting with other disciplines, ranging from biology and medical sciences to the humanities and social sciences. This muddles the perception and self-understanding of psychiatry as a specific, clearly demarcated, and autonomous discipline. The history of psychiatry is less linear than that of other medical sciences and it cannot be written without constant references to other scientific fields, because all these fields always exert crucial influence. Psychiatry's striving for its own and stable legitimacy, has always been "contaminated" and subverted by the theories emerging in other scientific fields. Thus, in order to understand today's psychiatry, it is necessary to expose its connivance and dissension with these other disciplines, influencing psychiatry's theoretical situation and psychiatry's clinical and fundamental research.

The diencephalon, being the target of scientific approaches from different disciplines and perspectives, can be considered what the German philosopher and historian Hans-Jörg Rheinberger calls an "epistemic object":

> In following the development of *epistemic things* rather than that of concepts, topics, problems, disciplines, or institutions, the boundaries have to be crossed, boundaries of representational techniques, of experimental systems, of established academic disciplines, and of institutionalized programs and projects. In following the path of epistemic things, classifications have to be abandoned. Does this study belong to the history of cancer research? Of cytomorphology? Of biochemistry? Of molecular biology? Is it a prehistory of protein synthesis? All of these—and none (1997, p. 34; italics added).

Retracing the evolution of an "epistemic object" such as the diencephalon provides an opportunity to see the development of psychiatry in the first half of the twentieth century as being closely influenced by the ideas, concepts, and scientific findings of the disciplines outside psychiatry.

An analysis of the vicissitudes of an "epistemic object" helps to write the history of psychiatric neurosciences in a new way: instead of focusing on "overturns" or "heroes" of neurosciences, irrespective of the discipline concerned, it is essential to keep a reflexive position, by understanding better how current brain research has been influenced by questionings that came before the so-called neuroscientific revolutions. It is often said that psychiatry, as a clinical neuroscience is a "continuation" of "biological psychiatry." Certainly, the introduction of psychoactive drugs in the treatment of mental pathologies changed the perception (and self-perception) of psychiatry. Now it became a scientific enterprise because it possessed a therapeutic profile resembling other medical sciences. The transformations caused by these new drugs, from the mid 1950s onward, make it a kind of "pivotal period" that would mark the transition from a psychiatric practice without a scientific basis to one driven by the ambition to understand the neurochemical basis of mental pathologies. However, this way of presenting the history of psychiatry as if there were a clearly defined "before" and "after" the introduction of psychoactive drugs, hides the fact that within psychiatry, and long before the 1950s, a significant part of clinical practice and research was dedicated to the study of the relationship between the psyche and brain dysfunctions. For some features, current research in psychiatric neurosciences is just as close to studies undertaken on the brain at the time for shock therapies as to those measuring psychological and cerebral modification caused by psychoactive drugs. In order to avoid reductive simplifications, the historic epistemology of the attempts to link brain dysfunction and mental illness must reflect on the *recurrent* character of some issues that have run through the history of the so-called biological psychiatry and which are still on the agenda.

This is the reason why I have chosen to show how the examination of theories developed before the first use of psychoactive drugs in psychiatry can cast a new light on the principal stakes and questions faced by current psychiatric neurosciences. Indeed, no period in the history of psychiatry is exempt from some specific interest in a particular brain anomaly in the patients suffering from a particular mental disorder and a wish to link this particular anomaly to the etiology of the particular disorder. This recurrent approach has produced a large number of hypotheses on the link between the brain and the mental disorders for more than a century. Once the theories are considered solid enough, they offer the discipline an opportunity to affirm its affiliation to the biological sciences, providing an explanatory dimension to mental pathologies. Whether they focus on a dysfunction caused by brain damage, a neurochemical imbalance, or a molecular deficiency, these biological hypotheses instantiate, throughout the history of psychiatry, a recurrent questioning and hope inspired by a potential understanding of the relation between the mental and the brain.

In this chapter, I have focused on the "diencephalic hypothesis," as it falls within an often little-studied history of psychiatry and deserves close attention in order to understand the attempts to establish a relationship between brain dysfunction and mental disorder in the era of shock therapy. In a general manner, my research aims to shed new light on the conditions in which certain theories and hypotheses emerged, instead of focusing on the so-called revolutions that supposedly radically changed the history of psychiatry.

14.2 How the Diencephalon Became "interesting" for Psychiatry

I have chosen to do what historian of science Lorraine Daston calls a "biography" (2000) of the diencephalon, in order to clarify the conditions that made this area of the brain be of interest to different scientific communities, and to analyze how the observation of this particular scientific object evolved through these studies. Describing the emergence and course of a scientific object requires an understanding of the dynamics that facilitated the circulation of knowledge and a grasping of the specific constellations of interests (also outside psychiatry) that articulated themselves in this specific context. Thus, what is at stake is to figure out how a particular brain area became *sufficiently relevant* to be subjected to experimentation and therapeutic exploration. Following this approach does not imply neglecting the historical importance of particular individuals, or of specific collaborations between disciplines. Rather, the aim is to precisely analyze these various aspects through the historical vicissitudes of the diencephalon in psychiatry.

Whereas it was easy to identify the relevant psychiatric and neurological references to the diencephalon from the late 1930s to the mid 1950s, it was more difficult to understand why and how the diencephalon became specifically attractive for psychiatry. Indeed, it required an examination of studies performed in neurosurgery, endocrinology, anatomical pathology, and physiology. Far from having been "discovered" by psychiatrists, the so-called diencephalic model was built, step by step, thanks to the development of very diverse experimental approaches.

The experimental studies on the diencephalon by the Austrian physiologists Johann Karplus and Aloïs Kreidl from 1909 to 1911 mark the beginning of several investigations aiming to understand its role in the autonomic regulation. The stimulation of the diencephalon in living animals revealed various autonomic reactions such as an increase of pulse and blood pressure, pupillary dilatation, and contractions of the uterus and bladder. These findings encouraged the view of this brain area as a main autonomic center. The arrival of lethargic encephalitis during World War I motivated the study of a potential role of the diencephalon in emotional regulation. The characteristic symptoms of encephalitis lethargica were not restricted to drowsiness, fever, muscle contractions, and cranial nerve palsies; the patients or their relatives also observed mental changes, such as visual hallucinations, compulsive phenomena, or alterations of mood (Delay 1948; Grinker 1939; Lempérière 2004; Steck 1927). Some patients showed emotional reactions apparently resembling those of schizophrenia (Jelliffe 1927) or spontaneous fits of rage without apparent cause (Grinker 1939). The postmortem brain examinations often revealed lesions in the diencephalon (Delay 1946; Grinker 1939; Ingram 1939; von Economo 1930). The clinical manifestations of the disease in conjunction with neuropathological findings stimulated a surge of studies on the diencephalon in the second half of the 1920s. These series of studies were mainly performed on cats and dogs, using electrical or chemical stimulation. The results seemed to suggest that the diencephalon was a major entity in the regulation of waking and sleep, instincts, and emotions. The studies of two American physiologists, Walter Cannon and his disciple Philip Bard (Bard 1928, 1934; Cannon 1927, 1931), are in particular worth mentioning: in cats, in which almost the entire brain, with the exception of the diencephalon, had been removed, they observed an unusual anger. Cannon and Bard called this anger a *sham rage* and concluded that the source of this emotion was located in the diencephalon. These findings were replicated and strengthened by other studies, jointly pointing to a specific role of the diencephalon in evoking anger-like emotions (Bard 1934; Cannon 1931; Ingram 1939; Ranson and Magoun 1939).

In addition to animal experiments and postmortem studies, the contribution of neurosurgery in the promotion of the view of the diencephalon as an "emotional center" was also very significant (Beattie 1932; Cox 1937; Fulton and Bailey 1929). The work of two German neurosurgeons, Otfrid Foerster and Oskar Gagel (1931, 1932, 1933), suggested that during the operations for diencephalic brain tumors, one could observe in the patients emotional reactions similar to "euphoria characteristic of mania" (Delay 1948, p. 44). Moreover, it also seemed that the autopsies of the patients who had suffered from emotional problems frequently revealed a diencephalic tumor (Alpers 1937, 1940; Cox 1937; Fulton and Bailey 1929; Morgan 1939). In the mid 1930s, the diencephalon was considered not only as a main regulator of the autonomic system, but was also definitely considered as a major center of regulation of psychic functions (Fulton 1947).

This flourishing research with spectacular results in neurosurgery and physiology quickly attracted the attention of psychiatrists. It is in this context, that the American psychiatrist Roy R. Grinker developed a theory linking the diencephalon and psychosomatic disorders. To compare the effects of diencephalic stimulation in humans and animals, he created his own techniques of electrical stimulation of the diencephalon and observed a profound anxiety in patients whose diencephalon was stimulated: some wept uncontrollably, others saw their lives flash before their eyes, and some believed that the end of the world was approaching (Grinker 1938, 1939; Grinker and Serota 1938). In Europe, the French psychiatrist Jean Delay played an influential role in promoting the significance of the diencephalon for psychiatry. He published several books in which he underlined the key role of the diencephalon in maintaining emotional balance. Delay believed that alterations of the diencephalon could upset the instinctive-emotional balance and thereby generate different types of mood disturbance (Delay 1953), and accordingly, that psychiatric therapies should aim at rebalancing the functioning of the diencephalic area. Being a fervent supporter of shock therapies, Delay conducted many studies with electroshock to measure its effects on patients' brain, psyche, and body. The psychological and somatic reactions were very similar to those observed in diencephalic stimulation, which led him to believe that the action of shock therapy took place in the same areas that were stimulated or affected in the experimental and clinical studies. Thus Delay supposed that the effects of shock therapy corresponded to a stimulation of the diencephalic-hypophyseal centers (Delay 1953, p. 183).

This assumption aimed to be an explanation of the mode of action and efficacy of shock therapy for mental disorders. At the beginning of the 1940s, the numerous studies on shocks and their behavioral effects by Delay and his colleagues came to underscore the relevance of the diencephalon for psychiatry. The diencephalon became internationally recognized by several disciplines interested in brain function and emotional manifestations. This apparently successful focus on the diencephalon gave new hope to psychiatry in its pursuit of biological understanding of mental illness. It is thus not surprising to find multiple and lengthy passages devoted to the diencephalon in textbooks of psychiatry, neurology, and endocrinology published in the 1940s and the 1950s.

14.3 The Diencephalon: A Territory of Convergence

Although it is impossible and irrelevant to provide an exhaustive inventory of the research on the diencephalon and on emotion from the 1940s within the space of this chapter, it is important to draw attention to the main research areas that this part of the brain has motivated. Numerous studies published in Francophone, Anglophone, and Germanophone journals and handbooks, linked together mental pathology, somatic disorders, and diencephalic dysfunctions. Manic-depressive illness, schizophrenia, hysteria, catalepsy, but also Cushing syndrome or acromegalia are the pathologies that the psychiatrists, focusing on the diencephalon, were trying to better understand. The diencephalon was supposed to be implicated in all of these pathologies since almost all the patients suffering from one of them also showed disorders in their autonomic regulation (e.g., problems in regulating water and sugar metabolism, sleep disorders, sexual disorders, etc.). Dysfunction in the diencephalon could thus create both emotional and autonomic disorders. In this context, the borders between the psychic and the somatic symptoms were very fluid. The psychiatrists aimed to better understand their interconnections, guided by the view that the suffering subject must be understood as a whole system (Delay 1946a, 1946b, 1948; Ingram 1939; Morgan 1939; van Bogaert 1935).

The growing interest in the diencephalon is also linked with the rise of the psychosomatic current in the United States as well as in Europe (Weiss and Spurgeon 1943/1952). Published in 1939, the first issue of the journal *Psychosomatic Medicine* dedicated its first three articles to the diencephalon, imparting to this area of the brain the role of "psychosomatic relay," as Delay called it. In this particular context, an emphasis was put on case studies. Apart from experimentations on humans and animals, case studies were considered to be the best possibility to give new insights on the implication of the brain in the emergence of psychological and somatic disorders. If the number of cases presented in an article or a conference could vary between one and ten, some studies followed numerous cases during several years. Moreover, the same case was sometimes described in different journals (endocrinology, physiology, psychiatry, etc.). This permeability between the disciplines is particularly striking when looking at the bibliographies which follow the articles: the quoted references are never restricted to psychiatry. We can say that the diencephalon has become a "territory of convergence," a terrain attractive not only for psychiatry, which was one of the reasons why this area was so appealing for the followers of psychosomatic medicine.

14.4 Shock Therapy and Endocrinology

Other studies motivated by the interest in the diencephalon tried to relate potential mechanisms in the emergence of psychosis and the mode of action of shock therapy, thereby envisaging new therapeutic possibilities. Most of the studies which confer on the diencephalon the status of a common substrate of the emergence of psychosis, and thus the target of the shock therapy, are following Delay's research. It is interesting to analyze the minutes of the First International Congress of Psychiatry (*Comptes Rendus des séances du Premier Congrès Mondial de Psychiatrie*), which took place in Paris in 1950. During the congress, an Italian neuropsychiatrist, Ugo Cerletti, the creator of electroshock therapy, publicly acknowledged the role and influence of Delay in his own way of conceiving the action of electroshock. Indeed, Cerletti was convinced that his instrument specifically acted on the diencephalon. He also referred to his more recent research on "acroagonines," the substances supposed to appear just after the epileptic seizure triggered by the shock. After having injected this kind of substances—taken from pigs' brains—into the anxious patients, Cerletti observed a suppression of anxiety, sleep improvement, and a normalization of the weight (*Comptes Rendus des séances* 1952, vol. IV). He was convinced that further follow-up research was necessary in order to discover the composition of acroagonines, and to substitute them for electroshock. Cerletti's acroagonine research is proximate to the other studies, testing different substances on human behavior (sedatives, barbiturates, amphetamines, hormones, and alkaloids) carried out in the late 1940s. This kind of research interest reflects a new and henceforth relentless quest for "the" substance, effective in the treatment of mental disorders. Cerletti's effort was particularly interesting from a theoretical point of view because it was directly influenced by Delay's writings on the diencephalon and because it specifically aimed at creating a new biological psychiatric therapy, which could have a potential to restore the emotional and diencephalic imbalance in mental disorders.

The theories and empirical research on the diencephalic action of shock therapies were reinforced by the research on the endocrine system. Since the diencephalon is anatomically connected with the hypophysis, it was also considered as the main neuroendocrine "crossroad." In his research on stress, the Canadian endocrinologist Hans Selye showed that all the autonomic and psychic reactions related to the first stage of stress reaction ("alarm reaction") disappeared when the hypophysis or the entire diencephalon of animals was removed (Delay 1953; Selye 1956a, 1956b). Numerous studies tried then to compare the processes of shock therapies used in psychiatry with the stress processes described by Selye in order to detect a common site of action located in the diencephalon. Here, we find studies concerning the adrenocorticotropic hormone (ACTH) (Mote 1950): some major changes were observed in patients suffering from mental or somatic disorders who were treated with this hormone (Pincus and Hoagland 1950). Psychiatrists and physiologists then deduced that ACTH could potentially have similar therapeutic efficacy as electroshock, and several studies were carried out to compare both therapies (Delay et al. 1952, 1954). Although the relationship between psychiatry and endocrinology was only on an experimental level in the beginning of the 1950s, the attention it attracted can be well understood in the light of the potential benefits of a better comprehension of the complex interactions between the nervous and endocrine systems in regulation of behavior.

One might wonder how research on endocrine therapies in psychiatry or on "acroagonines" would have evolved if chlorpromazine was not introduced 2 years after the First International Congress of Psychiatry in 1950. Indeed, the interest for endocrinology will continue in the big field of neurotransmitters, the latter having modified the entire research approach in psychiatry. But it was not a coincidence that the endocrine therapies and the shock therapies were discussed at the same session of the International Congress. It obviously reflected the concerns of psychiatry on finding a drug with the same effects as biological shock therapy and a continuing interest in the diencephalon. Cerletti's work on acroagonines never materialized with an effective therapy and we can assume that the introduction of the new antipsychotics held back potential research on various substances.

14.5 Toward New Territories of Convergence

We have seen how the diencephalon, once "shared" by a part of the psychiatric community, has promoted the development of practices and encouraged new types of research. The experimental research as well as publications on this area were so prolific (Spiegel et al. 1951) that the implication of the effects of the diencephalon on mental disorders was qualified in 1950 with the terms such as "doctrine," "big current issue," or "the most successful current explanation for mental disorders" (Baruk 1955, p. 129). We can also see how the study of the diencephalon progressively fostered new hypotheses about the links between the brain and mental disorders. For example, the studies on lobotomy and its mode of action strengthened the idea that the diencephalon (and more precisely the thalamus) was included in a complex brain circuit, which regulated emotions (Yahn 1951). Most of the research carried out from the mid 1940s shared the idea that a brain area plays its particular role only in accordance with other structures of the brain. This conception will culminate with the great success of the limbic system theory (McLean 1949, 1955). But the main influence of the "diencephalic hypothesis" is on the first studies on chlorpromazine. It is indeed no coincidence that Delay, one of the biggest protagonists of the "diencephalic hypothesis," is today considered to be one of the "discoverers" of chlorpromazine. Without displaying the details of the first observations with chlorpromazine by the French surgeon Henri Laborit, and then by Delay and Deniker in psychiatry, it is important to understand that Delay and his colleagues were precisely trying to develop "a treatment which can act inversely to shock therapy" (1952b, p. 267). When reading the first reports from 1952, it explicitly appears that the interest in chlorpromazine is due to the fact that this substance probably acts on the same brain centers than electroshock, but provokes the opposite effect on the autonomic system. The diencephalon often appears in reports on chlorpromazine since it was assumed that chlorpromazine first acts on wake and sleep regulation inside the diencephalon. The research on this new treatment did not contradict previous assumptions on the diencephalon and shock therapy. Rather, the action of chlorpromazine and shock therapy were compared in order to better understand the stimulation or the resting that these therapies produced in the nervous system. In the articles published in psychiatry 10 years after the introduction of chlorpromazine, the issue about its action still remains open. Delay never ceased to repeat that psychoactive drugs modify the interactions between the cerebral cortex and the diencephalon.

We can thus talk about a "transition" of the "diencephalic hypothesis" of mental disorders: step by step and linked with the rise of the theories on neurotransmission, the diencephalon became partly "bereft" of its properties to the benefit of the limbic system. Eating and sexual behaviors, emotions, mood, sham rage, which were all previously attributed to the diencephalon, will in current retrospect pertain to the story of the "discovery" of the limbic system. In this new narrative, the structures of the diencephalon were partially integrated to the limbic system and still keep some of their originally described properties. However, we cannot say that the diencephalon gave way to the limbic system to explain the emotional process. Rather, from the mid 1950s, the roles of the different structures have been redistributed. Once this redistribution was completed, the influence of the diencephalon in psychiatry clearly decreased. However, one should not underestimate its influence on the first theories about the action of antipsychotic drugs. Actually, the theories on the diencephalon pertain both to the history of neurochemical hypotheses of mental disorders and to the history of the limbic system theories.

It is important to understand that if the diencephalon has been a neglected element in the history of psychiatry, this might be because it belongs to the construction of the history of a great number of medical disciplines and research fields: endocrinology, neurology, psychosurgery, psychosomatic medicine, behavioral disorders (manic depression, schizophrenia, Cushing's syndrome, hysteria among, etc.), shock therapy, neuroleptics, and the limbic system, to mention only some of them. Thus it is virtually impossible to delimit the distinctive features and the complexity of the roles of the diencephalon without taking a close look on these diverse histories and their influence on the development of biological psychiatry. Taking the diencephalon as a central theme allows us to rock the (too often) rigid narrative that states that psychiatry became scientific thanks to the discovery of neuroleptic drugs and to the development of neurochemical hypotheses on mental disorders. The aim is, on the one hand, to avoid the pitfall of a deceivingly simple chronology of the steps of the role ascribed to the diencephalon before the introduction of neuroleptics, and, on the other, to acknowledge that the narratives on the introduction of neuroleptics, constructed a posteriori, have contributed to masking the hypotheses on brain function proposed before the 1950s, and attempting to explain the development of mental disorders. This prior context that made the "discovery" of neuroleptics possible is indeed too often left out of these narratives. The theoretical work on the diencephalon shows, however, that numerous substances were experimented with before the 1950s in order to reveal the cerebral bases of behavioral disorders and to relieve these disorders by means of biological therapies.

If it is impossible to affirm that the first antipsychotic drugs were the most suitable substances to ease mental disorders, it remains, however, certain that these substances quite clearly contributed to the development of new hypotheses, which have considerably modified the landscape of biological psychiatry. Neither can it be said that there was a clean break between the anatomical and neurochemical models. The reading of the minutes of the *Colloque international sur la chlorpromazine et les médicaments neuroleptiques en thérapeutique psychiatrique* (International Congress on chlorpromazine and neuroleptic drugs), assembled in the journal *L'Encéphale* (1956), reveals that despite its promising effects on the behavior of a majority of the patients, antipsychotic drugs, as all the therapies that came before, did not allow a deeper understanding of the brain functioning of the individuals suffering from mental disorders. An entire session at this conference is dedicated to communications on the potential action modes of chlorpromazine, and here we find again at the center of the debate the diencephalic centers and the hypothalamo-hypophysary axis. Even if the meeting happened several years before the theories on chemical neurotransmission were accepted and contributed to the rise of new hypotheses on mental afflictions, already then one can perceive the first attempts to understand the effects of a chemical substance involved in neurotransmission. Serotonin, discovered to be present in the brain 2 years earlier, is mentioned on several occasions during the conference. Even though the "physiological role of this hormone remains unknown," it is assumed that the action of antipsychotic drugs "on the serotonin level in the brain is linked to its action on the psyche" (*Colloque international* 1956, p. 337). Moreover, the first studies on serotonin reveal its distinctive concentration in the middle of the diencephalon.

Therefore the question of the possible effect of chlorpromazine on serotonin circulation in this part of the brain is naturally addressed. At the *Congrès des Médecins Aliénistes et Neurologistes de France et des Pays de Langue Française* (*The Congress of Psychiatrists and Neurologists in France and the French speaking Countries*), in 1957, an entire session is devoted to the "New Chemotherapies in Psychiatry." Once more, it is striking to observe the extent to which the hypothalamus and the thalamus are present in the presentations. The introduction of chlorpromazine and other neuroleptic drugs induces a coexistence of a great number of theories focusing on the neuroendocrine system, the diencephalon, and the reticular formation, with the exception of some theories treating the cortex independently. This is the context from which the attempts to interpret the effects of the treatments on the substances progressively known as neurotransmitters emerge. In some discourses held at the time, like the one given by the North American psychiatrist, Winfred Overholser, at the International Conference on Chlorpromazine, one can note the desire to arrive at a better comprehension of the neurochemical nature of mental disorder:

> In the light of our knowledge of the psychic effects of the new drugs, would it be too extraordinary to think that some day, the psychoses called "functional" by lack of a better term, would be at least partially caused by endogenous chemical substances? They would affect the central nervous system; and we may even be able to establish the fact that the chemical antagonists having the function of therapeutic agents would be developed. There have been numerous swings of the pendulum concerning psychiatric treatment […]. It seems to me that the pendulum has yet another time oscillated towards the pharmacological era. This new era will bring psychiatry closer to the rest of the medical discipline and will make our patients more receptive to individual as well as group psychotherapy, and to other complementary therapies. It will increase our knowledge of brain functions, and more importantly, it will favor the return of our patients to health and to society. (*Colloque international* 1956, p. 319, author's translation)

14.6 The Posterity of the Diencephalon in Psychiatry

The diencephalon has undeniably played a role in the promotion of chlorpromazine. Therefore one can suppose that the theories on the diencephalon have contributed to the great changes influencing psychiatry between the mid 1950s and the end of the 1960s. Rather than mentioning "discoveries" and "revolutions" that would have disrupted a practice, until then characterized by "inefficient" and "inhuman" treatments (lobotomies, electric shocks, etc.), it is important to understand that the "new" biological psychiatry of the 1950s arrives in a gradual transition from two decades preceding the arrival of neuroleptics. As Jack Pressman, specialist in the history of psychiatry, emphasizes:

> The problem lies with the assumption that typically there exists a single "Eureka!" moment when a discovery bursts fully formed into a researcher's consciousness. More often, a researcher (or perhaps a scattered group of investigators) becomes

intrigued by an interesting set of experimental phenomena and begins to reshape available theories and definition to fit the unexpected results. The process is a continuing one, with new conceptions being shuffled and reshuffled among old ones until all the clunkers are discarded and a stable new framework survives. When a scientific community reaches consensus that a discovery has indeed occurred, after an interval of often considerable duration, its first action is to certify which experiments or ideas were the crucial stepping-stones that led to the current triumph. The lone surviving framework thus becomes a template with which to reorganize the prior scientific record into a coherent, rational tale of progress, a means of identifying which researches managed to get a piece of the puzzle "right". Such narratives of discovery, although edifying and ennobling, are an invitation to bad history. (Pressman 1998, p. 56)

If the diencephalon has virtually disappeared from the accounts of the "discovery" of neuroleptics, constructed a posteriori, the reason may be the need in the psychiatric community of promoting the idea of *a rupture with a less scientific past* and the belief in the beginning of a new era characterized by the use of "mind drugs." Once the transition was initiated, the diencephalon is less and less frequently mentioned for its role in emotional regulation, giving an advantage to theories with neurochemical explications to mental health problems and their origins.

In this context, the interest in brain structures, without totally disappearing, leaves room for studies on multiple networks and brain connections supposedly involved in emotional imbalance. However, it would be incorrect to think that the diencephalon has totally disappeared from the psychiatric landscape. Since the end of the twentieth century, the diencephalon is becoming again increasingly invested in psychiatric neurosciences: some abnormalities in the structures of the diencephalon, such as the thalamus and the hypothalamus, are indeed presumed to play a role in schizophrenia and borderline personality disorders. However, structural deficits, demonstrated by brain imaging techniques, ask for different interpretations by different prominent neuroscientists on their putative link to the manifest symptomatology of schizophrenia. Thus Bernhard Bogerts, reviewing the studies regarding the thalamus concludes that "clinical symptoms associated with dysfunction of the thalamus *resemble the negative symptoms of schizophrenia*" (1993, p. 433; italics added). In contrast, Nancy Andreasen seems to ascribe predominantly positive symptoms to the dysfunctional thalamus, with negative symptoms arising as coping mechanisms:

[The thalamus] plays a significant role in filtering, gating, processing, and relaying information. An abnormality in this structure could explain most of the psychopathology in schizophrenia [...] A person with a defective thalamus is likely to be flooded with information and overwhelmed with stimuli. That person may consequently experience the striking misperceptions that we refer to as delusions or hallucinations or may withdraw and retreat and display symptoms such as avolition. (Andreasen et al. 1994, pp. 296–297)

We can also note that a number of current studies recycle the theories developed in the era of the "diencephalic hypothesis": the interest is (indeed) still in the neurophysiology of the hypothalamo-hypophyseal axis as well as in the neuroendocrine interactions. This can be seen by the numerous publications and research projects aiming to understand if and how stress exposure is likely to increase the risk of developing mental illness (Ehlert et al. 2001; Scharnholz et al. 2014).

With the substantial development of psychiatric neurosciences, it appears as though we are assisting in an important proliferation of epistemic objects that are likely to raise interest in the field of psychiatry. Undeniably, the amygdale—which have been for some years the main focus in studies concerning the emergence of fear, area 25—a small structure highlighted by the American neurologist Helen Mayberg and considered having a major role in depression (Mayberg et al. 2005), or glutathione—an antioxidant supposedly deficient among schizophrenic subjects, all form a fertile ground for the development of hypotheses in the psychiatric neurosciences. The renewed interest in psychiatry for the diencephalon is perhaps the consequence of this increased number of epistemic objects and hence of a plurality of "levels of analysis" (see Turkheimer, Chapter 26, this volume), which makes possible a coexistence of studies focusing on brain structures and others on molecules or neuronal networks. In this context, one can suppose that the diencephalon and its connections with the rest of the brain could still be of increasing interest in the psychiatric neurosciences.

14.7 **Conclusion: A Recurrent Problematic?**

Mobilizing the psychiatric history of the diencephalon can be useful to foster a reflection on the current studies on brain structures, along with the increasing development of the psychiatric neurosciences. Until recently, the neurosciences were surely bringing hope that an understanding of the neurobiological and cerebral dysfunctions implicated in mental pathologies was "just around the corner," a view strongly entertained and publicized for the last 30 years. This optimism in neuroscientific progress, largely amplified and spread by the media, was hiding the historical truth that the hope of imminent understanding has always been with us. Psychiatry began to investigate the brain in the numerous ways available to it, long before the development of contemporary neurosciences. Despite the countless debates and controversies marking the history of psychiatry, its principal and dominant goal, which is to uncover the neurophysiological mechanisms of mental disorders, has never been a secret. Whether a biological reductionism is the only option, is another matter, beyond the scope of this chapter (see Parnas and P. Bovet, Chapter 23, this volume). At every step in this history, various neuroscientific targets, for example, "zones," "neurotransmitters," "molecules," "modules," or "brain circuits," crystallized and emblematized the reductive hopes and influenced psychiatry as a whole.

The currently dominant discourse in neuropsychiatry suggests that neuroimaging shows more and more precisely the anatomical and functional details of brain activity. However, we need an epistemological analysis in order to decide if one specific neurobiological hypothesis of mental disorders should be regarded as being more attractive than other hypotheses. Using the diencephalon as an historical example shows that the understanding of the cerebral bases of mental illness is characterized by a recurrent problem: the emphasis is invested on an area, a circuit, or a substance inside of the brain, in order to promote a new and unifying hypothesis for all endeavors to link brain and mental disorders. Extrapolating from the diencephalic story makes it impossible to predict how long certain areas of the brain or certain chemical molecules that are currently in vogue in science will continue to occupy the center stage. Looking at the theoretical work surrounding the diencephalon illustrates how this part of the brain was invested by diverse professionals in order to discover the biological bases of mental disorders. The diencephalic story also aims to facilitate a more general reflection on how the theories around brain dysfunctions responsible for mental disorders are successively generated and dismissed at a time when brain sciences increasingly invest the field of psychiatry. It is essential that students of science and technology analyze the development of psychiatric neurosciences with *a critical distance*, which may prevent the pitfalls of fascination or dismissal of brain sciences. In this regard, for example, a re-inscription of the advances of neurosciences in an already existing history would favor the elaboration of a constructive reflection. This would also encourage clinicians as well as researchers not to neglect the past that serves as a basis from which numerous new directions of research and questionings could and may emerge. Revisiting the history of psychiatry and its connections with brain research might put into perspective a certain type of naïve progressist discourse. Moreover it may instead stimulate a reflection upon the way certain efforts, made before the development of contemporary neurosciences, can be remobilized in order to fruitfully rethink the place of the clinic.

In 1987, the French psychiatrist Gladys Swain stressed the necessity to carry out a "historic analysis of the present," to make an effort to "treat the moment that we are living," and "to take *ourselves* as we take and treat any other moment of the past"; she adds later: "this program may appear quite evident. It is all but evident. History is always *the other* [...]. The historic gaze is painless the time it treats an almost dead matter and when it targets those who are no longer. When we apply it, it becomes surgical, and it hurts." (1987/1994, p. 265; italics added, author's translation). At present, rather than adopting a dogmatic reductionism or constructivism, without analyzing the contents of neuroscientific psychiatry, a constructive approach would be to continue the path proposed by Swain. This can be done, for example, by highlighting how the interests of actors from different disciplines converge toward the same scientific (epistemic) object, and how knowledge, theories, and practices are articulated within this particular object. To treat the present of psychiatric neurosciences as we would treat any other moment of the past would be a useful approach for the scientist trying to adopt a reflective position on how the brain sciences have reconfigured the field of psychiatry. In addition to highlighting the recurrence of certain issues which, in spite of the progress achieved in the study of the active brain, reflect the complexity of the etiology of mental disorders, such an approach would inspire a vital reflection on the connections between the clinical practice and the research in psychiatry.

References

Alpers, B. (1937). Relation of the hypothalamus to disorders of personality. Report of a case. *Archives of Neurology and Psychiatry*, 38(2), 291–303.

Alpers, B. (1940). Personality and emotional disorders associated with hypothalamic lesions. *Psychosomatic Medicine*, 2(3), 286–303.

Andreasen, N.C. (1997). The role of the thalamus in schizophrenia. *Canadian Journal of Psychiatry*, 42, 27–33.

Andreasen, N.C., Arndt, S., Swayze, V., et al. (1994). Thalamic abnormalities in schizophrenia visualized through magnetic resonance image averaging. *Science*, 266(5183), 294–298.

Bard, P. (1928). A diencephalic mechanism for the expression of rage with special reference to the sympathetic nervous system. *American Journal of Physiology*, 84(3), 490–515.

Bard, P. (1934). On emotional expression after decortication with some remarks on certain theoretical views. *The Psychological Review*, 41(4), 309–449.

Baruk, H. (1955). La thérapeutique en psychiatrie. In R. Leriche (ed.) *Somme de médecine contemporaine. La thérapeutique*, pp. 123–137. Monaco: Les Editions Médicales.

Beattie, J. (1932). Hypothalamic mechanisms. *The Canadian Medical Association Journal*, 26, 400–405.

Bogerts, B. (1993). Recent advances in the neuropathology of schizophrenia. *Schizophrenia Bulletin*, 19(2), 431–445.

Cannon, W. (1927). The James-Lange theory of emotions: a critical examination and an alternative theory. *The American Journal of Psychology*, 39 (1–4), 106–124.

Cannon, W. (1931). Again the James-Lange and the thalamic theories of emotion. *The Psychological Review*, 38 (4), 281–295.

Cerletti, U. (1950). Old and new information about electroshock. *American Journal of Psychiatry*, 107, 87–94.

Colloque international sur la chlorpromazine et les médicaments neuroleptiques en thérapeutique psychiatrique (Paris, October 20–22, 1955) (1956). *L'Encéphale*, 4.

Comptes Rendus des Congrès des Médecins Aliénistes et Neurologistes de France et des Pays de Langue Française, 1933 à 1955 (18 volumes). (1935–1957). Paris: Masson et Cie Editeurs

Comptes Rendus des séances du Premier Congrès Mondial de Psychiatrie, Paris, 1950. (1952). Volume IV. Thérapeutique biologique. Paris: Masson et Cie Editeurs.

Comptes Rendus du IVe Congrès Neurologique International, Paris, 1949. (1951). Paris: Masson et Cie Editeurs.

Cox, L.B. (1937). Tumors of the base of the brain: their relation to pathological sleep and other changes of the conscious state. *Medical Journal of Australia*, 24(1), 742–752.

Daston, L. (ed.) (2000). *Biographies of Scientific Objects*. Chicago, IL: The University of Chicago.

Delay, J. (1946a). *Les dérèglements de l'humeur*. Paris: Masson.

Delay, J. (1946b). *L'électro-choc et la psycho-physiologie*. Paris: Masson.

Delay, J. (1948). *La psycho-physiologie humaine*. Paris: PUF.

Delay, J. (1953). *Etudes de psychologie médicale*. Paris: PUF.

Delay, J., Bertagna, L., and Lauras, A. (1954). A.C.T.H. et cortisone en psychiatrie. *Annales médico-psychologiques*, 112(1), 536–541.

Delay, J., Deniker, P., and Harl, J.-M. (1952a). Utilisation en thérapeutique psychiatrique d'une phénothiazine d'action centrale élective (4560 RP). *Annales médico-psychologiques*, 110(2), 112–131.

Delay, J., Deniker, P., and Harl, J.-M. (1952b). Traitement des états d'excitation et d'agitation par une méthode médicamenteuse dérivée de l'hibernothérapie. *Annales médico-psychologiques*, 110(2), 267–273.

Delay, J., Deniker, P., Harl, J.-M., and Grasset, A. (1952). Traitement d'états confusionnels par le chlorhydrate de diméthylaminopropyl-N-chlorophénothiazine (4560 RP). *Annales Médico-psychologiques*, 110(3), 398–403.

Delay, J., Pichot, P., Perse, J., and Aubry, J,-L. (1952). Etude expérimentale des modifications psychologiques produites par les traitements à l'A.C.T.H. et la cortisone. *L'Encéphale*, 41, 393–406.

Ehlert, U., Gaab, J., and Heinrichs, M. (2001). Psychoneuroendocrinological contributions to the etiology of depression, posttraumatic stress disorder, and stress-related bodily disorders: the role of the hypothalamus–pituitary–adrenal axis. *Biological Psychiatry*, 57(1–3), 141–152.

Foerster, O. and Gagel, O. (1931). Ein Fall von sogennantem Gliom des Nervus opticus—Spongioblastoma multiforme ganglioides. *Zeitschrift für die gesamte Neurologie und Psychiatrie*, 136, 335–366.

Foerster, O. and Gagel, O. (1932). Ein Fall von Recklinghausenscher Krankheit mit fünf nebeinander bestehenden verschiedenartigen Tumorbildungen. *Zeitschrift für die gesamte Neurologie und Psychiatrie*, 138, 339–360.

Foerster, O. and Gagel, O. (1933). Ein Fall von Ependymcyste des III Ventrikels: ein Beitrag zur Frage der Beziehungen psychischer Störungen zum Hirnstamm. *Zeitschrift für die gesamte Neurologie und Psychiatrie*, 149, 312–344.

Fulton, J. (1947). *Physiologie du système nerveux (traduit de l'anglais par Camille Chatagnon)*. Paris: Vigot Frères.

Fulton, J. and Bailey, P. (1929). Contribution to the study of tumors in the region of the third ventricle. *Journal of Nervous and Mental Diseases*, 69, 1–25, 145–164, 261–277.

Grinker R. (1938). A method for studying and influencing cortico-hypothalamic relations. *Science*, 87(2247), 73–74.

Grinker, R. (1939). Hypothalamic functions in psychosomatic interrelations. *Psychosomatic Medicine*, 1(1), 19–47.

Grinker, R. and Serota, H. (1938). Studies on corticohypothalamic relations in the cat and man. *Journal of neurophysiology*, 1, 573–589.

Hess, W.R. (1949). *Das Zwischenhirn. Syndrome, Lokalisationen, Funktionen.* Basel: Benno Scwabe & Co.

Ingram, W.R. (1939). The hypothalamus: a review of the experimental data. *Psychosomatic Medicine*, 1(1), 48–91.

Jelliffe, S.E. (1927). The mental picture in schizophrenia and in epidemic encephalitis; their alliances, differences and a point of view. *American Journal of Psychiatry*, 83, 413–465.

Karplus, J. and Kreidl, A. (1909). Gehirn und Sympathicus. I. Zwischenhirnbasis und Halssympathicus. *Pflügers Archiv für die gesamte Physiologie des Menschen und der Tiere*, 129, 138–144.

Karplus, J. and Kreidl, A. (1910). Gehirn und Sympathicus. II. Ein Sympathicuszentrum im Zwischenhirn. *Pflügers Archiv für die gesamte Physiologie des Menschen und der Tiere*, 135, 401–416.

Karplus, J. and Kreidl, A. (1912). Gehirn und Sympathicus. III. Sympathicusleitung im Gehirn und Halsmark. *Pflügers Archiv für die gesamte Physiologie des Menschen und der Tiere*, 143, 109–127.

Lempérière, T. (2004). Histoire de la neuropsychiatrie. *Annales Médico Psychologiques*, 162, 39–49.

Mayberg, H., Lozano, A.-M., Voon, V. et al. (2005). Deep brain stimulation for treatment-resistant depression. *Neuron*, 45(5), 651–660.

McLean, P. (1949). Psychosomatic disease and the "visceral brain". Recent developments bearing on the Papez theory of emotions. *Psychosomatic Medicine*, 11(6), 338–353.

McLean, P. (1955). The limbic system ("visceral brain") in relation to central gray and reticulum of the brain stem. Evidence of interdependence in emotional processes. *Psychosomatic Medicine*, 18(5), 355–366.

Morgan, L.O. (1939). Alterations in the hypothalamus in mental deficiency. *Psychosomatic Medicine*, 1(4), 496–507.

Mote, J. (ed.) (1950). *Proceedings of the First Clinical ACTH Conference*. Philadelphia, PA: The Blakiston Co.

Pincus, G. and Hoagland, H. (1950). Adrenal cortical responses to stress in normal men and in those with personality disorders. *American Journal of Psychiatry*, 106(9), 641–650.

Pressman, J. (1998). *Last Resort. Psychosurgery and the Limits of Medicine*. Cambridge: Cambridge University Press.

Ranson S. and Magoun, H. (1939). The hypothalamus. *Ergebnisse der Physiologie, Biologischen Chemie und Experimentellen Pharmakologie*, 41, 56–163.

Rheinberger, H.-J. (1997). *Toward a History of Epistemic Things. Synthesizing Proteins in the Test Tube*. Stanford, CA: Stanford University.

Scharnholz, B., Gilles, M., Marzina, A., et al. (2014). Do depressed patients without activation of the hypothalamus–pituitary–adrenal (HPA) system have metabolic disturbances? *Psychoneuroendocrinology*, 39, 104–110.

Selye, H. (1956a). Stress and psychiatry. *American Journal of Psychiatry*, 113, 423–427.

Selye, H. (1956b). *The Stress of Life*. New York: McGraw Hill.

Spiegel, E., Wycis, H., Freed, H., and Orchinik, C. (1951). The central mechanism of the emotions (experiences with circumscribed thalamic lesions). *American Journal of Psychiatry*, 108, 426–432.

Steck, H. (1927). Contribution à l'étude des séquelles psychiques de l'Encéphalite léthargique (les formes délirantes et hallucinations). *Schweizer Archiv für Neurologie und Psychiatrie*, 21, 214–237.

Swain, G. (1987). Chimie, cerveau, esprit et société. Paradoxes épistémologiques des psychotropes en médecine mentale. *Le Débat*, 47, 172–183. (Published in G. Swain, (1994), *Dialogue avec l'insensé*. Paris: Gallimard.)

Van Bogaert, L. (1935). L'hystérie et les fonctions diencéphaliques. *Comptes Rendus des Congrès des Médecins Aliénistes et Neurologistes de France et des Pays de Langue Française*, 39, 169–229.

Von Economo, C. (1930). Sleep as a problem of localization. *The Journal of Nervous and Mental Disease*, 71(3), 1–5.

Weiss, E. and Spurgeon, O. (1943/1952). *Médecine psychosomatique. L'application de la psychopathologie aux problèmes cliniques de la médecine générale*. Paris: Delachaux & Niestlé.

Yahn, M. (1951). Le mode d'action de la leucotomie cérébrale (note sur la relation entre le physique et le psychique). *Annales Médico-psychologiques*, 112(2), 737–744.

Zondek, H. (1938). *Les affections des glandes endocrines (traduit de l'allemand par Marcel Filderman)*. Paris: Librairie Maloine.

Chapter 15

Some reflections on historiographic strategies for the neurosciences

Eric J. Engstrom

15.1 Historical (Dis)continuities

Emilie Bovet is right to insist that we pay greater attention to historical continuities and to question whether the so-called psychopharmaceutical "revolution" of the 1950s was as radically new and transformative as some observers contend. No doubt the retrospective construction of historical discontinuities can be put to effective use in decontextualizing historical origins and thereby imbuing those origins with an aura of timelessness, separate from and hence unsullied by a "less scientific past."

To avoid such "reductive simplifications" and "naïve" notions of scientific progress, Bovet proposes an alternative approach that uses the epistemic object of the diencephalon in order to explore certain recurrent themes within the history of biological psychiatry. Most prominently, Bovet argues that—to varying degrees throughout the twentieth century—the diencephalon has been mobilized in order to sustain the hopes of uncovering the neurophysiological foundations of mental disorders. She argues that by focusing our historical attention on the diencephalon and how it was invested with meaning and significance, we can trace the efforts of diverse professional actors in sustaining hopes of overcoming the divide between body and mind. By interpreting the diencephalon as the embodiment of these hopes, Bovet constructs lines of historical continuity that span the endeavors of researchers across the entire twentieth century.

15.2 Proleptic Rhetoric

Among other things, this observation points to an important characteristic of discourse within the medical sciences. It reminds us of how researchers often trade in the promise that scientific progress will bring ever better cures for our ailments, that is to say, how they deploy a distinctly anticipatory or "proleptic" rhetoric. In perpetually holding out the prospect of more effective future treatments, this rhetoric serves as an important motor for much of the discourse, to say nothing of its role in the distribution of resources within medical science. Other scholars have noted how this proleptic rhetoric tends to be sustained by successive waves of new technologies and instruments that have generated fascinating new images and invasive possibilities (microscope, electroencephalography, magnetic resonance imaging, etc.) (Hagner and Borck 1999). For Bovet, however, it is not so much technological innovation per se, but rather researchers shifting investments in the diencephalon that shape the proleptic rhetoric. Studying the diencephalon is revealing for what it illustrates about how the as-yet—and by now one must say chronically—unfulfilled promise of overcoming the division of mind and body has evolved.

15.3 Historiographic Interdisciplinarity

Contemporary neurosciences are no doubt heavily invested in this promise (Kandel and Squire 2000). Beyond that, however, they also understand themselves as being integrative, multidisciplinary endeavors. One of their hallmarks, it would seem, is disciplinary permeability and, conversely, a professional-political agenda of transcending disciplinary overspecialization. Put succinctly, the neurosciences themselves are in some sense constituted as territories of convergence. And so it strikes me that in construing the diencephalon as a "territory of convergence," Bovet is somehow instantiating the notion of transdisciplinary openness that characterizes the contemporary neurosciences. Just as the neurosciences understand themselves as territories of convergence, so Bovet interprets the diencephalon as a "territory of convergence." And along similar lines, the critique of the history of psychiatry as being not sufficiently interdisciplinary (i.e., too discipline bound) to account for the diencephalon, and hence needing a much broader historiographic perspective, seems likewise to adopt this integrative and doubtless very productive dogma of the neurosciences. And so in Bovet's analysis, (1) the neurosciences, (2) the diencephalon, and (3) psychiatric historiography itself have all been conceptualized as "territories of convergence."

Given such interpretive overlap, it is worth asking what the costs might be of pursuing a historiographic strategy that, in choosing to focus on the diencephalon as an "epistemic object," privileges interdisciplinary perspectives to the detriment of other—and especially disciplinary—ones. Attempting to transcend the limitations of overspecialization may be desirable in the interests of more effective contemporary neuroscientific research, but does that necessarily translate into a productive historiographic strategy? For choosing *not* to focus on disciplinary specificity seems not just to prefigure the outcome of the diencephalon as a "territory of convergence," but also to exclude evidence that might point toward territorial divergence. In other words, emphasizing the "circulation of knowledge" beyond psychiatry runs the risk of concealing or ignoring very real blockages, conflicts, and resistances. While Bovet emphasizes the expansive realm that the diencephalon draws together and incorporates, nothing is said about what it excludes, obviates, or displaces. What theories, practices, diagnoses, disciplines, and therapies *couldn't* be brought under the umbrella of the diencephalon? And what alternative "circulation of knowledge" and "constellation of interests" did it displace? It seems that only when our narratives are sufficiently robust to accommodate not just the convergences, but also these displacements will we be able to assess the fuller historical meaning and significance of the diencephalon.

References

Hagner, M. and Borck, C. (1999). Brave neuro-worlds. *Neue Rundschau*, 110(3), 70–88.

Kandel, E.R. and Squire, L.R. (2000). Neuroscience: breaking down scientific barriers to the study of brain and mind. *Science*, 290, 1113–1120.

Section 6
The history of psychiatry as interdisciplinary history

Chapter 16

Introduction to "On attitudes toward philosophy and psychology in German psychiatry, 1867–1917"

Kenneth S. Kendler

I seek here to illustrate continuity in the issues Engstrom illustrates in Chapter 17 about the career of Kraepelin in the late nineteenth century (with some attention also to that of Ziehen) and those that currently confront psychiatry early in the twenty-first century. In particular, I want to contextualize this chapter within the framework of what is arguably the most central of historical debates within psychiatry—the degree to which we view ourselves as a medical specialty focused on the brain versus on the mind. One of the several critical consequences of the position adopted on this question is how we relate to our colleagues in neurology/neuroscience on the one hand and psychology on the other. I began my psychiatric training in 1977 in a department famous for its psychoanalytic orientation but which was then in the process of moving rapidly into the world of biological psychiatry. As a resident, I was exposed to these competing paradigms having supervisors from both camps. Interestingly, no one then seemed very interested in teaching us about how a mind-based and brain-based view on psychiatric illness might coexist, and even (one might hope) cross-fertilize. Rather, the goals of my supervisors seemed mostly to "convert" me into their camp.

Certainly, the star of biological psychiatry was rising, fueled by the success, as shown in an influential series of double-blind controlled studies, of antipsychotic and antidepressant drugs and lithium. Equally important was the rising influence of neuroscience, in those ancient days restricted largely to the classical monoamine neurotransmitters: dopamine, serotonin, and norepinephrine. The ascendance of biological psychiatry at that time had another important ally. Psychoanalysts had in general derided psychiatric diagnosis as focusing only on "surface" phenomenon, while the real action was occurring at the level of dynamic intrapsychic processes. Starting first with the Washington University St. Louis school of psychiatry and their Feighner criteria (Feighner et al. 1972; Kendler et al. 2010), descriptive psychiatry—using "objective" operationalized criteria—made an increasingly vigorous come back in the United States that eventually produced, first, the Research Diagnostic Criteria (Spitzer et al. 1975) and then, DSM-III

(American Psychiatric Association 1980). The hero of this movement was Emil Kraepelin; and this group of biologically-oriented descriptive psychiatrists was proud to call themselves "neo-Kraepelinians" (Compton and Guze 1995). During this era, biological and descriptive psychiatry were allies seeking, together, to move psychiatry away from psychoanalytic dominance and toward a biological/descriptive brand of psychiatric research and practice.

In this insightful and wide-ranging chapter, the psychiatric historian, Engstrom, sheds light on the early phases of Kraepelin's career and reveals that the historical reality of this important figure is out of keeping with his reconstruction as the forerunner of modern biological psychiatry. As he writes, "Kraepelin was not the man he has become in our eyes." Ironically, as Engstrom relates, Kraepelin was himself reacting against an earlier phase of biological psychiatry in which the dominant paradigm was neuropathology. This movement was led by figures like Meynert and Wernike who developed highly speculative brain-based accounts of psychiatric illness that were overzealous in far outstripping what the science really then had to offer. We learn from Engstrom's essay that Kraepelin saw that not all the answers to psychiatric questions could come from brain-based perspectives. He writes, "Kraepelin was trying both to distance himself from research in pathological anatomy and to rehabilitate a psychological dimension to psychiatric research." Contrary to our current views of him as an "arch-neuropsychiatrist," Kraepelin was an advocate for the application of the then young science of psychology—lead by his former mentor, Wundt—to the problems of diagnosis and etiology of psychiatric illness. In the first flush of this young science, there was an excitement that "scientific psychology" could make advances where neuropathology had failed.

Future historians might profitably examine the similarities and differences between the time frames in the history of psychiatry that Engstrom examines here: the latter third of the nineteenth century and the latter third of the twentieth century. As Michels reviews elsewhere in this volume (see Chapter 20), the rise of the biological psychiatric paradigm in the last three decades of the twentieth century was related to declining influences of the psychoanalytic paradigm, which turned away from biomedical models toward more hermeneutic pursuits.

Interestingly, Engstrom notes that "Kraepelin criticized those brain researchers who had blazed a trail into neuropathology, but who had never found their way back to psychiatry." Exactly the same process is at work now with most neuroscientists actively pursuing the causes of psychiatric illness. Many have little training or interest in psychopathology. They see their job as finding basic molecular, cellular, or network processes that underlie psychiatric illness. The idea that they need to follow these "causes" back up into the mind–brain system to determine how they actually result in the symptoms of illness is rarely a concern (but see Kapur (2003), Mellor (1970), and Adams et al. (2013) for important exceptions).

Two recent examples illustrate efforts of the dominant descriptive-biological paradigm within American psychiatry to take up Kraepelin's task of explicitly trying to add psychological dimensions to psychiatric research. The ten personality disorders included in DSM-III (American Psychiatric Association 1980) were widely recognized to be an arbitrary list derived from a range of clinical traditions rather than from any systematic theoretical viewpoint. In discussions leading up to the revision of DSM-5, one focus was on revamping these personality disorder categories so as to map them onto the "Big Five" personality dimensions (Costa and Widiger 2002), long a favorite of many scholars in personality psychology. For a number of complex reasons, this effort failed. Moving from the world of psychiatric nosology to that of academic personality psychology was, at least at this first iteration, a bridge too far. On a more favorable note, a major research initiative of the US National Institutes of Mental Health has been the Research Domain Criteria (RDoC) that has been suggested as a focus of psychiatric research and might eventually replace DSM diagnostic categories. While RDoC has a complex genealogy, many of its central constructs derive from academic psychology including such key constructs as "attention," "arousal," "working memory," and "reward learning" (Cuthbert and Insel 2013).

So the reader of this chapter should have a keen sense of the irony regarding the historical transformation of the figure of Kraepelin. What this can teach us about the field of psychiatry is worth pondering. Kraepelin started as a pluralistic thinker who sought to expand the narrow confines of organic nineteenth-century neuropsychiatry with the exciting developments of the then young mind-based science of academic psychology. One hundred years later, he became the symbol of a narrowing of the focus of psychiatry toward a more biological direction. This narrowing turned the focus not back to neuropathology, but instead toward neurochemistry and psychopharmacology, and away from a different mind-based vision of the field—that of psychoanalytic psychiatry.

References

Adams, R.A., Stephan, K.E., Brown, H.R., Frith, C.D., and Friston, K.J. (2013). The computational anatomy of psychosis. *Frontiers in Psychiatry*, 4, 47.

American Psychiatric Association (1980). *Diagnostic and Statistical Manual of Mental Disorders* (3rd ed.). Washington, DC: American Psychiatric Association.

Compton, W.M. and Guze, S.B. (1995). The neo-Kraepelinian revolution in psychiatric diagnosis. *European Archives of Psychiatry and Clinical Neuroscience*, 245(4–5), 196–201.

Costa, P.T. and Widiger, T.A. (2002). *Personality Disorders and the Five-Factor Model of Personality* (2nd ed.). Washington, DC: American Psychological Association.

Cuthbert, B.N. and Insel, T.R. (2013). Toward the future of psychiatric diagnosis: the seven pillars of RDoC. *BMC Medicine*, 11, 126.

Feighner, J.P., Robins, E., Guze, S.B., Woodruff, R.A., Jr., Winokur, G., and Munoz, R. (1972). Diagnostic criteria for use in psychiatric research. *Archives of General Psychiatry*, 26(1), 57–63.

Kapur, S. (2003). Psychosis as a state of aberrant salience: a framework linking biology, phenomenology, and pharmacology in schizophrenia. *American Journal of Psychiatry*, 160(1), 13–23.

Kendler, K.S., Munoz, R.A., and Murphy, G. (2010). The development of the Feighner criteria: an historical perspective. *American Journal of Psychiatry*, 167(2), 134–142.

Mellor, C.S. (1970). First rank symptoms of schizophrenia. I. The frequency in schizophrenics on admission to hospital. II. Differences between individual first rank symptoms. *British Journal of Psychiatry*, 117(536), 15–23.

Spitzer, R.L., Endicott, J., and Robins, E. (1975). *Research Diagnostic Criteria for a Selected Group of Functional Disorders* (2nd ed.). New York: New York Psychiatric Institute.

Chapter 17

On attitudes toward philosophy and psychology in German psychiatry, 1867–1917

Eric J. Engstrom

> The hypothetical and changing character of fundamental psychiatric assumptions as well as the uncertainties that plague diagnoses based on systemic preconditions usually remain invisible to psychiatric practitioners. They become visible as soon as other sciences, that either ignore tacitly accepted professional conventions or deem them irrelevant, question psychopathological facts according to *their* rules.
>
> (Janzarik 1972, p. 588)

17.1 Introduction

Historians usually draw a distinction between phenomena that transpired at an earlier time (the past) and our record of those phenomena (history). Whereas the past confronts us with an ultimately unfathomable continuum of events and experiences, history involves our attempts to interpret and make sense of the residual traces of those events and experiences. And so to ask about the nature of historical change is to ask about how our record, our representation of the past has changed, and in particular how the narrative conventions we use to describe and interpret the past have evolved over time. The study of the shifting narrative conventions that historians use in studying the past is the task of historiography.

In the case of psychiatric historiography, there have been two especially prominent and influential narrative conventions that have dominated much historical research. The first, so-called Whiggish convention tells a story of psychiatry progressing mainly by force of its own dynamics and internal logics toward more salubrious resolutions of our experiences with mental anguish. This story is often cast in terms of the rise of a biomedical model of psychiatric illness and the falling away of older—and putatively benighted—religious or moral cultures that heretofore enveloped the phenomena of madness. In response to (and as a critique of) this general plot line, a second narrative convention has instead attributed much of the development in psychiatry to larger social, political, and economic forces. By these revisionist accounts, psychiatry's development was driven not so much by rational scientific discourse or empirically grounded evidence, but rather by "external" agendas that ultimately influenced the path taken by psychiatric science and that sometimes compromised its integrity.

Both of these narrative traditions have provided important perspectives on psychiatry's past and given us the interpretive wherewithal to explain the winding and contingent pathways it traversed from the mid nineteenth century to the present. But in tandem, their implicit internalist/externalist duality and their juxtaposition of "science" and "society" also manifest the very real interpretive limitations of both narratives. Revisionist historians interested in the coercive marginalization of the mad in the interests of social cohesion, public security, or economic rationalization are rarely attuned to shifts in conceptual understandings or to research perspectives brought on by technological innovations or institutional practices. And by the same token, Whiggish historians too often underestimate the cultural assumptions and social conditions of possibility that can underpin the truth-claims of psychiatric science.

One strategy for escaping the limitations of these competing narrative conventions involves shifting our attention away from both the minutiae of scientific research as well as the amorphous sweep of social forces and instead refocusing our attention on the psychiatric profession itself. As a profession, psychiatry can be understood as an intermediate site of governance, responsible in part for (among other things) setting standards of practice, adjudicating disputes, allocating resources and funding, reinforcing divisions of labor, and organizing disciplinary loyalties. At the same time, however, it is also an actor in a larger ecology of interest groups, including other professions, state regulators, corporate interests, and patient advocacy groups. Studying these and other aspects of the profession's structures and ecologies provides historians with a useful platform from which to link downward into the "internalist" dynamics that engage psychiatric researchers and practitioners, as well as upward into broader sociocultural forces that can impinge or expand the horizons of psychiatric practice. At this meso-level of analysis, between "science" and "society," it becomes easier to craft more plausible histories that incorporate both internalist and externalist perspectives (vectors) and that bridge the divide between Whiggish and revisionist narratives.

Certainly one of the challenges facing any study of the psychiatric profession involves how to interpret psychiatry's relationships with other regimes of knowledge and practice. Indeed, one common refrain trumpeted in a good portion of the contemporary literature is that narrow (and narrow-minded) disciplinary perspectives need to be overcome and that histories of psychiatry must instead be rewritten in ways that accommodate broader transdisciplinary exchange. For many reasons, it has become *au courant* to discount the history of disciplines or professions as being inherently deficient and incapable of accommodating the fuller diversity of past phenomenon. And indeed, historians of psychiatry have not generally written their histories in relational terms, as examinations of psychiatry's evolving interactions with its professional neighbors and other interest groups.

In this chapter I therefore intend to sketch out a relational or interdisciplinary history of psychiatry. I will examine in particular its interface with philosophy and psychology in late nineteenth-century Germany. I will begin by briefly considering the crisis afflicting mid-nineteenth-century philosophy and then draw on the work of several protagonists (Wilhelm Wundt, Emil Kraepelin, and Theodor Ziehen) to explore how that crisis influenced psychiatry. I will be asking how contemporaries interpreted the relationship between psychiatry and philosophy, exploring some of the exchanges that transpired across their disciplinary threshold, and hopefully illustrating how those exchanges contributed to some nontrivial historical developments. In particular, I will be arguing that much of Emil Kraepelin's early research encountered a well-entrenched, antimetaphysical bias within his profession and that that research involved deploying experimental methods used in the neighboring fields of philosophy and psychology in order to introduce psychological dimensions into the overwhelmingly neuropsychiatric research paradigms of his day.

17.2 Philosophy's Crisis of Identity after 1833

In his landmark study of the history of nineteenth- and early twentieth-century philosophy in Germany, Herbert Schnädelbach (1983, p. 88) argued that by the mid nineteenth century philosophical impulses and arguments were exerting ever less influence over scientific discourse and idealistic philosophy was losing its "monopoly over definitions of what constituted science." As never before, industrialization was reinforcing the important influence of science and technology as productive societal and economic forces—that were increasingly molding the lives of citizens throughout Germany and Europe. Concepts such as specialization, mechanization, materialism, progress, and objectivity characterized fundamental structural (and functional) shifts in mid-nineteenth-century science. Scientific developments were evolving in leaps and bounds and contributed decisively to a growing "belief in the pervasive authority and normative power of science," that is, in a kind of scientism that seemed to make philosophy appear not just "impotent and irrelevant," but also plunged it into a "crisis of identity." According to Schnädelbach, this crisis of identity went hand in hand with an "exclusion of metaphysics" (*Ausgrenzung der Metaphysik*), especially in the natural sciences.

In Germany, this crisis of identity manifested itself across a variety of psychiatric domains: in the acrimonious disputes between so-called mentalists and somaticists (Kutzer 2003); in critiques of older, deductive "systems" and "schemata" and the insistence on new, inductive, and empirically open scientific research; in the theoretical abstinence and pragmatic orientation of the profession's premiere journal, the *Allgemeine Zeitschrift für Psychiatrie* (Engstrom 2003a, pp. 37–38); in the displacement of psychological themes by neuropathological ones at professional meetings (Schmiedebach 1986, p. 158); and in the shift away from metaphysical notions of the soul toward Griesinger's concepts of "mental tone" (*psychischen Tonus*) and "individual psychology" (*Ich-Psychologie*).

Over a relatively short span of time in the mid nineteenth century, the "exclusion of metaphysics" manifested in these trends became deeply ingrained in the consciousness and memory of psychiatric professionals, indeed it became dogma for entire generations of psychiatric practitioners (Kraepelin 1918; Birnbaum 1928). Taking stock of the historical development of his profession in the 1920s, the Berlin psychiatrist Theodor Ziehen (1927) described early nineteenth-century philosophy's "strange proximity" and its "dominant influence over psychiatry," only then to juxtapose it to subsequent decades in which psychiatrists had come to reduce philosophical problems "to a minimum" and "assiduously avoid epistemological arguments and conclusions." Ziehen hailed this philosophical abstinence as a thoroughly positive development: without a doubt, the exclusion of philosophy had only served to promote scientific progress in psychiatry. It had paved the way for a new era of neuropsychiatry.

With hindsight, historians have written about this period (glowingly) as the dawn of the first era of biological psychiatry (Shorter 1997, pp. 69–112), as well as (more skeptically) the "triumph of somatic positivism" (Schmiedebach 1986, p. 241). But what they have often overlooked is that psychiatric practitioners were not only looking to neuroanatomy and neurophysiology to explain their patients' illnesses. Indeed from the very outset, some clinical skeptics had insisted that alienists had already "dissected and rummaged around in enough psychiatric cadavers" (Kahlbaum 1863, p. 60); and indeed the somatocerebral convictions of many neuropsychiatrists would ultimately come to be denounced as "brain mythology" (Gruhle 1932, pp. 17–18; Kraepelin 1887, pp. 7–12). Not least because of this skepticism and increasingly from the 1880s—as the therapeutic breakthroughs of neuropathological research kept not materializing—many practitioners also looked outward to "scientific psychology" in search of answers to the challenges facing their post-metaphysical science.

That psychiatrists never completely abandoned philosophy can be seen in debates in the 1870s about Wilhelm Griesinger's legacy (Engstrom 2003a, pp. 51–87; Sammet 1997; Verwey 2004). Soon after Griesinger's premature death in 1868, he too fell victim to efforts to banish philosophy from psychiatry and his work was attacked for its "strongly aprioristic and speculative" approach (Westphal 1868, p. 766). In his defense, Griesinger's advocates argued that most of the progress that he had brought to psychiatry transpired "not in spite of his philosophical tendencies, but because of them" and that it was really only thanks to Griesinger that a "theory of psychological action" ("*Theorie des psychologischen Geschehens*") had been introduced into medicine (Lazarus 1868, p. 776). By this account, it had not been philosophy per se, but rather the "raw, common, unscientific empiricism" of early nineteenth-century romantic psychiatry and alienists like J.C.A. Heinroth that, for decades, had "hobbled and obstructed" psychiatry's development. Remarkably and contrary to much historiographic literature, at the end of the 1860s, some of Griesinger's most dedicated supporters placed their hopes for the future of psychiatry neither in clinical empiricism, nor in neuropathology, but rather in the psychological implications of Gustav Fechner's *Elements of Psychophsics* (Heidelberger 2004; Robinson 2010; Schnädelbach 1983, pp. 101–102).

17.3 The "New Psychology" and the Psychiatric Legacy of Wilhelm Wundt

In the minds of many contemporaries, philosophy's identity crisis would be overcome by turning to scientism and psychologism, that is, by transforming philosophy into a natural science and installing psychology as its lodestar. In this vein, a fair number of philosopher-psychologists sought to either save or inherit philosophy's traditional place as the "queen of the sciences." They envisioned psychology as a "natural science of the mind" (*geistige Naturwissenschaft*) and above all as an "integrative science" (*Integrationswissenschaft*) that might bridge the widening gap between the natural sciences and the humanities (*Geisteswissenschaften*) (Leibbrand and Wettley 1961/2005, pp. 567-70; Schnädelbach 1983, pp. 96-97, 125).

A prominent example of this new, empirically oriented psychology was the Marburg neo-Kantian Friedrich Albert Lange, whose *History of Materialism* (1866) attempted to ground Kantian epistemology on psychophysiological foundations (Mayerhofer and Vanecek 2007). Lange's "psychology without the soul" jettisoned both Heglian idealism and the philosophical psychology of Johann Herbart, replacing them with a so-called somatic method to study the laws of mental process and to account for their organic and physiological foundations (Teo 2002). Powerfully influenced by Gustav Fechner's psychophysics and admired by Wilhelm Wundt, Lange's experimental method and psychophysical parallelism inspired a generation of budding philosophers qua psychologists in the 1860s and 70s (Green 2009; Guillin 2004; Huemer and Landerer 2010).

Recently, Mitchell Ash (2005) has summarized concisely several of the features that united the proponents of this new psychology: (1) their scientific reputations rested on what Lorraine Daston has called "instrumental rationality"; (2) in their writings they drew on physiological analogies and metaphors (machines, organisms, psychical energy) to describe mental processes; (3) they tended to abstain or at least remain vague about the relationship between body and mind and adopt a stance of psychophysical parallelism; (4) they used methods described as "experimental"; and (5) they tended to restrict their subject matter to objects and fields that could be examined using natural scientific methods and instruments such as psychophysics, sensory psychology, attention span, and retention/memory.

No doubt Germany's most prominent representative of this new psychology was Wilhelm Wundt (1832-1920), who by the late 1870s was perhaps the most influential experimental psychologist in the world (Araujo 2012; Hatfield 1997; Wong 2009). His reputation was based on his book *Principles of Physiological Psychology* (1874). Wundt had finished writing that book in Zurich, where he had succeeded Albert Lange in the chair for inductive philosophy and from where he would soon depart to take up a position in Leipzig (Ziche 2008). Wundt's treatise applied the mathematics of Gustav Fechner's psychophysics to neurophysiology: by quantifying and computing sensations, Wundt believed that he could mathematically describe conscious mental representations and processes.

In countless experiments conducted in his laboratory in Leipzig, Wundt was guided by the basic "empirical hypothesis" of psychophysical parallelism: "Just as body and soul (*Leibliches und Seelisches*) run parallel to each other, so too should the laws that govern them" (Schneider 1990, p. 57; Weygandt 1901; Wundt 1894). As Mai Wegener (2009) has emphasized, psychophysical parallelism was a strategy used by Wundt (and many others) in distancing himself from natural philosophy, and especially from notions involving an "organ of the soul" and its implicit assumption of a causal linkage (*Wechselwirkung*) between body and soul.

Wundt was wary about using experimental methods to study mental illness, as his scathing critique of contemporary discourse on hypnotism illustrates. He rejected categorically any notion of a subconscious or double consciousness—be it within the individual or within larger collective social groups (Gödde 1999; Nicholls and Liebscher 2010). From at least 1874, he treated everything outside of consciousness in physiological terms (Araujo 2012, p. 4). Accordingly, Wundt described French debates on hypnotism as "part phantasy, part dilettantish hypnotism-cult" that was mistakenly being identified with "experimental psychology" (Peiffer 2004, p. 728). For Wundt, hypnotism belonged not in the "laboratory of the psychologist, but rather on the hospital ward"; it was of no fundamental significance to experimental psychology: "Hypnotic sleep was like any other abnormal condition. It was just as inappropriate to base all of psychology on hypnotism, as it was to base it on dreams, mania or paralytic dementia" (Wundt 1911, p. 18). And so Wundt's own understanding of the domain of experimental psychology's applicability clearly stopped well short of the gates to psychiatry.

But others were far less reserved in applying the new psychology in psychiatric contexts. Far more so than historians have generally appreciated, Wundt's experimental psychology had a marked impact on psychiatric research in Germany at the end of the nineteenth century and numerous psychiatrists began conducting research in experimental psychology, among others Robert Sommer, Friedrich Jolly, Otto Binswanger, Wilhelm Weygandt, Theodor Ziehen, and Emil Kraepelin. Reflecting in hindsight on its impact, Oswald Bumke remarked that younger psychiatrists could hardly imagine the enormous hope that psychiatrists had placed in it. According to Bumke, natural scientific psychology had, "at least for a few decades, freed us from the drivel of brain-mythological and pseudo-philosophical metaphysics" (Bumke 1928, p. 6). The psychiatric promise of experimental psychology lay first and foremost in the potential it harbored for developing new diagnostic techniques that would allow practitioners to measure their patients' mental abilities. And this promise manifested itself in the fact that by 1910 laboratories for experimental psychology had been established in numerous university psychiatric clinics across Germany, including the clinics in Munich and Heidelberg where Wundt's most loyal student (Emil Kraepelin) worked, as well as in Berlin, where one of his most trenchant critics (Theodor Ziehen) held the chair in psychiatry (Kuchta 1988; Ringer 1969, pp. 312–315).

17.4 Emil Kraepelin

The enormous influence of Emil Kraepelin (1856–1926) on psychiatric nosology is commonly put down to the clinical methodology that he introduced as a means of isolating specific categories of madness. According to advocates and detractors alike, his unique powers of observation and empirical research techniques were decisive factors in his delineation of the endogenous psychoses, especially his distinction between dementia praecox and manic-depressive insanity. So it is hardly surprising—and certainly not without some justification—that we have come to view Kraepelin as a clinical nosologist. But Kraepelin was not the man he has become in our eyes. In fact, in 1887 he was not a clinical nosologist at all. On the contrary. A far more apt description of him at this point in his career would be that of an experimental psychologist and psychiatric diagnostician. Indeed, his foremost concern throughout the 1880s—and beyond—seems to have been the accuracy of his diagnostic techniques, rather than any ultimately lasting taxonomic validity. While Kraepelin was convinced that he could hone the accuracy of his clinical observations and measurements, he was equally sure that his nosology would ultimately be displaced and overtaken by the march of scientific progress.

A clear manifestation of his concern for diagnostic accuracy was his abiding passion for experimental psychology. As a young psychiatrist working in Wundt's laboratory in the early 1880s, he conducted numerous psychophysical experiments designed to test mental ability and the effects of pharmacological and other stimulants. He later built laboratories in Dorpat/Tartu, Heidelberg, and Munich and founded a journal (*Psychologische Arbeiten*) dedicated to research in experimental psychology. For well over 40 years, up to the very end of his career, Kraepelin conducted research in experimental psychology and remained convinced of its importance for the development of psychiatric science.

Kraepelin's inaugural lecture at the university of Dorpat/Tartu in 1887 can help illustrate the importance of experimental psychology in his early research agenda (Kraepelin 1887). The lecture's significance lies in helping us to reconstruct Kraepelin's early research priorities and the historical context in which he set them. Specifically, and perhaps most strikingly, the lecture illustrates how Kraepelin was trying both to distance himself from research in pathological anatomy and to rehabilitate a psychological dimension to psychiatric research. In one of the remarkable passages of that lecture, Kraepelin flatly contradicted Wilhelm Griesinger's maxim that mental illness was a brain disease. Although Kraepelin paid glowing tribute to Griesinger and his somatic legacy, he also believed that Griesinger's students—and neuropathologists in general—had made two fundamental errors. First, they had been too eager to draw clinical conclusions from their laboratory research. The result had been all too speculative effusions—especially on the part of Theodor Meynert—about the causal linkage between psyche and soma. Second, Kraepelin criticized those brain researchers who had blazed a trail into neuropathology, but who had never found their way back to psychiatry. In his view, the failings of romantic medicine had driven many researchers to opposite extremes and led them to adopt positions of "naive materialism." As a result, large swaths of their pathoanatomic research had become irrelevant or only peripherally significant to psychiatry proper.

It is in the context of these failings of cerebral pathology that Kraepelin situated his own research agenda. His skepticism toward the approaches of Theodor Meynert, Carl Westphal, Carl Wernicke, and others reflects an important shift away from the mechanistic and materialist assumptions that had pushed psychiatry toward pathological anatomy from the mid century onward. While Kraepelin never doubted the somatic origins of madness, he did insist that pathological anatomy and physiology were themselves incapable of grasping the complexity of the psyche. Reflecting the psychophysical parallelism of his mentor Wilhelm Wundt, Kraepelin therefore insisted that psychological experimentation was an essential tool in helping to explain mental processes. He argued that because Wilhelm Wundt had transformed psychology into a natural science, psychiatrists could now embrace it unreservedly and thus move the study of mental processes to the fore of psychiatric research (Kraepelin 1895, 1897).

Historians have adopted different interpretations about the significance of Wundtian experimental psychology on Kraepelin's nosology, some attempting to link them more closely, others to disassociate them from each other (Burgmair et al. 2003; Engstrom 2003b; Engstrom and Weber 2005). Traditional interpretations of Kraepelin's work have generally ignored the psychological experiment, coming to view it as little more than an awkward appendage to his larger oeuvre (Birnbaum 1928; Gaupp 1939; Gruhle 1929). Likewise, Paul Hoff (1992, p. 121) argues that it had little direct nosological impact, serving instead largely as a means to shore up and legitimize psychiatry's natural scientific credentials. By contrast, others have tended to stress its formative influence on Kraepelin's nosology. Their aim, unlike those who admire Kraepelin's work as a clinical nosologist, has been to downplay the clinical side of his nosology and emphasize instead its origins in premises drawn from laboratory practice. For example Volker Roelcke interprets Kraepelin's uses of Wundtian experimental methods as indicative of a biological reductivism that effectively ignored or marginalized social and biographical dimensions in psychiatric diagnosis (Roelcke 1999). And the historian of psychology Helmut Hildebrandt goes so far as to ground the entirety of Kraepelin's nosology on experimental psychology and Wundt's concept of apperception (Hildebrandt 1993).

Of course, from the perspective of clinical medicine, Kraepelin's hopes of integrating experimental findings into his broader nosological scheme were never fulfilled. His enormously influential textbook was all but silent on the relevance of the psychological experiment to psychiatric practice. Hence, it is not surprising that it has been largely purged from historical memory, while at the same time his pragmatic and useful taxonomy was readily canonized by clinical psychiatry (Janzarik 1972, p. 589).

Kraepelin's legacy as a nosologist has therefore done much to obscure his efforts to establish psychological methods as part of the psychiatrist's diagnostic repertoire. Indeed, most historical interpretations have been retrospectively nosological. That is to say, the significance of Kraepelin's experimental research has been assessed against the monumental backdrop of what his nosology later *became*. By interpreting experimental psychology's significance—or lack thereof—simply in relation to his nosology, these interpretations have to some degree fallen victim to hindsight, that is, to the inflated legacy of that nosology.

What these interpretations tend to miss is that Kraepelin was initially rather skeptical about the prospects of clinical research and nosological validity. As admirable an aim as demarcating categories of psychiatric illness may have been, he found most of these endeavors to be rife with "speculation." He lamented the "labyrinth of clinical signs" and the sharp "divergence of efforts at clinical classification" that plagued clinical research. And so he argued that, for the immediate future, research efforts would best be directed *not* toward the construction of disease categories or nosologies, but rather toward the supposedly more modest goals of delineating clinical symptoms and breaking complicated psychological processes down into their component parts. As Paul Hoff (1994) has pointed out, Kraepelin considered himself much more of a diagnostician than a nosologist: as paradoxical as it may sound in our neo-Kraepelinian age, Kraepelin would have agreed with those who later sought to "denosologize" his legacy.

Put succinctly, Kraepelin's research agenda in the late 1880s had, first and foremost, diagnostic aspirations. As a medical scientist and researcher, he was more concerned about the empirical accuracy of his clinical techniques than he was about the larger, often contested, and to his mind ultimately ephemeral taxonomic architecture built upon those empirical foundations. He hoped that his experimental methodology would enhance diagnostic accuracy and reliability and thereby—among its many other advantages (Engstrom 2003b)—bring greater scientific rigor to psychiatric practice. Just as other branches of medicine deployed arrays of physical and chemical tests to establish the *status praesens* of their patients, so Kraepelin (1895, p. 69) hoped to deploy psychological tests and procedures that would ensure—as he would later put it—a "rapid psychological mapping of the individual." Of course, Kraepelin never succeeded in achieving this goal. But situating diagnostic concerns at the forefront of his early research agenda suggests that deficiencies of psychiatric practice were paramount in his thinking at this time.

Kraepelin also recognized the real limitations of the very laboratory methods he espoused—methods that could capture only a snapshot of symptoms at one given moment in patients' lives and that depended on those patients' cooperation for success. Yet far from constricting his clinical perspective, these and other limitations prompted him to widen his later research agenda to include more intensive anamnestic and catamnestic assessments (Berrios and Hauser 1988; Engstrom 2005; Weber and Engstrom 1997). In other words, Kraepelin's early experimental research is likely to have been a catalyst for his later clinical research in Heidelberg in the sense that it evoked greater recognition of the importance of disease course and outcome and thereby prompted him to expand the breadth of available information about patients beyond what laboratory tests could provide. Accordingly, a more apt interpretation of the origins of Kraepelinian psychiatry would have experimental psychology neither dismissed entirely nor posited as the wellspring of his clinical research, but instead viewed as a necessary and formative prerequisite to his later emphasis on disease course and outcome, both of which came to define his work as one of the most influential nosologists of the twentieth century.

17.5 Theodor Ziehen

Lest one assume that Kraepelin was the only prominent academic psychiatrist seeking to rehabilitate psychological perspectives, the case of Theodor Ziehen (1862–1950) is also instructive. Ziehen held the chair in psychiatry at the University in Berlin from 1904 to 1912. Unlike Kraepelin, however, Ziehen was probably Wundt's most vehement psychiatric critic. In the introduction to his *Leitfaden der physiologischen Psychologie* (1893, p. iii) Ziehen rejected the "Wundtian doctrine so dominant in Germany" and instead proclaimed himself an advocate of English association psychology. Ziehen's critique was directed at the two cornerstones of Wundt's philosophy: apperception and psychophysical parallelism. According to Ziehen, Wundt had too often simply attributed complex mental processes to the work of apperception. Through his writings, Ziehen hoped to demonstrate that apperception was "superfluous" and that all psychological phenomena could be explained without recourse to it (Ziehen 1893, pp. iii, 2). Attacking Wundt's psychophysical parallelism, Ziehen argued that the search for parallel processes of cerebral physiological phenomena had contributed to a "hypothetical elongation" of the psychological causal sequence (*psychologische Kausalreihe*) (cf. Wegener 2009, p. 279). Openly contemptuous of Wundt's work, Ziehen (1893) dismissed such notions as "animistic" and considered Wundt's psychophysical parallelism to be a figment of his imagination.

Ziehen's sharp attack prompted Wundt to write a lengthy article on mental causality and the principle of psychophysical parallelism (Wundt 1894; Ziehen 1895). The article was published at the height of wider contemporary debates—involving most prominently Wilhelm Dilthey and Hermann Ebbinghaus—about the distinction between the natural sciences and humanities (*Geisteswissenschaften*). His research having turned increasingly away from experimental psychology and toward so-called *Völkerpsychologie*, Wundt now sought to stake out more clearly the place of psychology within the humanities: he began to distance himself from what he considered to be a materialistic appropriation of psychophysical parallelism and moved instead to reemphasize psychology's proximity to philosophy. As useful as psychophysical parallelism had been in helping to demarcate the new psychology from natural philosophy, Wundt now reinterpreted it to express not a causal disjunction between psyche and soma as he had in his earlier writings, but rather their mutual interaction or *Wechselwirkung* (Wegener 2009 pp. 300–302).

Although Ziehen rejected Wundtian notions of psychophysical parallelism and apperception, he nevertheless adopted the experimental methodology of Wundt's "inductive philosophy," using it to explore his own somatically grounded theory of association (Ziehen 1904). Ziehen's "physiological psychology" embedded mental processes deeply into the brain, postulating the existence of "perception cells" (*Empfindungszellen*), "representation cells" (*Vorstellungszellen*), "memory cells"

(*Erinnerungszellen*), and "motor cells" (*motorische Zellen*) that were interconnected in a network of association fibers (Ziehen 1902, p. 4). For Ziehen, mental processes corresponded with "the meanderings [*Wandern*] of physiological stimuli from the spheres of sensation to the motor region" (Ziehen 1904). And accordingly his experiments were designed to test theories of association as well as the neurological and cerebral reflexive arc (*Reflexbogen*). Measuring perceptions, mental representations, the association of ideas, and motor actions comprised the core of his experimental research. He studied the entire spectrum of stimuli (tactile, acoustic, gustatory, and visual stimuli) and organized his psychodiagnostic approach around these stimuli (Ziehen 1900, p. 24).

As mentioned earlier, Wundt thought his experimental methodology ill-suited to the study pathological conditions. Ziehen, however, insisted that psychiatrists couldn't do without it: "There can be no science of psychiatry without the science of psychology" (Ziehen 1900, p. 4). What's more, Ziehen considered this fact to be grounded in history. In his inaugural lecture at the University of Berlin, he described how, following phases of alienists' "naive psychological observations" and the subsequent turn to neuropathology, a new, third historical era had now arrived—an era that continued the tradition of neuropathology, but that "replaced old naive psychological observation with the experimental-psychological examination of patients in accordance with modern physiological psychology" (Ziehen 1904). By circumscribing experimental psychology within anatomy and physiology, Ziehen sought to ensure that psychology would not again fall back "under the sway of metaphysics" (Ziehen 1900, p. 4).

What's remarkable about Ziehen's inaugural lecture is that he—like Kraepelin and other advocates of the new psychology—were ultimately attempting to draw psychology into neuropsychiatry. Neither he nor Kraepelin went as far as Freud in reintroducing the notion of a subconscious, for to have done so would, to his mind, have jeopardized psychiatry's recent and hard-won status as a medical science. Nevertheless, his aim was to compensate for the strong neuropathological predominance within contemporary psychiatric research. Accordingly, Ziehen was decidedly critical of localization theories. In the programmatic first issue of the journal *Monatsschrift für Psychiatrie und Neurologie* which he cofounded in 1897, he sought to "oppose premature schematization of incomplete anatomic findings," especially Paul Flechsig's efforts to locate centers of association and cognition in the brain. While sensations and representations depended on certain regions of the brain, "in no way did they actually inhabit a *region* of the brain" (Ziehen 1912, p. 53).

It would no doubt be going too far to speak of a "psychologization of psychiatry." But it was precisely the strength of somatic paradigms—coupled with their relatively meager therapeutic results as well as various other problems of psychiatric practice (Engstrom 2003a, pp. 123–127)—that helped facilitate greater interest in contemporary psychological methods and perspectives. The aim of Ziehen and other representatives of the new psychology was to overcome the powerful legacy of antipathy toward natural philosophy. The dispute over the status of psychology within psychiatry and the strategies deployed to overcome resistance to it, has received relatively little attention in psychiatric historiography. But there is no doubt that the dispute was remarkably acrimonious. Ziehen considered Kraepelin's experimental research to be "genuinely bad" and a "caricature of Ebbinghaus's well-known work" (Ziehen 1896, p. 248). And in turn, by the early 1920s, Ziehen's critics were celebrating the demise of his association theory and the "blind, senseless ... and arbitrary" cerebral connectivity that it preached (Binswanger 1924, p. 409). Amongst Kraepelin's students, Ziehen had the reputation of an "arrogant, superficial know-it-all, completely ignorant of all psychiatric things"—or at least that was the view of Kraepelin's close colleague and former assistant, Robert Gaupp (Gaupp 1903; cf. also Engstrom 2010, p. 790).

17.6 Conclusion

By way of conclusion, it's worth giving this "know-it-all" Theodor Ziehen the last word. In an article on the relationship between psychiatry and philosophy, Ziehen (1927, pp. 341–342) concluded that while "psychiatry and cerebral pathology couldn't do without psychology, they tended to fare better without philosophy." At the same time, however, Ziehen stressed that psychiatrists and philosophers were working on opposite sides of the same divide, studying the same material and psychological processes. Ziehen hoped that that divide wouldn't become a "Chinese wall," but rather a wall equipped with a small interdisciplinary door or *Zwischentür*.

Although Ziehen's interdisciplinary door in the wall between psychiatry and philosophy may have been shrinking in the second half of the nineteenth century, it continued to bear more traffic than most historians of psychiatry have come to assume. And to the degree that we fail to account for the traffic between psychiatry and its disciplinary neighbors such as philosophy and the new psychology, our histories will remain unable to account for the full complexity of the historical evidence. In this vein, I have sought to illustrate how the development of Emil Kraepelin's psychiatric nosology confronted and was shaped by internal resistances that his neuropsychiatric colleagues had marshaled in order to banish the specter of metaphysics and to reinforce psychiatry's somatic credentials within medical science. In overcoming those resistances, however, Kraepelin drew on the external practices and methods of nascent experimental psychology. In doing so, he was working to relativize the importance of cerebral pathology and to expand the purchase of the "new psychology" amongst his own professional peers. It was not least because this "new psychology" that Kraepelin was perhaps better positioned than others to overcome, in the words of Werner Janzarik (1972, p. 588), "tacitly accepted professional conventions" and to reassess some of the fundamental psychiatric assumptions and diagnostic uncertainties of his age.

References

Araujo, S.F. (2012). Why did Wundt abandon his early theory of the unconscious? Towards a new interpretation of Wundt's psychological project. *History of Psychology*, 15(1), 33–49.

Ash, M.G. (2005). The uses and usefulness of psychology. *Annals of the American Academy of Political and Social Science*, 600, 99–114.

Berrios, G.E. and Hauser, R. (1988). The early development of Kraepelin's ideas on classification—a conceptual history. *Psychological Medicine*, 18, 813–821.

Binswanger, L. (1924). Welche Aufgaben ergeben sich für die Psychiatrie aus den Fortschritten der neueren Psychologie. *Zeitschrift für die gesamte Neurologie und Psychiatrie*, 91, 402–436.

Birnbaum, K. (1928). Geschichte der psychiatrischen Wissenschaft. In O. Bumke (ed.) *Handbuch der Geisteskrankheiten* (Vol. 1), pp. 11–49. Berlin: Springer.

Bumke, O. (1928). Ziele, Wege und Grenzen der psychiatrischen Forschung. In O. Bumke (ed.) *Handbuch der Geisteskrankheiten* (Vol. 1), pp. 1–10. Berlin: Springer.

Burgmair, W., Engstrom, E.J., and Weber, M.M. (eds.) (2003). *Emil Kraepelin: Dorpat, 1886–1891.* Munich: Belleville.

Engstrom, E.J. (2003a). *Clinical Psychiatry in Imperial Germany: A History of Psychiatric Practice.* Ithaca: Cornell University Press.

Engstrom, E.J. (2003b). La messende Individualpsychologie: sur le rôle de l'expérimentation psychologique dans la psychiatrie d'Emil Kraepelin. *Psychiatrie—Sciences Humaines—Neurosciences*, 1(2), 40–46.

Engstrom, E.J. (2005). Die Ökonomie klinischer Inskription: Zu diagnostischen und nosologischen Schreibpraktiken in der Psychiatrie. In C. Borck and A. Schäfer (eds.) *Psychographien*, pp. 219–240. Zurich: Diaphanes.

Engstrom, E.J. (2010). Neurowissenschaften und Hirnforschung. In H.-E. Tenorth (ed.) *Geschichte der Universität Unter den Linden, 1810–2010*, pp. 777–797. Berlin: Akademie Verlag.

Engstrom, E.J. and Weber, M.M. (2005). The directions of psychiatric research by Emil Kraepelin 1887. *History of Psychiatry*, 16(3), 345–364.

Gaupp, R. (1903). Robert Gaupp to Willy Hellpach, 25 April 1903. Generallandesarchiv Karlsruhe, N69 Hellpach 282.

Gaupp, R. (1939). Die Lehren Kraepelins in ihrer Bedeutung für die heutige Psychiatrie. *Zeitschrift für die gesamte Neurologie und Psychiatrie*, 165, 47–75.

Gödde, G. (1999). *Traditionslinien des "Unbewußten": Schopenhauer, Nietzsche, Freud.* Tübingen: Edition Diskord.

Green, C.D. (2009). The curious rise and fall of experimental psychology. *History of the Human Sciences*, 22(1), 37–57.

Gruhle, H.W. (1929). Kraepelins Bedeutung für die Psychologie. *Archiv für Psychiatrie und Nervenkrankheiten*, 87, 43–49.

Gruhle, H.W. (1932). Geschichtliches. In O. Bumke (ed.) *Handbuch der Geisteskrankheiten* (Vol. 9/5), pp. 1–30. Berlin: Springer.

Guillin, V. (2004). Théodule Ribot's Ambiguous positivism: philosophical and epistemological strategies in the founding of French scientific psychology. *Journal of the History of the Behavioral Sciences*, 40(2), 165–181.

Hatfield, G. (1997). Wundt and psychology as science: disciplinary transformations. *Perspectives on Science*, 5(3), 349–382.

Heidelberger, M. (2004). *Nature from Within: Gustav Theodor Fechner and His Psychophysical Worldview.* Pittsburgh, PA: University of Pittsburgh Press.

Hildebrandt, H. (1993). Der psychologische Versuch in der Psychiatrie: Was wurde aus Kraepelins (1895) Program? *Psychologie und Geschichte*, 5, 5–30.

Hoff, P. (1992). Emil Kraepelin and philosophy: the implicit philosophical assumptions of Kraepelinian psychiatry. In M. Spitzer, F.A. Uehlein, M.A. Schwartz, and C. Mundt (eds.) *Phenomenology, Language and Schizophrenia*, pp. 115–125. New York: Springer.

Hoff, P. (1994). *Emil Kraepelin und die Psychiatrie als klinische Wissenschaft: Ein Beitrag zum Selbstverständnis psychiatrischer Forschung*. Berlin: Springer.

Huemer, W. and Landerer, C. (2010). Mathematics, experience and laboratories: Herbart's and Brentano's role in the rise of scientific psychology. *History of the Human Sciences*, 23, 72–94.

Janzarik, W. (1972). Forschungsrichtungen und Lehrmeinungen in der Psychiatrie: Geschichte, Gegenwart, forensische Bedeutung. In H. Göppinger (ed.) *Handbuch der forensischen Psychiatrie* (Vol. 1), pp. 588–662. Berlin: Springer Verlag.

Kahlbaum, K. (1863). *Die Gruppierung der psychischen Krankheiten und die Einteilung der Seelenstörungen*. Danzig: A.W. Kafemann.

Kraepelin, E. (1887). *Die Richtungen der psychiatrischen Forschung: Vortrag, gehalten bei der Übernahme des Lehramtes an der kaiserlichen Universität Dorpat*. Leipzig: Vogel.

Kraepelin, E. (1895). Der psychologische Versuch in der Psychiatrie. *Psychologische Arbeiten*, 1, 1–91.

Kraepelin, E. (1897). *Ueber geistige Arbeit* (2nd ed.). Jena: Fischer.

Kraepelin, E. (1918). Hundert Jahre Psychiatrie: Ein Beitrag zur Geschichte menschlicher Gesittung. *Zeitschrift für die gesamte Neurologie und Psychiatrie*, 38, 161–275.

Kuchta, G. (1988). *Beiträge namhafter Kliniker der deutschen Medizin zur Beförderung der psychologischen Ausbildung der Ärzte zwischen 1860–1945*. Medical Dissertation, University of Leipzig.

Kutzer, M. (2003). "Psychiker" als "Somatiker"—"Somatiker" als "Psychiker": Zur Frage der Gültigkeit psychiatriehistorischer Kategorien. In E.J. Engstrom and V. Roelcke (eds.) *Psychiatrie im 19. Jahrhundert: Forschungen zur Geschichte von psychiatrischen Institutionen, Debatten und Praktiken im deutschen Sprachraum*, pp. 27–47. Basel: Schwabe.

Lange, F.A. (1866). *Geschichte des Materialismus und Kritik seiner Bedeutung in der Gegenwart*. Iserlohn: Baedeker.

Lazarus, M. (1868). Rede auf W. Griesinger. *Archiv für Psychiatrie und Nervenkrankheiten*, 1, 775–782.

Leibbrand, W. and Wettley, A. (2005). *Der Wahnsinn: Geschichte der abendländischen Psychopathologie*. Munich: Karl Albers. (Work originally published in 1961.)

Mayerhofer, H. and Vanecek, E. (2007). *Friedrich Albert Lange als Psychologe und Philosoph: Ein kritischer Geist in den Auseinandersetzungen des 19. Jahrhunderts*. Frankfurt/M: Lang.

Nicholls, A. and Liebscher, M. (eds.) (2010). *Thinking the Unconscious: Nineteenth-Century German Thought*. Cambridge: Cambridge University Press.

Peiffer, J. (2004). *Hirnforschung in Deutschland 1849 bis 1974: Briefe zur Entwicklung von Psychiatrie und Neurowissenschaften sowie zum Einfluss des politischen Umfeldes auf Wissenschaftler*. Berlin: Springer.

Ringer, F. (1969). *The Decline of the German Mandarins: The German Academic Community, 1890–1933*. Cambridge, MA: Harvard University Press.

Robinson, D.K. (2010). Fechner's "inner psychophysics." *History of Psychology*, 13(4), 424–433.

Roelcke, V. (1999). Laborwissenschaft und Psychiatrie: Prämissen und Implikationen bei Emil Kraepelins Neuformulierung der psychiatrischen Krankheitslehre. In C. Gradmann and T. Schlich (eds.) *Strategien der Kausalität. Konzepte der Krankheitsverursachung im 19. und 20. Jahrhundert*, pp. 93–116. Pfaffenweiler: Centaurus.

Sammet, K. (1997). *"Ueber Irrenanstalten und deren Weiterentwicklung in Deutschland": Wilhelm Griesinger im Streit mit der konservativen Anstaltspsychiatrie 1865-1868*. Hamburg: Lit.

Schmiedebach, H.-P. (1986). *Psychiatrie und Psychologie im Widerstreit: Die Auseinandersetzung in der Berliner Medicinisch-Psychologischen Gesellschaft, 1867–1899* (R. Winau and H. Müller-Dietz, eds.). Husum: Matthiesen.

Schnädelbach, H. (1983). *Philosophie in Deutschland, 1831–1933*. Frankfurt: Suhrkamp.

Schneider, C.M. (1990). *Wilhelm Wundts Völkerpsychologie: Entstehung und Entwicklung eines in Vergessenheit geratenen, wissenschaftshistorisch relevanten Fachgebietes*. Bonn: Bouvier.

Shorter, E. (1997). *A History of Psychiatry: From the Era of the Asylum to the Age of Prozac*. New York: John Wiley & Sons.

Teo, T. (2002). Friedrich Albert Lange on Neo-Kantianism, Socialist Darwinism, and a psychology without a soul. *Journal of the History of the Behavioral Sciences*, 38(3), 285–301.

Verwey, G. (2004). *Wilhelm Griesinger: Psychiatrie als ärztlicher Humanismus*. Nijmegen: Arts & Boeve.

Weber, M.M. and Engstrom, E.J. (1997). Kraepelin's diagnostic cards: the confluence of empirical research and preconceived categories. *History of Psychiatry*, 8, 375–385.

Wegener, M. (2009). Der psychophysische Parallelismus: Zu einer Diskursfigur im Feld der wissenschaftlichen Umbrüche des ausgehenden 19. Jahrhunderts. *Zeitschrift für Geschichte der Wissenschaften, Technik und Medizin*, 17, 277–316.

Westphal, C. (1868). Nekrolog. *Archiv für Psychiatrie und Nervenkrankheiten*, 1, 760–774.

Weygandt, W. (1901). Zur Frage der materialistischen Psychiatrie. *Zentralblatt für Nervenheilkunde und Psychiatrie*, 24, 409–415.

Wong, W. (2009). Retracing the footsteps of Wilhelm Wundt: explorations in the disciplinary frontiers of psychology and in *Völkerpsychologie*. *History of Psychology*, 12, 229–265.

Wundt, W. (1874). *Gründzüge der physiologischen Psychologie*. Leipzig: Engelmann.

Wundt, W. (1894). Über psychische Causalität und das Princip des psychophysischen Parallelismus. *Philosophische Studien*, 10, 1–124.

Wundt, W. (1911). *Hypnotismus und Suggestion* (2nd ed.). Leipzig: Wilhelm Engelmann.

Ziche, P. (2008). *Wissenschaftslandschaften um 1900: Philosophie, die Wissenschaften und der nichtreduktive Szientismus*. Zurich: Chronos.

Ziehen, T. (1893). *Leitfaden der physiologischen Psychologie in 15 Vorlesungen*. Jena: Gustav Fischer.

Ziehen, T. (1895). Review of Wilhelm Wundt's *Über psychische Causalität und das Princip des psychophysischen Parallelismus*. *Zeitschrift für Psychologie und Physiologie der Sinnesorgane*, 8, 453–457.

Ziehen, T. (1896). Review of E. Kraepelin (ed.) *Psychologische Arbeiten*, vol. 1.1. *Zeitschrift für Psychologie und Physiologie der Sinnesorgane*, 10, 247–252.

Ziehen, T. (1900). *Ueber die Beziehungen der Psychologie zur Psychiatrie.* Jena: Gustav Fischer.

Ziehen, T. (1902). *Psychiatrie für Ärzte und Studierende* (2nd ed.). Leipzig: S. Hirzel.

Ziehen, T. (1904). Die Entwicklungsstadien der Psychiatrie. *Berliner Klinische Wochenschrift,* 41.29, 777–780.

Ziehen, T. (1912). *Über die allgemeinen Beziehungen zwischen Gehirn und Seelenleben.* Leipzig: Barth.

Ziehen, T. (1927). Psychiatrie und philosophie. *Monatsschrift für Psychiatrie und Neurologie,* 63, 336–345.

Chapter 18

Interdisciplinarity versus compartmentalization: an eternal dilemma in psychiatry

Yuji Sato

18.1 Remembrance of the Things Past in Psychiatry

In discussing the history of psychiatry as an interdisciplinary history in Chapter 17, Eric Engstrom called our attention firstly to the three most productive and academically wide-ranging figures in late nineteenth-/early twentieth-century German psychiatry and psychology, namely Wundt, Kraepelin, and Ziehen. As Engstrom pointed out, the achievements of these three major figures, in particular those of Kraepelin, are understood today in a much more parochial and limited way than was previously the case. Engstrom's chapter makes it abundantly clear that one of the most illuminating lessons a good history of psychiatry can teach us is how little we psychiatrists in the twenty-first century have learned from the vast reservoir of trials and errors, proposed and discarded hypotheses, and pregnant perspectives, of our predecessors in the field.

Secondly, Engstrom reminded us of the critical importance of interdisciplinary collaboration; his point was made with regard to the history of psychiatry as an interdisciplinary enterprise, but beyond this, I was impressed by the highly interdisciplinary nature of the intellectual perspectives of Wundt, Kraepelin, and Ziehen. As a medical student I was naïve enough to regard psychiatry as the most interdisciplinary specialty within medicine, encompassing as it does the natural, humanistic, and social sciences. I soon came to recognize my naïveté when I learned of the huge extent to which subspecialization and intellectual compartmentalization go on even in a single subspecialty within psychiatry, for example, clinical psychopharmacology. The fact that, despite occasional rivalry and acrimony, interactions between psychology, philosophy, and psychiatry clearly took place amongst the then leading figures of mainstream German academia indicates firstly that in those days researchers were not impossibly inundated with exponentially increasing amounts of scientific information in a given subspecialty, and secondly that the walls between the different disciplines and specialties were still not so high and thick as to prohibit toing and froing through "an interdisciplinary door" (*Zwischentüren*). In modern scientific research, these walls are unfortunately an untoward and invariable epiphenomenon of advances and developments. Thirdly, the zeitgeist in academia in those days seems to have allowed for the presence of polymaths and dilettantes (in the good sense of the word), neither of which are highly regarded today.

18.2 **Interdisciplinarity Wanes, Compartmentalization Waxes**

The interdisciplinarity (Frodeman et al. 2010; Moran 2010) and its quintessential significance for psychiatry need, in my view, to be further elaborated on in the context of the theme of this volume, that is, the nature and sources of historical change. As Engstrom has pointed out repeatedly, psychiatry has since its inception been destined to grapple with extremes and contradictions, perhaps reflecting the Cartesian dualism, or worse, Manichean dichotomy inherent in the field: soma against psyche, objectivity versus subjectivity, qualitative research versus quantitative research, or *nomothetische* versus *idiographische Forschung*—binary examples are almost endless. Although this dichotomous tension manifests itself in different forms in psychiatry, one thing is clear: this tension, or everlasting conflict, has no simple solution, and having, or pretending to have, a prima facie straightforward, universal solution simply implies neglect and repression of the tension, which in fact remains intact and will sooner or later burst. Unfortunately this pretense, that is, the habit of hailing one aspect at the expense of another, is all too common amongst psychiatrists. A fairly recent example might be Nancy Andreasen and other neuroscientists (Andreasen 1997), who enthusiastically proclaimed that psychiatry, along with neurology, can be renamed clinical neuroscience (Editorial 1997), because neuroscience has developed in a way that makes psychiatry merely part of its field of application. In this vein, Kraepelin seems to have been a rare exception in that he once attempted to establish diagnostic accuracy (reliability), later moving on to focus more on taxonomic validity; he does not appear to have overly favored either of these extremes over the other.

Tolerating this intellectual tension is always a difficult challenge, and only a few exceptional scholars have dared try—perhaps only those endowed with what the poet John Keats called negative capability (1817/1970). Gustav Fechner, to whom Wundt owed so much, may be another example of someone who was fairly successful in internalizing these conflicts, though in his case this seems to have been possible via the Dr. Jekyll and Mr. Hyde manner in which he published, under the pseudonym of Dr. Mises, works that were deeply inimical to his psychophysics, such as *Nanna oder über das Seelenleben der Pflanzen* (1848)—surely the spiritual life of plants cannot be within the scope of his psychophysical research?

Solution by division, or splitting in psychoanalytic parlance, of this sort can be generational: one may very well recall the Nobel-laureate immunologist who ferociously denounced psychoanalysis (Medawar 1972), only for his daughter, Caroline Garland, to later become a leading psychoanalyst.

At any rate, if these conflicts and tensions are never to be divorced from psychiatry, it is essential to at least acknowledge them, and then establish one's own perspectives that allow one to "hold" the conflicts and contradictions without violently discarding them. In order to do so, interdisciplinary collaboration, or coexistence, of extreme views seems to be the only feasible path forward. In short, listening to others, in particular those from outside one's own specialty, should make one self-conscious, critical, and humble, and thus hopefully enhance one's intellectual honesty and level-headedness.

18.3 Historical Changes in Interdisciplinary Permeability

A schematized representation of interdisciplinary toing and froing through *Zwischentüren* as a metaphor for permeability between disciplines is shown in Figure 18.1.

Suppose there is an academic discipline α, from which concept A is transported through the "interdisciplinary door" into another discipline ψ, which signifies psychiatry here. As Figure 18.1 suggests, it is very often the case that concept A, on being transported through the door, is modified, intentionally or unintentionally, into concept B, which is slightly different from the original concept A. Concept B thus modified may further undergo alteration within discipline ψ into concept C. Concept C may occasionally be transported yet again through the door into discipline α, whereupon concept C transforms into concept D thanks to the transportation itself. If permeability of the door disappears or decreases, or if the door itself is severely damaged or lost, there is a great risk that the interrelatedness of concepts A, B, C, and D becomes difficult to trace and fully understand, with the result that the concepts are mistakenly interpreted as distinct and completely different from each other. A good conceptual history is perhaps the only method by which the original relationships among these concepts can be elucidated so that the misunderstanding is cleared up. The original conceptualization of operational definition by the American physicist Bridgman, its reification and

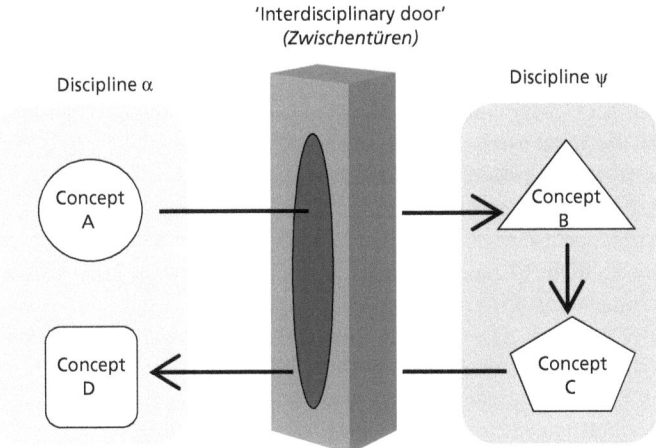

Fig. 18.1 "Interdisciplinary door" and disciplinary permeability.

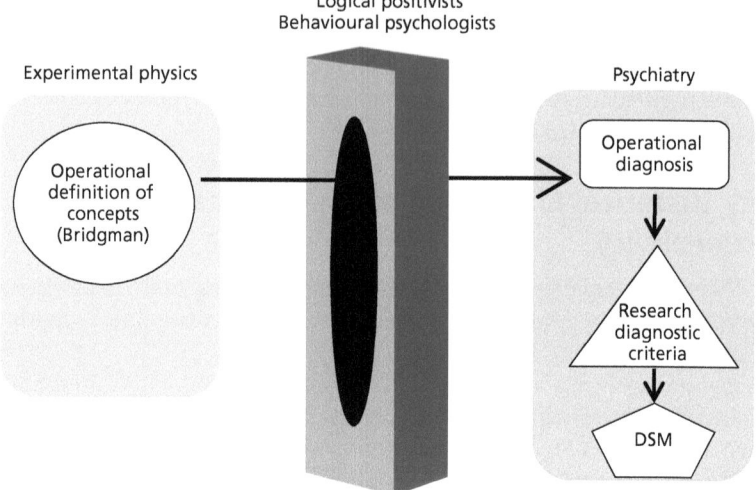

Fig. 18.2 Conceptual history of operational diagnosis.

indoctrination by logical positivists and behavioral psychologists, and its subsequent transportation into psychiatry to give birth to operational diagnosis (see Parnas and P. Bovet, Chapter 23, this volume) is a good example of how conceptual history can be most aptly explained by this model of the interdisciplinary door and its demise (Figure 18.2).

In conclusion, in order for psychiatry to survive as a meaningful discipline in medicine and to serve its patients better, it desperately needs to be supplied, however intermittently, with interdisciplinary and cosmopolitan oxygen to escape its stifling intellectual milieu. I am indebted to Engstrom for supplying me with a sufficient amount of such oxygen to help me survive at least my flight back to Tokyo. I hope that more oxygen will be supplied on a long-term basis from our learned colleagues for years to come in order to keep psychiatry sound.

References

Andreasen, N.C. (1997). Linking mind and brain in the study of mental illnesses: a project for a scientific psychopathology. *Science* 275, 1586–1593.

Editorial. (1997). The crisis in psychiatry. *The Lancet*, 349, 965.

Fechner, G.T. (Dr. Mises) (1848). *Nanna oder über das Seelenleben der Pflanzen*. Leipzig: Leopold Voss.

Frodeman, R., Klein, J.T., and Mitcham, C. (eds.) (2010). *The Oxford Handbook of Interdisciplinarity*. Oxford: Oxford University Press.

Keats, J. (1970). *Letters of John Keats: A Selection* (R. Gittings, ed.) Oxford: Oxford University Press. (Work originally published in 1817.)

Medawar, P. (1972). *Hope of Progress*. London: Methuen.

Moran, J. (2010). *Interdisciplinarity* (2nd ed.). New York: Routledge.

Section 7
Psychiatry and psychoanalysis in the United States

Chapter 19

Introduction to "The development of psychoanalysis in the context of American psychiatry"

Kenneth S. Kendler

In Chapter 20, Michels undertakes to recount for us what has to be one of the foremost stories in twentieth-century American psychiatry—the rise of psychoanalytic influence to a central place within both the clinical practice of psychiatry and in academic psychiatric departments, and its subsequent decline. Despite the fact that Freud never wanted psychoanalysis to be part of psychiatry and did not particularly like America or Americans, one of the apogees of psychoanalytic influence within medicine was reached through psychiatry in the United States for decades from the 1930s to the 1960s.

To give a sense of the magnitude of psychoanalytic dominance of key departments of psychiatry, let me relate a brief personal story. In 1981, I attended, as a psychiatry resident, a seminar given by one of the world's leading basic psychopharmacologists, a psychiatrist then in his late 40s. He told us a story of his first years as a faculty member at Yale University some 15 years earlier, then as now, one of the premier psychiatric departments in the United States. He was advised by several members of the department that he should enter into psychoanalytic training. When he said he had neither the time nor interest to undertake this, they said that it would be difficult for him, without psychoanalytic training, to be promoted within the department. He ignored the advice and went on to a stellar career. I recall then being struck at what this story said about psychoanalytic dominance in academic US psychiatry well into the 1960s.

Michels reviews for us the multiple influences on this historical process. These include: (1) the internal developments within psychoanalysis starting from the antipsychiatry views of Freud and the subsequent hermeneutic turn of the field; (2) the initial sense that psychoanalysis could bring psychiatry closer to general medicine, especially through its theories of psychosomatic disorders; (3) the intellectual fascination of the field and its early promise to provide a true key to our inner mental life; (4) the success of psychoanalytically informed treatment of traumas in World War II; (5) the failure of its psychosomatic theories to be supported by subsequent research; (6) the increasing success of psychopharmacological treatments that provided viable alternatives to psychoanalysis; (7) the limited evidence for the efficacy of psychoanalytic treatment, especially for the more severely psychiatrically ill; (8) the move within academic psychiatry toward a greater research focus often with a biological bent coupled with, as Michels outlines, the fundamental lack of interest of psychoanalysis in etiologic or treatment research and its resulting failure to develop a strong research program; and (9) the unique locus of psychoanalysis being in independent training institutes. Certainly, this incomplete list provides much material for historical work about internal and external influences on the relationships between psychiatry and psychoanalysis.

Michels' essay emphasizes the two kinds of knowledge available to psychiatry, as famously articulated by Jaspers (1963) (with roots from Dilthey and Weber), understanding and explanation. He makes clear that, as the biological basis of psychiatry became increasingly researchable, academic psychiatry took a strong research turn toward third-person-based explanation in psychiatry. At the same time, psychoanalysis moved in another direction emphasizing its fundamentally hermeneutic character and focusing entirely on understanding. However, to be clear, psychoanalysis did not emphasize simple empathic understanding but rather the discovery, in the clinical encounter, of variations on a particular series of "story lines" of human development articulated by psychoanalytic theory.

Although the influence of psychoanalysis on psychiatry is surely in decline (and I would argue properly so), it has made some noteworthy contributions. Michels comments on the contribution of psychoanalysis to personality theory and especially in the area of borderline personality that has become a disorder of substantial clinical and research focus. Much of the modern concept of schizophrenia spectrum disorders, especially what we now called schizotypal personality disorder, began with psychoanalytic theorizing. Some of the important phenomenological contributions to psychiatry emerged from psychoanalysts. Finally, psychoanalysis made contributions to a humanizing of psychiatry as an advocate for the importance of understanding the subtleties of human experience that are not well captured by operationalized diagnostic criteria. In a field at risk of dominance by a reductionist biological (or perhaps more accurately a molecular neuroscience) perspective, we should strive not to lose this pluralistic richness: that we can and should be seeking both explanation and understanding.

Reference

Jaspers, K. (1963). *General Psychopathology* (7th ed., J. Hoenig and M.W. Hamilton, trans.) Chicago, IL: University of Chicago Press.

Chapter 20

The development of psychoanalysis in the context of American psychiatry

Robert Michels

20.1 Introduction

Psychoanalysis does not have an obvious relationship to psychiatry. It is not particularly interested in psychiatric illnesses, but rather in how people adapt, how they cope with stress, including the stress of illness, and including the stress of psychiatric illnesses, rather than in the illnesses themselves. It is interested in the person's mind, not his body or even his brain. Psychoanalysis began outside of psychiatry, and Freud, himself a neurologist, not a psychiatrist, never saw it as part of psychiatry.[1]

20.2 Psychoanalysis in America

The middle of the twentieth century brought major changes. Several American psychiatrists went to Vienna to study with and be analyzed by Freud. More importantly, many prominent European psychiatrist-analysts fled central Europe and settled in the United States. Freud himself wanted psychoanalysis to be independent from psychiatry and not restricted to physicians. He dreaded that it might, some day, become a chapter in a textbook of psychiatry. His view prevailed in much of the world. However, American psychoanalysts both native and immigrant were attracted by the prestige of psychiatry and medicine, and opposed his antimedical

---

[1] Freud's only visit to the United States in 1909 was hosted by psychologists, not psychiatrists. Jung, a psychiatrist, was invited to the same conference, and was better known than Freud by American psychiatrists. Unlike Freud he had worked with Bleuler in Zurich, had conducted empirical research employing his word association methods on schizophrenic patients, and had published in English. Soon after the conference Freud and Jung had a falling out, and Freud became annoyed with two leading American psychiatrists who were enthusiastic about psychoanalysis—Smith Ely Jelliffe and William Alanson White—who maintained strong ties to Jung. Freud disliked America and Americans, and he returned to Vienna to develop his new science, viewing American psychoanalysis as an embarrassment. He had little contact with American psychiatry, then or afterward (Barnett 2013).

and antipsychiatric stance. For more than half a century they succeeded in excluding nonpsychiatrists from the American Psychoanalytic Association and tying psychoanalysis to psychiatry and to medicine. They constituted an elite group whose status in American psychiatry, medicine, and society was enhanced by the exclusion of nonpsychiatrist analysts, an exclusion that only came to an end with a lawsuit filed by a group of psychologists that was not settled until 1988.

The success of psychoanalysis in the world of psychiatry was remarkable. For several decades it dominated American psychiatry. As psychoanalysis arrived on the scene, psychiatry had become increasingly alienated from the rest of medicine, and surprising though it seems to a contemporary reader, psychoanalysis was hailed as promising closer ties to medicine and to science. Through its prominence in psychosomatic medicine it meant a return from rural asylums for the insane to the teaching wards of general hospitals. It offered an intellectually fascinating theory that promised a new understanding of mental life that seemed far more scientific than that provided by the humane and perhaps clinically helpful but theoretically unimaginative "nondynamic" psychiatry. It provided a counterpart to the somewhat disreputable physical treatments of convulsive therapies and lobotomies that were frightening to the public. Perhaps most importantly, it arrived with a reputation for clinical efficacy. Nonpsychiatrist physicians who had received brief psychiatric training with a psychoanalytic orientation and then placed in the front lines of World War II returned home with stories of great therapeutic success in treating traumatized soldiers. They were enthusiastic about their clinical experience and wanted to train as psychiatrists and psychoanalysts. The result was that psychiatry, and particularly psychoanalytic psychiatry, was increasingly accepted by the public and by general medicine, and psychoanalysis was increasingly influential in psychiatry (Hale 2000; Shorter 1997).

Psychiatry's enthusiasm for psychoanalysis faded over the next few decades. The scientific hypotheses of psychosomatic medicine generated a body of respected empirical research; however, this research largely demonstrated that strong psychoanalytic "specificity" theories about somatic disorders were not confirmed. The theories of psychoanalysis were interesting, but they failed to generate a body of empirical research, were criticized for being unscientific, and came to be seen as historic relics rather than scientific theories. Lobotomies and convulsive treatments were viewed with distaste but biologic psychiatry, beginning in the 1950s, replaced them with successive waves of psychopharmacologic treatments that were much more palatable to the public and increasingly came to compete with psychotherapy and psychoanalysis for the same population of patients. Perhaps most importantly, the psychodynamic psychotherapies that seemed so effective in treating the self-limited traumatic syndromes of the battlefield were much less effective when applied to the chronic mentally ill, while it became clear that their efficacy in treating acute trauma had little do with their psychoanalytic theoretical foundation. Psychoanalysis had seemed to promise a strategy for developing a scientific psychiatry, but it failed to deliver on that promise and the sociocultural factors that supported its role faded away.

20.3 Psychoanalysis and the Academic World

Before its decline, psychoanalysis had come to dominate academic as well as clinical psychiatry. Forty years ago psychoanalysts had been appointed as chairs at most major US medical schools, including Columbia, Yale, Stanford, University of California San Francisco, Pittsburg, Western Reserve, Dartmouth, and Brown. (None have psychoanalyst leaders today.) Psychiatry was entering its golden age in academic medicine, and psychoanalysis was already at the peak of its golden age in psychiatry. However, they were not quite in phase with each other, and as academic psychiatry gained increasing status, its dominant theme shifted first to social psychiatry and then to biological psychiatry and neuroscience, while the influence of psychoanalysis waned.

Psychoanalysis seemed much more relevant to psychiatric practice and education than to psychiatric research. In the 1950s, American academic psychiatry was dominated by its educational mission. Beginning the 1960s, as academic psychiatry matured and moved closer to other fields of academic medicine, it became more like them as its research mission became increasingly prominent. Success was no longer measured by student enthusiasm or recruitment into the field, but rather by research support and publications. Psychiatric research made immense strides, largely biologic research—first psychopharmacology, and later neuroscience, genetics, and brain imaging. Psychological research, and particularly research in psychotherapy, was much less prominent, and in psychoanalysis almost nonexistent. As academic psychiatry developed its scientific base its new leaders were more likely to be neuroscientists or biologic psychiatrists than psychoanalysts.

20.4 One Psychoanalysis or Many?

Psychoanalysis itself was changing simultaneously, independently of, and largely unrelated to the developments in psychiatry. Freud's death in 1939 ended an era in which there had been a single accepted criterion for what was truly "psychoanalytic" and initiated a period of pluralism that continues to this day. Freud's early theories had been strongly biologic; they speculated about what was going on in the patient's mind and brain and emphasized constitutional determinants of behavior, innate drives that somehow led to mental events. His theories were also, of course, psychological, mentalist, but even these were formulated in ways that were comfortable to those familiar with the positivist scientific thinking of the day and suggest the possibility of eventual neurobiologic reductionism. Freud believed that his method led to the discovery of previously existing although unconscious and therefore undetectable psychological phenomena, and that exposing them to the patient's consciousness would be curative. He had himself tried to construct neurobiologic models of his psychology, but even though he eventually gave these up, this was not because he thought that they were inherently inappropriate, but rather because he thought that they were premature. The necessary neuroscientific knowledge base did not exist at the end of the nineteenth century. However, he had no doubt that mental life would someday be understood as the reflection of underlying neurobiologic processes. With today's neuroscience he would probably be an enthusiastic fan of "neuropsychoanalysis" and eager to make another attempt at his project for developing a scientific brain-based psychology. He did not want psychoanalysis to be a branch of psychiatry, but was quite comfortable seeing it as biological, and ultimately reducible to the functioning of the nervous system (Makari 2008).

20.5 Psychoanalytic Research

Why didn't American academic psychiatry, during its period of psychoanalytic leadership and its growing interest in research, develop a program of psychoanalytic research? Psychoanalysts were eager to be seen as scientific, and they cast their early theories in the language of science. However, they failed to develop a true scientific methodology and had little interest in testing their theories or in attempting to invalidate them. In fact, most of the theories that they embraced were not based on psychoanalytic data, but rather were borrowed from contiguous disciplines—initially neuroscience and cultural anthropology, later developmental psychology and linguistics. Psychoanalysts neither developed nor tested them, and in fact didn't treat them as scientific theories at all. Rather, they used them as tools in the clinical process of searching for meanings, as sources of metaphor. The analytic process came to be seen more and more as an interpretive endeavor, developing new meanings, rather than searching for previously existing but unrecognized facts. The analyst and the patient co-constructed narratives, rather than uncovering forgotten memories. Psychoanalysis moved closer to the humanities rather than the sciences, and much as its practitioners admired science, borrowed its concepts, and aspired to be seen as scientists, their daily work and their intellectual interests moved them away from science, medicine, and psychiatry, and toward hermeneutics. Their goal was understanding, not explanation.

Freud wanted to develop an objective science of human subjectivity, and he viewed the psychoanalyst as a neutral observer of the patient's words and acts, data from which might be inferred the patient's inner experience. Contemporary psychoanalysts are not as confident in the analyst's neutrality or objectivity, and increasingly see the analyst's interpretations as reflecting the analyst's own subjectivity while relying on the analyst's countertransference as an important contributor to the data. This shift, from the patient's words and acts to the analyst's experience and reactions, moves psychoanalysis even further from the rest of psychiatry, medicine, and Popperian science.

I have mentioned the strong psychoanalytic interest in the theories and discoveries of adjacent sciences, if not in their methods. There has also been pressure within the psychoanalytic community for research on the treatment itself—its effectiveness, its indications, and so on. However this pressure has largely come from those concerned with public health, health policy, and economics. Clinical psychoanalysts have shown little interest in this kind of endeavor—the studies required would be long, expensive, and difficult, and relate to the sciences of biostatistics and evaluation of treatment outcome, not to those of interest to psychoanalysis. Clinicians anticipated little from the results that would enrich their daily work. They had no doubt that their treatment worked, and had more confidence in the wisdom of their elders than in systematic empirical studies that explicated whether or how it worked. Studies of its effectiveness might be of interest to skeptics or to those concerned with public policy, but not to practicing psychoanalysts. Clinical psychoanalysts want to enrich their repertoire of potential interpretations, not to learn what percentage of their patients might be expected to improve by what percent on scales of psychopathology.

However, there is another reason that a research tradition in psychoanalysis has not developed, one that I believe is more important and has little to do with the potential value of empirical research but is embedded in the social structure of the profession. Most professional education occurs in university settings, and university cultures have a strong commitment to research. Faculty advancement depends on research productivity, and academic leaders are selected for their research, not their clinical or educational excellence. Psychoanalysis is different and virtually unique. Freud was suspicious of universities; he feared that they would attack and destroy his fragile creation, and psychoanalysis developed and largely continues outside of them. Psychoanalytic education is conducted in freestanding institutes, collections of practitioners with no full-time faculty, often meeting only at nights or on weekends, devoted to study and teaching, but with little interest, time, or reward for research, and indeed research activity is often regarded with suspicion. Kernberg has compared these institutes to trade schools or seminaries (Kernberg 1986). The result is that psychoanalytic research is almost, although not quite, an oxymoron.

20.6 Psychoanalytic and Psychiatric Research

Nevertheless, this is not to say that psychiatric research has had no impact on psychoanalysis, or psychoanalytic research any impact on psychiatry, only that the impact has largely been sociocultural rather than scientific. Psychoanalysts have been wary or unenthusiastic about psychopharmacology but surprisingly interested in brain imaging. It is as though they finally see a strategy for fulfilling Freud's goal of finding the neurobiologic basis of mind. Studies of brain function related to mental events, or changes in brain function before and after psychotherapy, are popular. There are societies and journals of "neuropsychoanalysis" with, for reasons I have explained, "old fashioned" or "classical" analysts being enthusiastic, while "modern," "relational," "interpersonal," or "hermeneutic" analysts viewing them as a step backward.

To a lesser extent, there has even been an impact of the small world of psychoanalytic research on contemporary psychiatry. I will cite three examples. First, in the last few decades psychoanalysis has been particularly interested in serious personality disorders, impaired patients who are not seen as psychotic and are seen as possible candidates for psychoanalytic psychotherapy. The concept of borderline personality was developed by psychoanalysts, several "evidence-based" treatments have been developed and even tested by psychoanalytic groups, and the phenomenology, course, and outcome have all been studied by psychoanalysts. Finally, the DSM-5 conducted field trials that demonstrated the high interrater reliability of this diagnostic category, much higher in fact than the reliability of major depressive disorder (Freedman et al. 2013). For a psychoanalytically conceived and defined entity to become a respected member of DSM-5 is the ultimate sign of recognition in American psychiatry. Second, studies of the effectiveness of all psychiatric treatments have routinely been based on the relief of core symptoms at treatment termination or shortly thereafter. The psychoanalytic research community has argued that this is too narrow a scope—patients suffer from many problems in addition to their core symptoms, their work, their play, and their families suffer as well, and their life trajectories are altered. Also, the termination of treatment provides all too brief a period of follow-up to assess treatment outcome—the critical question is not whether a symptom can be relieved at the end of a course of treatment but whether the course of the patient's life can be improved. The psychiatric research community has accepted these critiques, and broader outcome measures and longer-term follow-up are more and more accepted. Finally, the psychoanalytic interest in infancy and childhood, the parent–infant relationship, and early development has spilled over and awakened a broad psychiatric interest in early development and the possibility of a preventive psychiatry. The direct observation of infants largely grew out of the importance of the hypothesized experience of infants in psychoanalytic theory.

20.7 Conclusion

Psychoanalysis grew out of the traditions of clinical medicine, the doctor–patient relationship, long seen as the art of humanistic practice. Freud tried to develop a systematic objective method for studying subjective experience, and by doing so to transform this art into a science. Psychiatry of the time was an early natural science, based upon the careful description of phenomena, but with barely an attempt at explanation, on observation, but not experiment, with little capacity to formulate testable hypotheses, let alone to test them. Psychoanalysis seemed to offer the potential of an explanatory model and thus a more scientific basis for psychiatry. This captured the enthusiastic support of the psychiatric community, support which was enhanced by an important sociocultural factor—the rewards in status for psychiatrist-psychoanalysts that resulted from their close relationship to medicine. However, the early scientific promise of psychoanalysis was not realized. It never developed an empirical research tradition, and the world of psychiatry became disillusioned, particularly with the failure of psychoanalysis to demonstrate relevance to the understanding or treatment of major psychiatric disorders. Biological models offered a much more robust scientific basis for psychiatry along with the possibility of new and effective treatments for major disorders. Psychoanalysis moved on to less psychiatric, less medical, and less scientific interests—intersubjectivity, relationships, and hermeneutics. Social determinants such as the academic culture dictated psychiatry's need for a strong scientific base and thus its recognition that it had to move on from its flirtation with psychoanalysis to more vital links to more scientifically based approaches. At the same time psychoanalysis recognized that its subject matter led it to approaches and traditions of inquiry that had little to do with the natural sciences. Today psychiatry offers the hope of a powerful scientific approach to psychiatric disorders, while psychoanalysis offers a rich model for understanding subjective experience and human interactions. Some psychiatric problems are best treated by understanding subjective experiences in the context of human interactions, and thus there remains an overlap, albeit a modest one.

However, as long as psychiatry is interested in the people who have diseases, and how they adapt to them, as well as in the diseases themselves, and as long as psychoanalysis recognizes that the realities of the brain and the body are important contributors to human experience there will be a fruitful and mutually enriching dialogue between them. In many ways the question may be not what will the relation be between psychoanalysis and psychiatry, but rather as medicine increasingly shifts its focus from diseases to people, will psychoanalysis offer medicine a strategy for considering patients as people as well as containers of pathology?

References

Barnett, A.J. (2013). The Psychoanalytic Review: 100 years of history. *Psychoanalytic Review*, 100(1), 1–56.

Freedman, R.F. Lewis, D.A., Michels, R., Pine, D.S., Schultz, S.K., Tamminga, C.A., et al. (2013). The initial field trials of DSM-5: new blooms and old thorns (editorial). *American Journal of Psychiatry*, 170(1), 1–5.

Hale, N.G. (2000). American psychoanalysis since World War II. In R.W. Menninger and J.C. Nemiah (eds.) *American Psychiatry After World War II*, pp. 77–102. Washington, DC: American Psychiatric Press Inc.

Kernberg, O.F. (1986). Institutional problems of psychoanalytic education. *Journal of the American Psychoanalytic Association*, 34, 799–834.

Makari, G. (2008). *Revolution in Mind*. New York: Harper.

Shorter, E. (1997). The psychoanalytic hiatus. In *A History of Psychiatry*, pp. 145–189. New York: John Wiley and Sons.

Chapter 21

Decline of psychoanalysis to the advantage of what?

Josef Parnas

In Chapter 20, Professor Michels gives a good overview of the pendulum-like swing of psychoanalytic influence in US psychiatry, from its rapid rise and culmination in the 1950s to its swift decline, in parallel with the explosive rise of biological psychiatry and the introduction of the DSM-III. At the summit of psychoanalytic domination, a membership of the American Psychoanalytic Association was required in order to become a chairman of a major US psychiatric academic institution. Today, US psychoanalysis continues its existence mainly in the extra-academic, quasi-monastic circles (aka psychoanalytic institutes). Michels proposes several reasons for the decline of psychoanalysis. His chapter, read in a more general perspective, touches upon psychiatry's self-understanding as an academic-clinical discipline and may therefore invite a wide range of potential reflections, not only on the nature of psychoanalysis as a theory and practice but also on the status of psychiatry in general.

I will restrict myself to a brief extension of the "psychoanalytic story" to Europe and then address some of Michels' major claims on the reasons behind the decline of psychoanalysis in the US and its current status. I need first to disclose my professional standing with respect to psychoanalysis. As a young intern and resident I was very attracted to the Jungian approach, read a lot of Jung, and invested 2 years in Jungian self-analysis, while as a part of my official training, I received supervision in Freudian-oriented psychodynamic psychotherapy. My clinical contact with psychotherapy ended by the end of my residency, when I joined an epidemiological-genetic research team. I am in no way a scholar on psychoanalysis.

The history of psychoanalysis in Europe is somewhat similar to its American counterpart, but much less dramatic. Naturally, we are subject to globalization and strong American cultural and scientific influences. In more general terms, however, the Europeans are probably less disposed than their transatlantic cousins (because of Europe's cultural and political heterogeneity) to enthusiastically join in a collective action, guided by a single, unifying pragmatic goal (e.g., a project of lunar landing, the Artificial Intelligence Program, elimination of cancer from the list of causes of death, or the Research Domain Criteria (RDoC) project) and therefore less likely to experience pendulum-like swings of the scientific and theoretical orientations. In the specific context of psychiatry, Jaspers' phenomenology acted as a buffer between competing scientific and intellectual orientations. There was among psychiatrists a tacit consensus that *some sort of phenomenologically oriented approach* to the "psychiatric object" was a necessary starting point, irrespectively of one's specific scientific or theoretical agenda (see also Parnas and P. Bovet, Chapter 23, this volume). Psychoanalysis in Europe was never a dominating academic force, and, as in the United States, its influence diminished over the last decades. Yet it did not vanish completely: dynamically oriented psychotherapy still belongs to a psychiatric training curriculum in many places and there exist psychotherapeutically oriented academic inpatient facilities. As in the United States, we have radically decoupled clinical skill and expertise from the mechanisms of academic promotion. Also in Europe, there exist extra-academic psychoanalytic institutions. Nonetheless, despite a strong domination of biological psychiatry, Europe has retained a certain intellectual diversity in the psychiatric academia, as the funding by the University of Copenhagen of the conference behind this book testifies to.

Now, I will turn to Michels' analysis of the mechanisms behind the decline of psychoanalysis in the United States. Michels' narrative seems to fit into a certain accepted schema, ruling our professional self-image and strongly defended at the slightest sign of dissent. It is a widely propagated claim of an unprecedented, revolutionary progress of biological psychiatry (see also Sato, Chapter 35, this volume). In this narrative, psychoanalysis failed because it was, for various reasons, unable to convert itself into an empirical science and compete with the emerging biological psychiatry on a comparable or compatible footing. According to Michels, "Psychiatric research made immense strides, largely biologic research—first psychopharmacology, and later neuroscience, genetics, and brain imaging." He concludes that the "Biological models offered a much more robust scientific basis for psychiatry along with the possibility of new and effective treatments for major disorders." However, this optimistic self-understanding of psychiatry begins today to crumble and loosen its grip. A "gaping disconnect" between the brilliant progress in basic neurosciences and molecular biology and "their almost complete lack" to translate into something useful in clinical psychiatry is becoming glaringly apparent (Hyman 2010, 2012; Insel et al. 2010). This alarming stagnation of clinical psychiatry was one of the justifications behind the launching of the RDoC project. All available biological treatments had been so far discovered more or less "by chance" and not due to "strident efforts" of biological psychiatry, working on a "robust scientific basis." As far as "biological models" *of psychiatry* are concerned, it is perhaps not too much to say that they have distinguished themselves by attracting money and producing publications rather than by providing us with an increasingly accurate representation of the mind–brain system in mental pathologies (see notably Kendler, Chapter 32, this volume). That a dysfunctional thalamus can be ascribed a central role in the formation of *both* positive *and* negative symptoms of schizophrenia (see E. Bovet, Chapter 14, this volume) testifies to the protean nature of current pathogenetic models in psychiatry. In other words, the spectacular reversal of the positions of biological psychiatry and psychoanalysis in the United States cannot be fully accounted for by their respective scientific merits or veracity. A full account should also include a sociological and anthropological approach, studying the processes of belief formation and dissemination. In Europe, biological psychiatry, psychiatric genetics, and psychiatric epidemiology have existed since the end of the nineteenth century, and as already mentioned, the European psychiatric academia is still theoretically diversified, albeit increasingly less so. I cannot fully agree with Michels' suggestion that the task of biological psychiatry is to deal with the core of the disease, whereas the hermeneutic approach is a useful tool in dealing with maladaptive copings or other, derivative problems. It is simply too early to say. I fail to see that in mental illness, coping and disease can be neatly (ontologically) separated into clearly distinct domains. The "explanatory gap," which is our inability to conceive how something mental-experiential arises from the physical substrate, is at the root of our difficulties in constructing coherent hypotheses of symptom formation and thus also of pathogenetic models (see also Berrios, Chapter 5, this volume).

The interdisciplinary nature of psychiatry flows from the explanatory gap and we need to include this interdisciplinarity into our self-understanding. Acknowledging the complexity (not only technological but also theoretical) of the "psychiatric object" is a better defense against the renewed attacks from a reborn antipsychiatry movement and increasing skepticism about our profession (Katschnig 2010) than perpetuating a promise of an imminent or ultimate biomedical solution.

However, it is impossible to disagree with Michels' conclusion that psychoanalysis, so to say, eliminated itself by neglecting empirical research, although it did stimulate the development and emergence of several other modified forms of psychotherapy. The Freudian metaphysics of the mind relied, in my view, on a sort of common-sense mechanical metaphor. Many European psychiatrists received it critically from the outset (e.g., Jaspers 1913/1963). From my personal, phenomenological perspective, the limitations of *classic* psychoanalysis comprised its fundamentally inadequate descriptive approach, epistemologically problematic status of the "Unconscious" (as an inaccessible, *additional representational domain*), its predominant focus on the *content* of experience (the *what* of experience) and a corresponding inability to deal with the psychopathological forms or *structures* (the *how* of experience) (Parnas and Zahavi 2002).

What I think was truly important about psychoanalysis but is badly missing in the contemporary managerial, checklist-based clinical psychiatry, was considering the patient as another human being, occupied by *human* concerns, irrespective of the strangeness of their manifestations. It is well known that efficacy research in psychotherapy is extremely difficult and it is especially cumbersome to determine the proportion of variance that may be ascribed to the therapy's theoretical framework. Paul Meehl once observed that any plan to conduct a large-scale psychotherapeutic study always has to confront the following, very mundane problem: when he was sometimes asked for advice concerning a referral to psychotherapy, he looked into his notebook and would only be able to find a couple of names that he trusted as competent therapists. From a clinical point of view, it is impossible not to be impressed by the encounters with patients who seem to crucially benefit from psychotherapy. Professor Elyn Saks (2007), in her well-known, first-person account of schizophrenia, puts it this way: "While medication had kept me alive, it was psychoanalysis that had helped me find a life worth living" (p. 175).

References

Hyman, S.E. (2010). The diagnosis of mental disorders: the problem of reification. *Annual Review of Clinical Psychology*, 6, 155–179.

Hyman, S.E. (2012). Psychiatric drug discovery: revolution stalled. *Science Translational Medicine*, 4, 1–5.

Insel, T.R., Cuthbert, B., Garvey, M., Heinssen, R., Kozak, M., Pine, D., *et al.* (2010). Research Domain Criteria (RDoC): toward a new classification framework for research on mental disorders. *American Journal of Psychiatry*, 167(7), 748–751.

Jaspers, K. (1963). *General Psychopathology* (7th ed., J. Hoenig and M.W. Hamilton, trans.) Chicago, IL: University of Chicago Press. (Work originally published as *Allgemeine Psychopathologie: Ein Leitfaden für Studierende, Ärzte und Psychologen*. Berlin: Springer, 1913.)

Katschnig, H. (2010). Are psychiatrists an endangered species? Observations on internal and external challenges to the profession. *World Psychiatry*, 9, 21–28.

Parnas, J. and Zahavi, D. (2002). The role of phenomenology in psychiatric classification and diagnosis. In M. Maj, W. Gaebel, J.J. López-Ibor, and N. Sartorius (eds.) *Psychiatric Diagnosis and Classification*, pp. 137–162. Chichester: John Wiley & Sons Ltd.

Saks, E.R. (2007). *The Center Cannot Hold. A Memoir of My Schizophrenia*. London: Virago Press.

Section 8
The operational revolution

Chapter 22

Introduction to "Psychiatry made easy: operation(al)ism and some of its consequences"

Kenneth S. Kendler

Josef Parnas has had, through much of his career, a focal interest in psychopathology. He has lived and worked within both the European traditions of descriptive and phenomenological psychiatry, and in the world of academic genetic and diagnostic research. The latter required a familiarity with and use of operationalized diagnostic criteria. Indeed, his work on the early symptoms of schizophrenia (e.g., Parnas et al. 2005) is a prominent example of empirically rigorous work that spans these two often disconnected subfields within psychiatry.

Parnas and his colleague, Pierre Bovet (P&B), are thus well equipped to provide a historical and conceptual/philosophical critique of operationalized criteria (OC) for psychiatric disorders. The adoption of OC surely represents one of the most important developments in psychiatric nosology in the last 50 years. Working as I do in both research and clinical psychiatric settings, I can attest to the fact that the vast majority of US psychiatric trainees, clinicians, and researchers, now, could hardly imagine any other way to approach psychiatric diagnosis. The triumph of OC, at least in US academic centers, has been nearly complete.

As is so often the case, this development of OC has upsides to it and downsides. P&B are correct that at least in more official US circles, the official version of OC adoption is triumphalist, seeing it as an unadulterated virtue. One would hear establishment figures who claim (with naïveté) that OC for psychiatric disorders "guarantee a reliable, context- and culture-immune understanding and use of the diagnostic criteria." But this attitude is not universal. I recently addressed the directors of psychiatric residency training programs from all over the United States in their annual meeting. I raised concerns about the "impoverishment of psychopathology" in US psychiatric training programs. Taking an approach not very different from points made by P&B, I argued that many young American psychiatrists felt that once the specific DSM criteria for any given disorder had been evaluated, that was all the questions they needed to ask. Equally importantly, the excess DSM focus on our training meant that young psychiatrists—already in a generation not known for its love of reading—had very little motivation to read the classics of descriptive psychiatry. Their limited world view does not see (much) beyond DSM. Both from comments during the talk and afterwards, it was clear that many of the residency directors shared these concerns.

However, OC do have some important virtues. Reliability is critical for any diagnostic procedure. Mental health clinicians with a reasonable degree of training can often reliably assess many of the important symptoms and signs of clinical psychiatric illness. But how we put those signs and symptoms into diagnoses was, prior to the introduction of OC, much more variable. History show us that, left to our own devices, each major teacher of psychiatry likes to develops his (or her) own diagnostic system. The result is diagnostic chaos where disorder X according to Professors A, B, and C, are somewhat similar but differ in some important ways. That problem—a serious one to the clinical but, especially, to the scientific progress of the field—has been substantially ameliorated by the use of OC.

One point that P&B might have insufficiently emphasized is that psychiatric symptoms differ dramatically in their complexity and, hence, the degree to which they fit easily into an OC framework. Many symptoms such as weight loss, insomnia, and tolerance to alcohol fit without much difficulty. Even somewhat more complex constructs such as "recurrent use of alcohol in situations where it is physically hazardous," "low energy or fatigue," "loss of pleasure in all or almost all activities," and "reckless disregard for safety of self or others" can, with some training, be relatively well captured by OC. But as P&B point out, for other constructs, the fit is considerably more problematic. "Delusions" is a far subtler construct as are several of the criteria for borderline personality disorder such as "identity disturbance: markedly and persistently unstable self-image or sense of self." This problem is a familiar one both to those who develop structured interviews and those who have to train interviewers for research, which includes trying to reliably assess these much subtler comments. The ease with which key aspects of psychopathology can be fitted into an OC framework differs widely.

P&B provide an incisive history of operationalism from the physicist Bridgeman through the Vienna Circle and logical positivism, and then to behaviorism in psychology. Having known personally some of the key developers of OC within psychiatry (Guze, Spitzer, and Winokur), I can, with some confidence, say that none of them were knowledgeable about this history. For better or worse, OC arose from a distinctly pragmatic strain within American psychiatry. Two influences were noteworthy in discussions with these founding figures. One was the previous use of OC for medical disorders especially rheumatic conditions disorders (Cohen et al. 1971; Jones 1944). The second was the strong reaction against psychoanalytic psychiatry with its near complete lack of interest in diagnosis, viewing it as a "preoccupation" with the unimportant "surface features" of psychiatric illness. Given the pragmatic orientation of the OC developers in the United States and their lack of the continental intellectual/philosophical traditions, it is little surprise that they used the OC without an appreciation of its history, clearly articulated by P&B. One of the chief virtues of this chapter is that it sets the OC "revolution" in its appropriate historical/conceptual context and effectively counterbalances the excessively triumphalist "official" version of its adoption.

Let me close with two points. First, I do not fully agree with P&B's view that psychiatric nosology is in a deep state of crisis. The path to DSM-5 certainly proved rockier than anyone predicted. A number of the injuries received in the public eye by organized US psychiatry were, in my view, partly self-inflicted. The effort could have been better coordinated with a stronger emphasis on rigorous and carefully implemented criteria for change. However, at the time of this writing, DSM-5 has now been in print or published for 9 months. The intense media coverage has ceased. The document itself does not represent radical departures from prior traditions and some (but not all) of the proposed changes are rather well empirically supported. I do not wish to argue that "all is well." There have been important adverse effects of the "DSM revolution." Critics of psychiatric nosology remain active and have some legitimate targets. But the system is not in current danger of collapse.

Second, there is another "deep" philosophical issue lurking at the corners of this discussion. Succinctly, do we think that diagnostic criteria (à la DSM-5 or ICD-11) "index" or "constitute" the disorder? I believe (but have not asked) that most senior psychiatric nosologists even in the United States would opt for the "index" option. They would, I hope, also note that these criteria reflect one fallible set of indices that we will try, with time, to improve upon. But many junior psychiatrists and trainees act as if the criteria "constitute" the disorder. That is, the presence or absence of the criteria are "all you need to know" about the condition. It is this assumption about the DSM that, perhaps largely unconsciously, has driven the "impoverishment of psychopathology" which reflects one of worst sequelae of the adoption of OC.

References

Cohen, A.S., Reynolds, W.E., Franklin, E.D., Kulka, J.P., Ropes, M.W., Shulman, L.E., et al. (1971). Preliminary criteria for the classification of systemic lupus erythematosus. *Bulletin on the Rheumatic Diseases*, 21(9), 643–648.

Jones, T.D. (1944). The diagnosis of rheumatic fever. *Journal of the American Medical Association*, 126(8), 481–484.

Parnas, J., Handest, P., Jansson, L., and Saebye, D. (2005). Anomalous subjective experience among first-admitted schizophrenia spectrum patients: empirical investigation. *Psychopathology*, 38(5), 259–267.

Chapter 23

Psychiatry made easy: operation(al)ism and some of its consequences

Josef Parnas and Pierre Bovet

23.1 Introduction

The introduction of polythetic diagnostic criteria and the so-called operational definitions of such criteria in the DSM-III (American Psychiatric Association 1980) and in its subsequent editions (DSM-IIIR, -IV, -IV-TR, and -5, henceforth DSM-III+), and replicated in the ICD-10 in 1992, reflects perhaps the most profound transformation of clinical and scientific psychiatry in the twentieth century.

Psychiatric diagnosis, prior to this based on textbook narrative prototype-descriptions and a process of matching the individual patient's clinical picture to such prototypes, was replaced by an explicit process of identifying a sufficient number of relevant symptoms and signs, representing allegedly "operational criteria" of the category in question. The "operational revolution" in psychiatry is an example par excellence of a profound scientific change that happened at the intersection of certain specific sociohistorical circumstances, novel theoretical ideas, conceptual and empirical crises and developments, cultural, linguistic, and political transformations, and a strong activism of a few, influential professionals. In other words, we witness here a multitude of "decision vectors" at play (see Solomon, Chapter 8, this volume).

The notions of "operational diagnoses" and "operational criteria" have acquired an exalted status among psychiatrists (Sato and Berrios 2001). Beginning at the undergraduate level, a student of psychiatry is trained to believe that whatever is called "operational" guarantees a high degree of objectivity needed by a scientific and evidence-based psychiatry. Given this mesmerizing effect of the adjective "operational," it is striking to realize that most psychiatrists are simply unaware of what the term "operational" actually signifies. The contemporary diagnostic manuals (DSM-III+, ICD-10) do not provide any precise definition of this term and are mute on its origins and introduction in psychiatry. As Sato and Berrios (2001) conclude: "One of the central innovative features of DSM [i.e., operational criteria] has not received much academic concern, as though the adjective 'operational' hints at some *basso continuo* that regulates whole music yet remains inconspicuous."

In this chapter, we will try to explicate the issue "operational." We will trace its origins and permutation before and after its introduction in psychiatry. We cannot dissociate the issue of operationalism from the closely related, epistemological problems confronting psychiatry today. Therefore, we will also summarize *some* of the consequences of operationalism.

This chapter is written from a perspective of psychiatric clinicians-researchers, with a bent for epistemology, philosophy of mind, and phenomenology (Parnas and Bovet 1991, 1995). We have both experienced firsthand the operational transformations in psychiatry during our professional careers, which also include international teaching of psychopathology and research collaborations.

23.2 The Origins of Operationalism

It is customary to trace back the roots of operationalism in psychiatry to the neo-positivist philosopher Carl Hempel and his lecture at a conference of the American Psychiatric Association (APA) in 1959 (Zubin 1961). Actually, however, it was a renowned Harvard high-pressure physicist and Nobel Prize laureate, Percy W. Bridgman, who some 30 years earlier urged the scientific community to change its attitude toward concepts, advocating "the operational character of concepts" (Bridgman 1927), a proposal foreshadowed in the writings of American pragmatists such as Charles Peirce and William James.

At the beginning of the twentieth century, physics was marked by a profound intellectual turbulence, stirred by the epoch-making arrivals of Einstein's relativity theories and of quantum physics, novelties that forever buried the, until then, prevailing Newtonian paradigm:

> It was a great shock to discover that classical concepts, accepted unquestioningly, were inadequate to meet the [situation of physics after Einstein's theories of relativity], and the shock of this discovery has resulted in a critical attitude toward our whole conceptual structure [...] We should now make it our business to understand so thoroughly the character of our [...] [conceptual] relations to nature that another change [...] such as that due to Einstein, shall be forever impossible. (Bridgman 1927, pp.1–2)

Bridgman noted that many concepts in physics have been defined in terms of their *preconceived* properties, such as Newton's Absolute Time, "flowing equably without regard to anything external," but that, often, no such properties can actually (experimentally) be found in nature. Thus, the attitude toward concepts has to change: a concept is only fixed (i.e., its meaning unequivocally determined) when the *operations by which it is determined* are fixed.

"In general, we mean by any concept nothing more than a set of operations; *the concept is synonymous with the corresponding set of operations*" (Bridgman 1927, p. 5). Bridgman points out that for instance, "the concept of length" equals the set of procedures by which it is measured. But the set of operations appropriate to measure length will vary when measuring the length of an ordinary static, middle-size object, an object moving at a very high velocity, a very large object, a stellar distance, or a length at subatomic level. Not only will the set of operations be different, but also the set of *accompanying assumptions,* necessary to validate the measurement, will vary (e.g., assumptions about simultaneity, about the Euclidean character of space, or about the field equations of electrodynamics). Outside the domain in which a given concept has been operationally defined, one might be forced to replace the original operations by others (e.g., replacing a measuring rod with a radar).

> [However], we must recognize in principle that *in changing the operations we have really changed the concept,* and that to use the same name for these different concepts over the entire range is dictated only by considerations of convenience. (Bridgman 1927, p. 23, our italics)

The motivation for Bridgman's proposal was to secure an incremental scientific progress by liberating scientists from potentially damaging interferences from unwarranted, often implicit or unconscious, metaphysical assumptions ("speculative abstractions," such as Newton's Absolute Time), hindering empirical progress.

The philosophers and scientists of the so-called Vienna Circle, promoting logical positivism (logical empiricism), quickly picked up Bridgman's ideas, which were both positively and negatively received. Defining concepts by operations appeared to facilitate implementation of the verifiability criterion of meaning. It also seemed to solve the problem of potential theory-, habit-, or language-derived contaminations of scientific, "observational" statements about the world. However, a critique was also articulated almost immediately (and later) by some prominent members of the Vienna Circle (e.g., Carnap), who considered "Bridgman's analysis as an ultimately unworkable oversimplification of the extremely intricate problem of meaning" (Green 1992, p. 296).

Nevertheless, many American psychologists, who considered Bridgman's ideas as an appropriate philosophy of science on which the emergent behaviorism might be founded, welcomed them warmly (an example of an operationalist solution to defining the concept of "intelligence," would be the following *operational* definition: "Intelligence is what is measured by the IQ-tests"). They converted Bridgman's operational *attitude,* a pragmatic and antimetaphysical proposal, into a dogmatic full-blown philosophy of science, which they named "operationism" (operationalism):

> The revolution that will put an end to the possibility of revolutions is the one that defines a straightforward procedure for the definition and validation of concepts. [...] Such a procedure is the one, which tests the meaning of concepts by appealing to the concrete operations by which the concept is determined. We may call it *operationism.* (Stevens 1935, p. 323)

This outcome actually frightened Bridgman: "I feel as if I have created a Frankenstein, which has certainly gotten away from me. *I abhor the word operationalism or operationism, which seems to imply a dogma or at least a thesis of some kind*" (Bridgman 1961, p. 76, our italics). In our opinion, Bridgman was rather inclined to antirealism, emphasizing the primacy of subjective experience and intrinsic incompleteness of empirical knowledge. His position seemed to be close to *phenomenalism*, a philosophical claim that statements about reality are reducible to statements about sense data.

23.3 Operationalism meets the Psychiatric Audience

Joseph Zubin and the APA organized in February 1959 a conference discussing the problems involved in the field studies of mental disorders. The conference was prompted by the unsystematic application of the international classification of mental disorders. Stengel, a major British expert on classification, expressed concern that the chapter on mental disorders in the ICD (released by the World Health Organization (WHO) in 1956) was the only section to be either *ignored* or *simply rejected* in many countries (Freedman et al. 1986).

The conference gathered approximately 40 leading American and European specialists in epidemiology and/or psychopathology such as E. Essen-Möller, B.G. Greenberg, P.H. Hoch, A.B. Hollingshead, M. Kramer, A. Lewis, Ø. Ødegaard, P. Pichot, E. Stengel, D. Wechsler, and J. Zubin.

Carl Hempel, a professor of philosophy at Princeton University (the only participant not involved professionally in health issues), delivered the main introductory lecture on the problems of taxonomy. Although Hempel's direct influence on the construction of the DSM-III (vide infra) was very limited (K.S. Kendler and R. Spitzer, personal information), his lecture is crucial to the story because of its strong impact on many of the attending participants (Zubin 1961). Hempel, a logical positivist, emphasized the idea of unity of science and (ultimately) a *nomological regulation* of scientific concepts (i.e., the use of concepts becoming anchored by their role in the laws of nature). Hempel introduced the concept of "operational definition" by exposing Bridgman's ideas in his own way:

> An operational definition for a given term is conceived as providing objective criteria by means of which any scientific investigator can decide, for any particular case, whether the term does or does not apply to that case. To this end, the operational definition specifies a testing "operation" T that can be performed on any case to which the given term could conceivably apply, and a certain outcome O of the testing operation, whose occurrence is to count as the criterion for the applicability of the term to the given case. Schematically, an operational definition of a scientific term S is a stipulation to the effect that S is to apply to all and only those cases for which performance of test operation T yields the specified outcome O. (Hempel 1961, p. 8)

Using an example from mineralogy, Hempel proposed, one could define mineral X as "being *harder*" than mineral Y if X can make a scratch on Y but not the other way round. The concept "harder" is here precisely defined by the result of a specific procedure or *operation* (tracking a sharp point of X under pressure over the surface of Y) that can be applied by anyone and repeated at any time or place. Yet Hempel realized that this method of defining would not be suitable for the vast majority of descriptive terms in psychiatry. He therefore suggested that "if the insistence on an *operational* specification of meaning for scientific terms is not to be unduly restrictive, the idea of operation has to be taken in a very liberal sense which does not require manipulation of the objects under consideration; the mere observation of an object [...] must be allowed to count as an operation." Of course, Hempel explicitly excluded any "reference to introspective and subjective" data (Hempel 1961, pp. 10–11).

Hempel departed from Bridgman *in two fundamental ways* (Sato 1997; Sato and Berrios 2001). "Mere observation" is, of course, *in stark contrast with the centrality of Bridgman's insistence on a specified set of operations* (procedures) or action rules. Second, Hempel conceded that a mere filling out of a checklist of observable characteristics might count as operational definition of a concept:

> Consider the checklist of characteristics, which Sheldon gives for dominant endomorphy. [It] includes such directly observable features as roundness and softness of body, [...] short neck, [...]. This is a *satisfactory way* of determining the concept of predominant endomorphy. (Hempel 1961, p. 10, our italics)[1]

For Bridgman, however, it was the very *act of observation itself*, and *not the characteristics to be observed*, that should count as "operation."

Needless to say that a psychopathology, based on the checklists of "directly observable features" and excluding the subjective realm, would become heavily behaviorist.

Shortly after the conference, Stengel proposed in the WHO *Bulletin* the introduction of "operational definitions" as a principle that would reduce the difficulties in psychiatric classification (Stengel 1959).

23.4 The Making of the DSM-III

At this point, it is necessary to sketch the general scientific, sociological, and political context prevailing during the 1960s and the 1970s in the United States (described in detail by Wilson (1993)) in order to understand why the DSM-III was able to transform American psychiatry so radically and so rapidly.

---

[1] It is worth recalling that Hempel also stressed that "clear and objective criteria of application are not sufficient," and that in order to be scientifically useful, concepts must lend themselves to "the formulation of general laws or theoretical principles which reflect uniformities in the subject matter under study" (Hempel 1959, p. 14), and gave as an example of such theoretical underpinning Kretschmer's typological system. Moreover, he stressed that only some terms could be operationally defined (trying to define everything would lead to infinite regress), and their use was dependent on implicit pre-understanding of a web of other concepts. Hempel also suggested that in practice, objects often resist to be classified in terms of a yes-or-no, an either-or matter, and that many "recent typological systems have replaced a strictly classificatory procedure by an *ordering* one," thus foreshadowing a dimensional approach to classification. It may also be added that one of the participants, Dr. A. Lewis, proposed *different* classification systems for different purposes: a "public" system, for disease statistics and cross-country comparisons, and "private" systems, for specific and varying purposes of psychiatric research groups (A. Lewis, in Zubin 1961, p. 34.)

During the post-World War II years, the psychosocial model (bringing together conceptions of Freud and Meyer) became predominant in American psychiatry (see also Michels, Chapter 20, this volume). The main assumption of the psychosocial model was that the transition from mental well to ill being is fluid; anyone, if exposed to severe enough environmental trauma, may fall ill. Mental illness was thus essentially seen as a *reactive psychological process*. The most renowned spokesman of the psychosocial model was Karl Menninger, who regarded the descriptive diagnoses as irrelevant and considered the syndromes described by Kraepelin to be reducible to a single and fundamental psychosocial process: *a failure of the individual to adapt to environmental stressors*. The psychosocial model became influential in a large variety of social practices: child rearing, education, management of human resources in industry and business, and so on. However, this large horizontal dissemination of the psychosocial model turned out to be also the source for its decline. Attacks came from within the profession, because the model did not lead to visible progress in research. The need for a nosological change became increasingly evident due to the availability of efficient psychotropic drugs (antipsychotics, antidepressants, and lithium salts), believed to be selectively effective in specific disorders. Particularly lithium salts (approved by the US Food and Drug Administration in 1970) proved dramatically effective in the treatment of bipolar disorder and made the *differential diagnosis of psychotic conditions to be of paramount importance*.

Other academic fields also voiced dissatisfaction with the psychosocial model: if mental illness is purely psychosocial, why should it remain the reserved province of medicine? The movement of antipsychiatry amplified this critique: if the boundary between normal and abnormal is fuzzy, then psychiatric diagnoses are arbitrary and can hardly be called diseases. Mental illness is a "myth" (Szasz 1961). Finally, the financial restrictions of the mid 1970s began to force psychiatry to be more accountable for its practice.

It is in this specific climate that the results from the US–UK Diagnostic Project (Cooper et al. 1972) created shock and impetus for change. The project, comparing American and British diagnostic habits, demonstrated that American psychiatrists grossly overdiagnosed schizophrenia at the expense of affective psychosis. It also demonstrated that using shared diagnostic criteria and standardized diagnostic questionnaires made the American diagnoses more similar to those of British psychiatrists. Another shock came from Rosenhan's study (1973). He sent out eight normal subjects to present themselves at different psychiatric hospitals with a single complaint of an unelaborated verbal hallucination. All were hospitalized and, although they behaved normally during their whole admission, all were discharged with the diagnosis of "schizophrenia in remission."

The change emerged from a group of psychiatrists at Washington University in St. Louis, who did not share the nosological disinterest of their peers. The group organized regular seminars for discussing ways of improving psychiatric diagnosis (Kendler et al. 2010). This effort was initiated by Edwin Gildea in the 1950s, and came to include G. Winokur, E. Robins, S. Guze, R. Woodruff, and R. Munoz. The group, eventually labelled as the "neo-Kraepelinians," advocated a biological-reductive research program to identify biological substrates of psychiatric "diseases," "carving nature at its joints." Their work culminated with the publication of the so-called "Feighner"- or "St. Louis" citeria (Feighner et al. 1972), subsequently elaborated and modified by Spitzer et al. (1978) as Research Diagnostic Criteria. These were the first, internationally famous, examples of "operationally defined" diagnostic criteria, which played an important role as the forerunners of DSM-III.

The group of people surrounding Robert Spitzer in New York, and involved in the forthcoming remake of psychiatric diagnosis (including the Europeans R. Kendell and E. Stengel), was in a close and continuous contact with the St. Louis circle. Being explicitly designed for research purposes, the Feighner and the RDC criteria overemphasized reliability (at the expense of validity), because the exclusion of false-negatives was considered less prejudicial than the inclusion of false-positives. Ultimately, a de facto fusion (still influential today) occurred between the operational project and the neo-Kraepelinian reductive research program, the former serving as the means for the latter. Spitzer became the head of the Task Force on Nomenclature and Statistics at the APA with the purpose of constructing the DSM-III. Unfortunately:

> The principles guiding the task force's work were in place from the very beginning. These guiding principles were never debated among the task force members, not only because of their common adherence to "operational" principles applied to descriptive psychiatry but also because of their common vision of where the profession should move in the future. [...] *Nearly every issue related to the development of DSM-III that was to become a controversy within the profession was decided without controversy by the task force at the beginning.* (Wilson 1993, p. 405, our italics)

These principles can be summarized as follows: etiology should not serve as a classificatory principle unless it was clearly known; diagnosis should be made on the basis of selected criteria for that diagnosis; the diagnostic criteria should favor the directly or easily observable features (requiring a minimum of inference, i.e., an essentially behaviorist agenda), and the phrasing of the criteria should be made in a simple, nontechnical language (assumed to assure unambiguity); "psychosis" and "neurosis" were not useful as classificatory principles but only as adjectives; mental disorders should be defined narrowly rather than broadly. The diagnostic system should be "a-theoretical." In fact, *no psychopathological-phenomenological framework* was applied *for describing subjectivity* (e.g., à la Jaspers), which might have had the potential to conceptualize psychopathological phenomena more precisely and to connect them into larger, clinically meaningful wholes. The single symptoms/signs came to be considered as mutually independent entities, co-occurring in a given diagnostic entity either due to an empirical, syndromatic contingency or inherited from tradition.

Up to the end of 1975, operational criteria were supposed to only be listed under the heading of "Suggested Criteria." They "*would not replace but merely supplement* the narrative definitions of the diagnostic categories" (Spitzer et al. 1975, p. 1190, our italics):

The use of specified criteria does not eliminate clinical judgment. *The proper use of such criteria requires a considerable amount of clinical experience and knowledge of psychopathology* because the criteria involve clinical concepts rather than a mere enumeration of complaints or observations of atomistic behaviors. [...] In any case, the criteria that may be listed in DSM-III would be 'suggested' only, and any clinician would be free to use them or ignore them as he saw fit. (Spitzer et al. 1975, p. 1191, our italics)

Unfortunately, this precaution did not survive into the published version of the DSM-III.

The risk of impoverishment of psychopathology was largely underestimated and even unforeseen. Only few, isolated voices (e.g., Faust and Miner 1986; Schwartz and Wiggins 1986, 1987a, 1987b) argued that the type of logical empiricism endorsed by the DSM-III was a regression to earlier, obsolete, and for psychiatry, quite inadequate views of scientific enterprise.

The DSM-III spread surprisingly quickly across the United States. Basically, DSM-III seemed to contain everything that a textbook of psychiatry needed to contain. It offered a shortcut to psychiatry by providing an easily readable, lay-language text, free of lengthy, descriptively rich, and conceptually demanding passages. For a pragmatically- and simplicity minded (US and international) audience, it was a gift.

23.5 "Operationalism" goes International: The ICD-10

The situation in European psychiatry during those years was significantly different from its transatlantic cousin's. Although with heterogeneous "schools of thought" (especially the French nosology differed significantly from the rest of Europe (Sartorius et al. 1990)) and linguistic differences, psychiatry in Europe was firmly, even if sometimes implicitly, based on the basic tenets of phenomenological psychopathology ("phenomenological" in the continental sense of the term), outlined and disseminated by, for example, Karl Jaspers, Kurt Schneider, Pierre Janet, Eugène Minkowski, and Henri Ey. Phenomenology seemed to have functioned as a conceptual and clinical *buffer* between different schools and pressures, preventing radical, pendulum-like swings of theoretical orientation. In many countries, psychoanalysis, biological psychiatry, psychosomatic and epidemiological research, and a newly beginning social psychiatry coexisted more or less peacefully. The majority of European academic psychiatrists of that time were multilingual, and eager to read scientific papers in various languages. For example, Manfred Bleuler, in his 1978 book, apologized for what he considered "regrettable limitations":

I did not have adequate knowledge of foreign languages. I was able to read efficiently only those papers that were originally written in German, English, or French, and with some considerable effort the Italian ones as well. [...] In other languages I had to depend on summaries [...] [those] that were particularly vital to my work [...] I had translated for my use. (Bleuler 1978, p. 49)

The influence by American science, culture, and, in particular, of the English language was very strong in those years in Europe and worldwide. Publishing in English, a new *lingua franca*, was increasingly regarded as being more prestigious and "international" than publishing in German or French. The high-ranking journals became increasingly the English-language journals.

Two influential British psychiatrists, Erwin Stengel (participant of the 1959 conference) and Robert Kendell, pushed for the adoption of operational definitions in psychiatry: "All diagnoses should be explicitly shorn of their aetiological implications and regarded simply as 'operational definitions' for certain types of behaviour" (Kendell 1975, p. 93).

The WHO's International Pilot Studies on Schizophrenia, involving several international centers (Jablensky and Sartorius 2008) also contributed to the project of common nosology. Thus, there emerged a consensus that a shared international nomenclature was needed to overcome parochial tendencies, improve statistical and epidemiological comparisons, facilitate research communication, and standardize the diagnostic, clinical, and treatment options.

The ICD-10, published in 1992, mimicked the essential tenets of the DSM-III (despite some differences). Most psychiatrists saw it as a step in the right direction, as a useful *guide* for making diagnoses more uniform. It was not anticipated that the ICD-10 would acquire a dogmatic influence and become an exclusive source of knowledge for psychiatrists in training, replacing the textbooks and seminal treatise descriptions, obviating a serious study of psychopathology, thus repeating the US experience with the DSM-III (Andreasen 2007).

23.6 What is "operational" in Operational Psychiatric Diagnoses and Diagnostic Criteria?

It is now time to determine in what sense psychiatric diagnoses and criteria are "operational." We will try to make *explicitly audible* the implicit *basso continuo* to which Sato and Berrios (2001) refer. We will examine to what extent the operations in psychiatry are consistent with the fundamental ideas of operationalism, that is, "operational" as equal to the specification of *measurement procedures rules* or *action rules*. We will ignore here Hempel's suggestion that "observation of an object" may count as "operation," because this modification empties the concept of "operation" of all its epistemological or scientific meaning.[2]

---

[2] Hempel's claim that "the criteria of application for a term may well be specified by reference to certain characteristics which can be ascertained *without any testing procedure more complicated than direct observation*" was a *regression* to earlier and quite problematic ideas of logical empiricism, the problems to which Bridgman's proposal was a solution. In brief, logical empiricism originally claimed that the world may be faithfully described by simple, atomic, "observational" or "record" statements (*Beobachtungssätze, Protokollsätze*). The problem of such descriptions, pointed out by the critics, was that no linguistic statements are "theory-free" (Parnas and Sass 2008). Bridgman's "operational

The polythetic diagnosis in the DSM-III+/ICD-10 is based (with inclusion and exclusion criteria) on a list of symptoms and signs ("criteria"), believed to be characteristic for a diagnostic category in question. A specific *number* of symptoms or signs detected from a given list in a given patient is *sufficient* to arrive at a diagnosis. We can say that the *operation* involved in the diagnostic process consists of "symptom counting" (McHugh 2012); for example, in a given case, *counting up* to, say, number five, gives us the correct diagnosis. Although *counting* is a *mental operation*, the operational nature of the diagnostic category itself depends on whether the counted component criteria lend themselves to operational definitions.

Are, then, the diagnostic criteria "operational" in any significant, epistemological sense? The answer to this question is a clear-cut *no*. The operational definition, as a measurement rule whose execution links the concept with its referent in reality in a clear-cut, unambiguous way (e.g., like the notion of "harder" in mineralogy, vide supra), is simply *inapplicable*, and therefore *unapplied*, to the vast majority of psychiatric terms. Instead, the symptoms and signs (criteria) are described in a common-sense, lay language at "the lowest order of inference" (American Psychiatric Association 1980, p. 7), although such desideratum was not implementable throughout the entire manual: "For some disorders, however, [...] a much higher order of inference is necessary" (American Psychiatric Association 1980, p. 7). The DSM/ICD definitions are disconnected from any phenomenological or conceptual considerations that existed in the classical texts and textbooks of psychopathology and that are frequently necessary to clarify more precisely the meaning of the term in question (e.g., formal thought disorder[3]). Phrased otherwise: psychiatric terms are impossible to define unequivocally as simple atomic entities but nearly always require an embededness in a conceptual/theoretical and ostensive context (e.g., with prototypical examples and discussions of their limits (Nordgaard et al. 2013; Parnas et al. 2013)). This was, in fact, an issue briefly touched upon in the discussion following Hempel's 1959 lecture (Zubin 1961, pp. 34–35). The authors of DSM-III/ICD-10 mistakenly believed that a simplistic approach to what in Europe is known as psychiatry's (notorious) "problem of description" (Nordgaard and Parnas 2013), would guarantee a reliable, context- and culture-immune understanding and use of the diagnostic

---

definitions" were specifically intended to solve this problem of hidden, unwarranted metaphysical contaminations of scientific concepts.

[3] To be able to identify clinically significant manifestations of formal thought disorder (yet less severe than the level stipulated for schizophrenia in the DSM-IV) requires not only a lot of supervised training but also acquisition and certain mastery of relevant theoretical issues, for instance, semantic-grammatical distinction, terms related to the nature of concepts (e.g., vagueness, concreteness, difference between organic and schizophrenic concreteness, metaphor, metonymy, etc.), and some knowledge about intersubjective and pragmatic aspects of discourse (the word "Monicagate," coined by a journalist to describe Bill Clinton's affair, is not considered as a schizophrenic neologism, whereas the word "nervebite," coined by a patient suffering from a neuralgic facial pain, would be, even though these two words have similar linguistic structure).

criteria (Mishara 1994; Mishara and Schwartz 2010). For example, *delusions* are defined in the DSM-5 as "fixed beliefs that are not amenable to change in light of conflicting evidence." Apart from the likelihood that half of humanity harbors beliefs so defined, the definition is hardly useful for the training of psychiatrists or as a quick, disambiguating diagnostic reference aid.[4] And consider such (DSM-IV) criteria as "identity disturbance … with unstable self-image or sense of self" or feeling "restless … or keyed up or on edge," or "a pattern of unstable and intense interpersonal relationships." All such features require forms of judgment and complex pattern recognition that cannot be taught or conveyed by a brief, ordinary language, common-sense descriptive statement (Nordgaard et al. 2013).

We are now left to examine the ordinary linguistic meaning of the term "operational." The online *Concise Oxford English Dictionary* (11th edition) gives the following definitions:

> Adjective operational: 1. In or ready for use: *the new laboratory is fully operational*; Relating to the routine functioning and activities of an organization: *the coffee bar's initial operational costs;* Relating to active operations of the armed forces, police, or emergency services: *an operational fighter squadron*. 2. *Philosophy*: Relating to or in accordance with operationalism.

In sum, since the adjective "operational" in psychiatry has nothing to do with philosophical operationalism, we end up with the conclusion that it simply, but *misleadingly*, means "easily applicable" or "ready for use."

23.7 *Selected* Consequences of the Operational Project

Today, more than 30 years after the introduction of the DSM-III, psychiatry again seems to confront a crisis. A chorus of critical voices, doubting the necessity of a new revision, or debating the justification for including/excluding/modifying certain diagnoses, surrounded the preparations for the release of the DSM-5. However, more general assessments of the DSM-III+ project have also been offered. Nancy Andreasen (2007), a prominent member of the Task Force on the DSM-III, published a paper on the "unintended consequences" of the DSM-III+ project. In the hindsight, she now believes that the operational project caused the "death" of American phenomenology (i.e., descriptive psychopathology):

---

[4] Two independent forensic psycho-diagnostic assessments of Anders Breivik (a Norwegian mass murderer who in 2011 bombed government buildings in Oslo, resulting in eight deaths, and then carried out a mass shooting on the island of Utøya, where he killed 69 people, mostly teenagers youths) resulted in the ICD-10 diagnoses of paranoid schizophrenia and narcissistic personality disorder, respectively. Clearly, no appeal to "operational definitions" could disambiguate the question whether Breivik was delusional or not (Melle 2013; Parnas 2013).

DSM-III and its successors [...] became universally and uncritically accepted as the ultimate authority on psychopathology and diagnosis. [...] Because DSM is often used as a primary textbook or the major diagnostic resource in many clinical and research settings, students typically do not know about other potentially important or interesting signs and symptoms that are not included in DSM. [...] DSM has had a dehumanizing impact on the practice of psychiatry. (Andreasen 2007, p. 111)

Hyman listed the counterproductive consequences of a complete monopolization of the editorial, funding, and research practices by the DSM-III+ categories, which, with the passage of time, naïvely came to be considered as unshakably valid (true) nosological entities (a process that Hyman calls "reification"), rather than taken for what they really were intended to be, namely heuristic or provisional proposals:

> As a result of its widespread acceptance, and the de facto reification of its diagnostic silos, the DSM-IV exerts far too much influence on the questions that scientists can ask and, in practice, do ask. [...] In the clinic, the limitations of the current [...] approach can be illustrated in three salient areas: (1) the problem of comorbidity, (2) the widespread need for "not otherwise specific (NOS)" diagnoses, and (3) the arbitrariness of diagnostic thresholds. (Hyman 2011)[5]

Many express a disappointment by the lack of advances in etiological and therapeutic knowledge, pointing to a "growing disconnect" between "the brilliant progress" of neurosciences and its "nearly complete failure" to translate into the diagnostic or therapeutic gains in psychiatry (Frances and Widiger 2012; Hyman 2010, 2012). There is an explosion of publications from a reborn antipsychiatry. Psychiatric academia is seen as becoming rapidly irrelevant to the concerns of clinicians (Kleinman 2012). In sum, serious concerns about the status and the future of psychiatry are being voiced (Katschnig 2010).

A prediction in the 1980s of rapid, groundbreaking discoveries is now replaced by a prospect of "gradual and painstaking work of many decades" (Frances 2013, p. 112), alas involving more of the same, only this time a more sophisticated approach, for example, studying "intracellular mechanisms" or "neural networks" (Hyman 2012). The recently launched Research Domain Criteria (RDoC)

---

[5] The concept of schizophrenia is perhaps a potential candidate case for the DSM-linked "reification" that may, very likely, have impeded clinical and research progress. First, the DSM-III+ criteria fail to reproduce the foundational, core (trait or fundamental) phenotypic features of the schizophrenia spectrum disorders (Parnas 2011, 2012a, 2012b). Second, a rigid framing of all research by the DSM-III+ criteria was certainly inappropriate given the ample empirical evidence that the number of patients diagnosed with schizophrenia, *within the same clinical sample*, varies considerably as a function of different, yet equally "reasonable," diagnostic criteria (Jansson et al. 2002; Jansson and Parnas 2007). One way of viewing a worldwide expansion of "prodromal research" (and a proposal of the diagnostic category of "attenuated psychosis syndrome" for DSM-5) is to consider this research as an attempt to overcome rigid (either/or) and clinically not useful boundaries of the schizophrenia concept in the DSM-IV/ICD-10.

proposal to study behavioral constructs with known neural bases (e.g., negative/positive valence systems, arousal/regulatory systems, etc. (Insel et al. 2010)) essentially suspends and defers the nosological concerns in the face of the difficulties posed by phenotype-guided research.

It is noteworthy that Andreasen's, Hyman's, and others' critiques do not consider the original operational project as having been *misconceived*. Rather, they believe that it was its fallible human execution that has gone astray. Thus, the critiques of the DSM+ (and suggested solutions) are all mute on what we believe are the *root theoretical problems of operational psychiatry*. These "inborn errors" could not avoid entailing the consequences described by Andreasen, Hyman, and others. Unfortunately, the theoretical issues continue to be disregarded. A proposal of Kendler et al. (2008) to establish a Conceptual Issues Work Group for DSM-5 was met with indifference or resistance and never materialized.

23.8 Epistemological Considerations

The root problem, in our view, is the *vast oversimplification of the ontology* (the nature of being) *and epistemology of the psychiatric object* (symptoms, signs (Parnas et al. 2013)), coupled with oblivion and/or ignorance of the resources already existing in the preoperational psychopathology and in contemporary phenomenology and philosophy of mind.[6]

Many psychiatrists believe that "the only reason most mental disorders are still defined by their clinical syndromes is that the human brain is an infinitely *more complex machine* ... [than] the heart, kidney, or liver" (Kendell 2002, p. 13, our italics). Kendell's equation of nephrology with psychiatry (*pace* complexity) is a prevalent, alas unquestioned, *category mistake*. In this model, the individual symptoms/signs are considered to be identical with specific configurations of dysfunctional neural networks (i.e., signals of dysfunction). There is no concern that biological reductionism, so successful in somatic medicine, may be in psychiatry facing the complications of what philosophers call the "explanatory gap" (Levine 1983), "the hard problem of consciousness" (Chalmers 1995) or some other, defiant distinctiveness of the ontology and epistemology of human consciousness (Parnas et al. 2013). In our view, a deplored lack of scientific progress is unrelated to a still insufficient resolution power of biotechnologies or the very existence of a phenotype-based classification. Rather, the stagnation is more fundamentally linked to a mismatch between the nature of phenomenal consciousness and the reductionistic-behaviorist epistemology inherent in the DSM-III+ operational project. This mismatch comprises inadequacy (or lack) of concepts, oversimplification of psychopathology, with deformed, insufficient, or arbitrary phenotypic distinctions, and coupled with an almost complete absence of empirical research

---

[6] A study of Bennett and Hacker's (2003) book on the philosophical issues involved in the sciences of mind would be a useful (and most likely highly rewarding) conceptual exercise in the education of psychiatrists.

that is not purely technology driven but also motivated by insights inspired by an intimate familiarity with the phenomenology of mental disorders (Urfer-Parnas et al. 2010).[7] In order to pursue the psychiatric etiological project of "naturalizing subjectivity," we need a prior, and serious study of the *explanandum* itself, i.e., consciousness and its pathologies. Indeed, "without some idea [...] of what the subjective character of experience is, we cannot know what is required of [...] [reductive] theory" (Nagel 1979).

23.8.1 The Object of Psychiatry: Pathologies of Subjectivity

The object of psychiatry is (and will remain) the patient's altered experience, expression, and existence, associated with "suffering in self and/or others" (Mishara and Schwartz 2010). We will therefore continue to need a clinical classification into which the brain enters in so far that it contributes to this suffering in *a medically relevant way* and not because the brain per se or *de jure* is of primary interest for psychiatry. The ontological status of subjectivity (consciousness) is unlike that of a *thing* or some other kind of, however complex, spatial, three-dimensional object (Parnas et al. 2013). Consciousness is a lived presence to itself and the world. "Psyche," writes Jaspers, is "not [...] an object [...] but 'being in one's own world', the integrating of an inner and outer world." Psyche does not consist of sharply separable, substantial intramental objects, exerting mechanical causality on each other. Rather, "it is (a) network of interdependent moments (i.e., nonindependent parts[8]) [...] founded on intentional intertwining, motivation and mutual implication, *in a way that has no analogue in the physical*" (Husserl 1977, section 37, our italics). In other words, in the physical domain, part-whole relations are determined by efficient (often mechanical) causality, whereas in the mental realm, part-whole relations are those of implication, motivation, entailment, etc. A rapidly emerging view in the philosophy of mind and neuroscience does not consider consciousness and cognition as being exclusively *confined to* the skull but rather as *extended*, that is, *constitutively including the physical and social Umwelt of the activity of the sentient organism*. On this view consciousness is "embodied, embedded, extended and enactive" (Clark 2008). Consciousness exhibits certain *structures*, crucially relevant for psychopathology, comprising intentionality (world-directedness), temporality, embodiment, self-awareness, and intersubjectivity (Parnas and Sass

---

[7] Only a small, and steadily shrinking fraction of those involved in neuropsychiatric research has any substantial clinical experience with psychiatric patients. It is striking that practically none of the neuropsychological tests currently in use in psychiatric research have been developed *inside of psychiatry*, for example, on the basis of reflections on the nature of mental disorders, but are imported from neurology or nonpsychiatric neuropsychology.

[8] Frequently proposed examples of "moments" (nondetachable parts) are color and extension. You cannot see a color without a surface and vice versa. They can only be detached in abstraction.

2008; Parnas and Zahavi 2002). Theoretically speaking, a psychiatric symptom is not a well-demarcated thing-like object, but rather a certain configuration that involves the flow of phenomenal consciousness, with its intentional contents and forms (structures). The symptoms are certain wholes of interpenetrating experiences, beliefs, expressions, and actions, all of them permeated by the patient's dispositions and by biographical (and not just biological) detail. The symptom individuates itself in the synchronic and diachronic *contexts* along all these dimensions, which combine into specific meaning-wholes. In short, a symptom/sign is not an entity "in itself"—easily or arbitrarily isolated out of the ongoing flow of consciousness, and described independently of its context. Rather, it may be best to consider the symptom in terms of a prototypical Gestalt.

23.8.2 Prototype and Gestalt

A prototype is a central example of the category in question (a sparrow is more typical of the category "bird" than is a penguin or an ostrich), with a graded dilution of typicality towards the borders of the category, where it eventually overlaps entities from neighboring categories. A prototype is *not just an example* (exemplar) but conveys a summary of the information on its internal configuration of properties, and in relation to neighboring prototypes (Murphy 2002). In psychiatry, we can use the concept of prototype-Gestalt in a narrow and a wide sense, neither one limited to perception but also involving more complex cognitions. In a narrow sense, a Gestalt is a *unity* or organization of phenomenal aspects that emerges from the relations between its experiential features (in terms of part-whole relations).[9] In a wider sense, the Gestalt transcends the experiential realm to entail a dynamic interplay of factors that extend throughout and beyond the organism (Weizsäcker 1986). One has to consider not just *a set of mental states*, but also the subject's pragmatic engagements in his physical and social environment. Detecting, for example, a delusion, which is a phenomenal Gestalt emerging from the interactions between numerous features (e.g., belief contents, their logical structures and mode of presentation, their ramifications, overarching belief framework, expressive/behavioral dimension, etc.) involves taking into account not only the contents of the patient's propositional statements but also his relational style, subjective experience, historical information, as well as relationships to other, potentially relevant Gestalts/prototypes. To competently use the concept of delusion, the psychiatrist must be familiar with a host of other prototypes and relevant background concepts (e.g., hallucination, passivity experience, overvalued idea, rationality, psychosis, etc.). It is tempting to quote Thomas Kuhn (1993) here: "Exposure to swans and geese plays an essential role in learning to recognize ducks" (p. 536). The concept of Gestalt/prototype is equally fit for description of symptoms and signs, and of larger entities, such as syndromes and diagnostic

---

[9] For a conceptual continuity between Gestalt theory, phenomenology, structuralism, and dynamic systems theory, see Petitot 2004.

categories. The prototypical approach also implies an intrinsic dimensionality of the diagnostic categories (Parnas and Gallagher in press).

The argument for a prototype-based approach is fundamentally linked to the fact that perception is (nearly) always apperceptively (conceptually) informed: perceiving something is to perceive it *as a something*, as a token or instance of a certain type,[10] an old insight of phenomenology and Gestalt psychology (Merleau-Ponty 1942), articulated against the classic empiricist view of the nature of perceptual experience as being accounted for by association of discrete, atomic "sense data." "A figure on a background is the simplest sensible given available to us" (Merleau-Ponty 1962, p. 4). We do not perceive an individual object as individual, that is, an autonomous and unfamiliar particular, but rather in terms of the type that implicitly includes it. The unknown is perceived in terms of the known, that is, in terms of "the general type that is activated in the particular perception" (Mishara and Schwartz 2010). This process, called *typification*, is intrinsic to all cognition and hence to the diagnostic process as well (Schwartz and Wiggins 1987a, 1987b). A natural unfolding of a comprehensive diagnostic assessment very much involves *reflective and critical questioning of typifications*, which become supported, modified, or discarded by explicitly elicited diagnostic information, progressively limiting the number of possible diagnostic options (Nordgaard et al. 2013). Yet typification as such can never be completely eliminated, even when assessing the most explicit kind of information, because it is an automatic and intrinsic aspect of our cognitive activity (Schwartz and Wiggins 1987a, 1987b; Westen 2012). It follows that the more knowledgeable and experienced is the psychiatrist, the greater and more refined is the conceptual (diagnostic) repertoire at his disposal (Jaspers 1913/1963).[11]

---

[10] Perception, and more generally, cognition, is *intentional*, that is, perception is always about something, it has a directionality towards its "intentional object." A distinction may be introduced here between *being conscious of* something and *being conscious that* something (Janzen 2008, p. 13). For example, I may be aware *of* a car passing by but not aware *that* it is a car (e.g., if I have been suddenly transported from a society where cars do not exist into a street of New York City). Similarly, a psychiatrist, listening to the patient's life history, may be aware *of* the patient's narrative but need not to be aware *that* the patient is talking about his profoundly insecure sense of basic identity (if the phenomenology of the sense of identity is unfamiliar to the psychiatrist). This latter example shows how experience and knowledge (i.e., conceptual framework) influence the content of perception.

[11] The psychiatrists assessing Anders Breivik noticed, with a certain perplexity, that Breivik had "a strange habit" of expressing himself in quantitative, percentage terms (e.g., "the mood today is at 30%"; "the wish to live dropped today by 10%"; "energy level today at 60%", etc.). The psychiatrists could not fit these statements into any specific psychopathological matrix (apart from qualifying this habit as "strange"). They were apparently unaware that this phenomenon is quite well described in classic psychiatric literature as a specific variant of the Gestalt of schizophrenic autism (Minkowski 1927, 1997; Parnas and Bovet 1991; Parnas et al. 2002). But autism was not included in DSM-III+: "Autism (is) perhaps a valid indicator of schizophrenia but (is) not used in the DSM-III criteria

An additional reason for taking prototypes seriously comes not from philosophy of mind or phenomenological psychopathology but from empirical cognitive research. A recent review of research on the mechanisms of concept formation, use, and understanding, suggests that *concepts are not constituted by a list of criteria* (which is called "the classical view") but are rather organized around *prototypes* (Machery 2009; see also Rosch 1973). Murphy (2002), in his seminal treatise on this issue, concluded that a "theory of concepts must be primarily prototype-based [...], within a broader knowledge representation scheme in which the concept is positioned both within a hierarchy and within a theoretical framework(s) appropriate to that domain" (p. 488).

23.8.3 Phenomenology

Psychopathological description, that is, individuation of experiential-expressive Gestalts that is not arbitrary or commonsensical but attempts to mirror the inherent distinctions of mental realm, is a task of phenomenology in its continental sense. It is a philosophically informed, systematic study of subjectivity that can be integrated into empirical research (Parnas and Sass 2008; Parnas and Zahavi 2002; Parnas et al. 2013). Phenomenological approach is mindful of implicit ideological prejudices, convictions of "natural attitude," premature objectivist- (strongly realist) or reductionist- assumptions, or of naïve tendencies to psychologize pathological phenomena. This suspending of explicit and implicit ontological dogmas and prejudices, called "phenomenological reduction" or "epoché," is *similar in spirit* to Bridgman's desideratum of cleansing scientific activity of interfering metaphysical influences.

23.8.4 Polythetic Diagnosis needs Prototypical Assistance

We will illustrate the issues described above by exposing some problematic aspects of polythetic diagnosis. For example, a major depression diagnosis in the DSM-IV is given when five or more symptoms out of a list of nine, of which at least one is "depressed mood" or "diminished interest or pleasure," are present for at least 2 weeks. It has been calculated that 227 different diagnostic combinations are possible following this definition (Østergaard et al. 2011). If the four criteria containing two symptoms ("weight loss or gain," "hypersomnia or insomnia," "agitation or retardation," and "feelings of worthlessness or inappropriate guilt") are split into their individual components, the total number of possible diagnostic combinations rises to 1497, without possible additional subdivisions (i.e., with or without psychosis, uni- or bipolar depression). We think that 1497 possible symptomatic combinations, coupled with their lack of temporal stability across relapses (Mann

---

because of its unreliability. [...] Autism probably is a basic feature of schizophrenia, but I do not know [...] how to define that concept operationally" (Robert Spitzer, in Klerman et al. 1984, p. 547).

2010), need some sort of connective, meaning conferring conceptualization. In the absence of extra-clinical markers, such conceptualization has to be articulated in phenomenological, prototypical-gestaltic terms. The example illustrates that assigning diagnosis by *counting symptoms,* while neglecting prototypical *quiddity* or *whatness* of the category in question (e.g., what *is* depression? What *does it mean* to be depressed?) may entail dubious validity of diagnostic categories and lead to absurd diagnostic practices (Parnas 2011, 2012a; Nordgaard et al. 2013).

23.8.5 Is the Structured Diagnostic Interview an Adequate Approach?

Another serious problem ensuing from the "operational revolution" is an almost universal use of structured interviews, considered to be the "gold standard" in research and, increasingly, in clinical work as well. Structured interviews consist of *preformed questions* asked in a *fixed sequence* ("do stick to the initial questions, as they are written …" (First et al. 2002)). This behaviorist purity of the stimulus-response paradigm ("publicly observable aspects of the behavior a subject shows in response to a specified publicly observable stimulus situation" (Hempel 1961, p. 11)) is assumed to be an adequate way of cutting through the complexities of experience and communication (reducing the "information variance"). The phrasing of the questions is as close as possible to the phrasing of the explored diagnostic criteria in order to minimize the "criterion variance." An implicit assumption behind the structured interviewing is that the symptom exists on analogy to a ripe fruit, hanging in the patient's consciousness, only waiting for a suitable push by a preformed interview question in order to fall down into a full view and naturally gravitate towards the corresponding diagnostic criterion. However, we also here face a theoretical and methodological singularity of psychiatry (Nordgaard et al. 2013, vide supra). Patients vary in their intellectual capacities, mastery of language and metaphor, their motivation, their impulse and ability to dissimulate, to entertain a "double book-keeping," etc. A symptom needs not to exist as a fully articulated, introspectible "mental object" but may exhibit a quasi-habitual, prereflective quality or even entail changes in the structure (form) of consciousness. Its reporting often involves recollection, imagination, and reflection. To adequately ask a relevant diagnostic question at a relevant moment requires a prior grasp of the conversational and situational *context*. All these (and countless other) reasons make the foundations of the structured interview something of an epistemological mystery. Our own empirical research demonstrated an extremely poor diagnostic performance of a fully structured interview (performed by a *for-the-purpose trained and certified*, freshly graduated clinical psychologist) in a sample of consecutive first hospital admissions (Nordgaard et al. 2012). Of 42 patients with a diagnosis of DSM-IV schizophrenia, only eight were so diagnosed by the fully structured interview. Extrapolating these results to a wider, psychiatric research context seriously questions the validity of research diagnoses and renders the celebrated diagnostic reliability empty of meaning.

23.9 Conclusions

It seems that psychiatry is facing a new crisis, which may become conductive to a "historical change," comparable in scope to that of the "operational revolution." Psychiatry will survive as a clinical-therapeutic activity because the patients will not vanish (Kleinman 2012). Yet, in order for psychiatry to survive as a *medical and academic profession*, the root theoretical issues selectively addressed above, need redressing, and urgently so. Briefly, psychiatry, because of the particular nature of its object, needs to regain its self-understanding as an intrinsically eclectic or *interdisciplinary*, and *scholarly* discipline, not only based on biology, but also upon a broad range of other sciences, including humanities. Psychiatry is *not now* and will probably *never be* "operational" in any philosophically pregnant sense. It needs to strengthen its psychopathological sophistication (Jablensky 2010) by integrating the insights and "rich descriptions" from the existing resources (see the initiative of Broome et al. 2012) and from contemporary studies of subjectivity. However, "rich description" cannot be just a literary exercise but needs to be disciplined by an epistemologically adequate conceptual-descriptive framework. In our view, it is phenomenological psychopathology that offers a potentially fruitful, integrative axis for a multitude of different levels of exploration of the psychiatric object (Parnas and Sass 2008). It is also indispensable for rehumanizing our praxis, which includes adequate communication with our patients.

References

American Psychiatric Association (1980). *Diagnostic and Statistical Manual of Mental Disorders* (3rd ed.). Washington, DC: American Psychiatric Association.

American Psychiatric Association (2007). *Diagnostic and Statistical Manual of Mental Disorders* (4th ed., text rev.). Washington, DC: American Psychiatric Association.

Andreasen, N.C. (2007). DSM and the death of phenomenology in America: an example of unintended consequences. *Schizophrenia Bulletin*, 33(1), 108–112.

Bennett, M.R. and Hacker, P.M.S. (2003). *Philosophical Foundations of Neuroscience*. Oxford: Blackwell Publishing.

Bleuler, M. (1978). *The Schizophrenic Disorders. Long-term Patient and Family Studies*. New Haven, CT: Yale University Press.

Bridgman, P.W. (1927). *The Logic of Modern Physics*. New York: Macmillan.

Bridgman, P.W. (1961). The present state of operationism. In P.F. Frank (ed.) *The Validation of Scientific Theories*, pp. 75–80. New York: Collier Books.

Broome, M.R., Harland, R., Owen, G.S., and Stringaris, A. (eds.) (2012). *The Maudsley Reader in Phenomenological Psychiatry*. Cambridge: Cambridge University Press.

Chalmers, D. (1995). Facing up to the problem of consciousness. *Journal of Consciousness Studies*, 2, 200–219.

Clark, A. (2008). *Supersizing the Mind: Embodiment, Action, and Cognitive Extension*. Oxford: Oxford University Press.

Cooper, J.E., Kendell, R.E., Gurland, B.J., Sharpe, L., and Copeland, J. (1972). *Psychiatric Diagnosis in New York and London*. London: Oxford University Press.

Faust, D. and Miner, R.A. (1986). The empiricist and his new clothes: DSM-III in perspective. *American Journal of Psychiatry*, 143, 962–967.

Feighner, J.P., Robins, E., Guze, S.B., Woodruff R.A. Jr, Winokur, G., and Munoz, R. (1972). Diagnostic criteria for use in psychiatric research. *Archives of General Psychiatry*, 26, 57–63.

First, M., Gibbon, M., Spitzer, R., and Williams, J.B.W. (2002). *User's Guide for SCID-I Structured Clinical Interview for DSM-IV-TR Axis I Disorders*. New York: New York State Psychiatric Institute, Biometrics Research Department.

Frances, A. (2013). The past, present and future of psychiatric diagnosis. *World Psychiatry*, 12, 111–112.

Frances, A.J. and Widiger, T. (2012). Psychiatric diagnosis: lessons from the DSM-IV past and cautions for the DSM-5 future. *Annual Review of Clinical Psychology*, 8, 109–130.

Freedman, A.M., Brotman, R., Silverman, I., and Hutson, D. (eds.) (1986). *Issues in Psychiatric Classification*. New York: Human Sciences Press.

Green, C.D. (1992). Of immortal mythological beasts: operationism in psychology. *Theory & Psychology*, 2, 291–320.

Hempel, C.G. (1961). Introduction to problems of taxonomy. In J. Zubin (ed.) *Field Studies in the Mental Disorders*, pp. 3–22. New York: Grune & Stratton Inc.

Husserl, E. (1977). *Phenomenological Psychology: Lectures from 1925*. (J. Scalon, trans.) The Hague: Martinus Nijhoff.

Hyman, S.E. (2010). The diagnosis of mental disorders: the problem of reification. *Annual Review of Clinical Psychology*, 6, 155–179.

Hyman, S.E. (2011). Diagnosing the DSM: diagnostic classification needs fundamental reform. *Cerebrum*, April 26. [Online] Available at: <http://dana.org/news/cerebrum/detail.aspx?id=32066>.

Hyman, S.E. (2012). Psychiatric drug discovery: revolution stalled. *Science Translational Medicine*, 4, 1–5.

Insel, T.R., Cuthbert, B., Garvey, M., Heinssen, R., Kozak, M., Pine, D., *et al.* (2010). Research Domain Criteria (RDoC): toward a new classification framework for research on mental disorders. *American Journal of Psychiatry*, 167(7), 748–751.

Jablensky, A. (2010). Psychiatry in crisis? Back to fundamentals. *World Psychiatry*, 9, 29.

Jablensky, A. and Sartorius, N. (2008). What did the WHO studies really find? *Schizophrenia Bulletin*, 34(2), 253–255.

Jansson, L.B., Handest, P., Nielsen, J., Sæbye, D., and Parnas, J. (2002). Exploring boundaries of schizophrenia: a comparison of ICD-10 with other diagnostic systems. *World Psychiatry*, 1, 109–114.

Jansson, L.B. and Parnas, J. (2007). Competing definitions of schizophrenia: what can be learned from polydiagnostic studies? *Schizophrenia Bulletin*, 33(5), 1178–1200.

Janzen, G. (2008). *The Reflexive Nature of Consciousness*. Philadelphia, PA: John Benjamins Publishing Company.

Jaspers, K. (1963). *General Psychopathology* (7th ed., J. Hoenig and M.W. Hamilton, trans.) Chicago, IL: University of Chicago Press. (Work originally published as *Allgemeine Psychopathologie: Ein Leitfaden für Studierende, Ärzte und Psychologen*. Berlin: Springer, 1913.)

Katschnig, H. (2010). Are psychiatrists an endangered species? Observations on internal and external challenges to the profession. *World Psychiatry*, 9, 21–28.

Kendell, R.E. (1975). *The Role of Diagnosis in Psychiatry*. Oxford: Blackwell.

Kendell, R.E. (2002). Five criteria for an improved taxonomy of mental disorders. In J.E. Helzer and J.J. Hudziak (eds.) *Defining Psychopathology in the 21st Century: DSM-V and Beyond*, pp. 3–18. Washington, DC: American Psychiatric Publishing.

Kendler, K.S., Appelbaum, P.S., Bell, C.C., Fulford, K.W. Ghaemi, S.N., Schaffner, K.F., et al. (2008). Issues for DSM-V: DSM-V should include a conceptual issues work group. *American Journal of Psychiatry*, 165, 174–175.

Kendler, K.S., Munoz, R.A., Murphy, G. (2010). The development of the Feighner Criteria: a historical perspective. *American Journal of Psychiatry*, 167, 134–142.

Kleinman, A. (2012). Rebalancing academic psychiatry: why it needs to happen—and soon. *British Journal of Psychiatry*, 201, 421–422.

Klerman, G.L., Vaillant, G.E., Spitzer, R.L., and Michels, R. (1984). A debate on DSM-III. *American Journal of Psychiatry*, 141, 539–553.

Kuhn, T.S. (1993). Metaphor in science. In A. Ortony (ed.) *Metaphor and Thought*, pp. 513–542. Cambridge: Cambridge University Press.

Levine, J. (1983). Materialism and qualia: the explanatory gap. *Pacific Philosophical Quarterly*, 64, 354–361.

Machery, E. (2009). *Doing without Concepts*. New York: Oxford University Press.

Mann, J.J. (2010). Clinical pleomorphism of major depression as a challenge to the study of its pathophysiology. *World Psychiatry*, 9(3), 167–168.

McHugh, P.R. (2012). Rendering mental disorders intelligible: addressing psychiatry's urgent challenge. In K.S. Kendler and J. Parnas (eds.) *Philosophical Issues in Psychiatry II: Nosology*, pp. 42–53. Oxford: Oxford University Press.

Melle, I. (2013). The Breivik case and what psychiatrists can learn from it. *World Psychiatry*, 12, 16–21.

Merleau-Ponty, M. (1942). *La Structure du comportement*. Paris: Presses Universitaires de France.

Merleau-Ponty, M. (1962). *The Phenomenology of Perception*. (C. Smith, trans.) London: Routledge.

Minkowski, E. (1927). *La Schizophrénie. Psychopathologie des schizoïdes et des schizophrènes*. Paris: Payot.

Minkowski, E. (1997). *Au-delà du rationalisme morbide*. Paris: Éditions L'Harmattan.

Mishara, A.L. (1994). A phenomenological critique of commonsensical assumptions in DSM-III-R: the avoidance of the patient's subjectivity. In J.Z. Sadler, O.P. Wiggins, and M.A. Schwartz (eds.) *Philosophical Perspectives on Psychiatric Diagnostic Classification*, pp. 129–147. Baltimore, MD: The Johns Hopkins University Press.

Mishara, A. and Schwartz, M.A. (2010). Who's on first? Mental disorders by any other name? *Association for the Advancement of Philosophy and Psychiatry Bulletin*, 17(2), 60–65.

Murphy, G.L. (2002). *The Big Book of Concepts*. Cambridge MA: The MIT Press.

Nagel, T. (1979). *Mortal Questions*. Cambridge: Cambridge University Press.

Nordgaard, J. and Parnas, J. (2013). A haunting that never stops: psychiatry's problem of description. *Acta Psychiatrica Scandinavica*, 127(6), 434–435.

Nordgaard, J., Revsbech, R., Saebye, D., and Parnas, J. (2012). Assessing the diagnostic validity of a structured psychiatric interview in a first-admission hospital sample. *World Psychiatry*, 11(3), 181–185.

Nordgaard, J., Sass, L.A., and Parnas, J. (2013). The psychiatric interview: validity, structure, and subjectivity. *European Archives of Psychiatry and Clinical Neuroscience*, 263(4), 353–364.

Østergaard, S.D., Jensen, S.O, and Bech, P. (2011). The heterogeneity of the depressive syndrome: when numbers get serious. *Acta Psychiatrica Scandinavica*, 124(6), 495–496.

Parnas, J. (2011). A disappearing heritage: the clinical core of schizophrenia. *Schizophrenia Bulletin*, 37, 1121–1130.

Parnas, J. (2012a). DSM-IV and the founding prototype of schizophrenia: are we regressing to a pre-Kraepelinian nosology? In K.S. Kendler and J. Parnas (eds.) *Philosophical Issues in Psychiatry II: Nosology*, pp. 237–259. Oxford: Oxford University Press.

Parnas, J. (2012b). The core Gestalt of schizophrenia. *World Psychiatry*, 11, 67–69.

Parnas, J. (2013). The Breivik case and "conditio psychiatrica." *World Psychiatry*, 12, 21–22.

Parnas, J. and Bovet, P. (1991). Autism in schizophrenia revisited. *Comprehensive Psychiatry*, 32, 7–21.

Parnas, J. and Bovet, P. (1995). Research in psychopathology: epistemologic issues. *Comprehensive Psychiatry*, 36, 167–181.

Parnas, J., Bovet, P., and Zahavi, D. (2002). Schizophrenic autism: clinical phenomenology and pathogenetic implications. *World Psychiatry*, 1, 131–136.

Parnas, J. and Gallagher, S. (in press). Phenomenology and the interpretation of psychopathological experience. In L.J. Kirmayer, R.B. Lemelson, and C.A. Cummings (eds.) *Revisioning Psychiatry: Cultural Phenomenology, Critical Neuroscience, and Global Mental Health*. New York: Cambridge University Press.

Parnas, J. and Sass, L.A. (2008). Varieties of "phenomenology": On description, understanding, and explanation in psychiatry. In K.S. Kendler and J. Parnas (eds.) *Philosophical Issues in Psychiatry: Explanation, Phenomenology, and Nosology*, pp. 239–277. Baltimore, MD: Johns Hopkins University Press.

Parnas, J., Sass, L.A., and Zahavi, D. (2013). Rediscovering psychopathology: the epistemology and phenomenology of the psychiatric object. *Schizophrenia Bulletin*, 39, 270–277.

Parnas, J. and Zahavi, D. (2002). The role of phenomenology in psychiatric classification and diagnosis. In M. Maj, J.J. Gaebel, N. Lopez-Ibor, and N. Sartorius (eds.) *Psychiatric Diagnosis and Classification*, pp. 137–162. Chichester: John Wiley & Sons Ltd.

Petitot, J. (2004). *Morphogenesis of Meaning*. Bern: Peter Lang AG.

Rosch, E.H. (1973). Natural categories. *Cognitive Psychology*, 4, 328–350.

Rosenhan, D.L. (1973). On being sane in insane places. *Science*, 179, 250–258.

Sartorius, N., Jablensky, A. Regier, D.A., Burke, J.D., and Hirschfeld, R.M.A. (eds.) (1990). *Sources and Traditions of Classification in Psychiatry*. Stuttgart: Hogrefe & Huber Publishers.

Sato, Y. (1997). *Operationalism in Psychiatry: A Conceptual History*. Dissertation. Department of Psychiatry, University of Cambridge.

Sato, Y. and Berrios, G.E. (2001). Operationalism in psychiatry: a conceptual history of operational diagnostic criteria. *Clinical Psychiatry* (Seishin Igaku), 43, 704–713.

Schwartz, M.A. and Wiggins, O.P. (1986). Logical empiricism and psychiatric classification. *Comprehensive Psychiatry*, 27, 101–114.

Schwartz, M.A. and Wiggins, O. P. (1987a). Diagnosis and ideal types: a contribution to psychiatric classification. *Comprehensive Psychiatry*, 28, 277–291.

Schwartz, M.A. and Wiggins, O.P. (1987b). Typifications. The first step for clinical diagnosis in psychiatry. *Journal of Nervous and Mental Disorders*, 175(2), 65–77.

Spitzer, R.L., Endicott, J., and Robins, E. (1975). Clinical criteria for psychiatric diagnosis and DSM-III. *American Journal of Psychiatry*, 132, 1187–1192.

Spitzer, R., Endicott, J., and Robins, E. (1978). Research Diagnostic Criteria. *Archives of General Psychiatry*, 35, 713–718.

Stengel, E. (1959). Classification of mental disorders. *Bulletin of the World Health Organization*, 21, 601–663.

Stevens, S.S. (1935). The operational basis of psychology. *American Journal of Psychology*, 41, 323–330.

Szasz, T. (1961). *The Myth of Mental Illness: Foundations of a Theory of Personal Conduct*. New York: Harper & Row.

Urfer-Parnas, A., Mortensen, E.L., and Parnas, J. (2010). Core of schizophrenia: estrangement, dementia, or neurocognitive disorder? *Psychopathology*, 43, 300–311.

Weizsäcker, V. von (1986). *Der Gestaltkreis. Theorie der Einheit von Wahrnehmen und Bewegen* (5th ed.). Stuttgart: Thieme.

Westen, D. (2012). Prototype diagnosis of psychiatric syndromes. *World Psychiatry*, 11, 16–21.

Wilson, M. (1993). DSM-III and the transformation of American psychiatry: a history. *American Journal of Psychiatry*, 150, 399–410.

World Health Organization (1992). *The ICD-10 Classification of Mental and Behavioural Disorders: Clinical Description and Diagnostic Guidelines*. Geneva: WHO.

Zubin, J. (ed.) (1961). *Field Studies in the Mental Disorders*. New York: Grune & Stratton.

Chapter 24

Hempel as a critic of Bridgman's operationalism: lessons for psychiatry from the history of science

Kenneth F. Schaffner and Kathryn Tabb

24.1 Introduction: The Complexity of Hempel

Pierre Bovet and Josef Parnas's insightful chapter provides a deeper look at the operationalist philosophy that so markedly influenced post-1980 psychiatry. Other scholars have framed discussions of contemporary psychiatry with in a history of the philosophical antecedents of DSM-III by citing Hempel's 1959 paper—reprinted as (Hempel 1965b)—but Parnas and Bovet further examine the influence of Percy Bridgman's 30-year-older book on the logic of modern physics (Bridgman 1927). This is salutary for three reasons, which we discuss briefly before turning to a critique of Bovet and Parnas's philosophical contribution.

First, several historical accounts of psychiatry have oversimplified and misrepresented Hempel's philosophical program (Kendell 1975; Stengel 1959). On this point the reader only need read Hempel's original papers, written in the 1950s prior to his celebrated 1959 essay, in order to appreciate the complexity and nuances of the evolving logical empiricism of that time (Hempel 1965a, 1965c; also see the recent assessment of Chang (2009)). Second, it was Bridgman who developed the early and influential approach that was incorporated with modification into the logical empiricist program represented by Hempel, and it was also Bridgman who provided the strongest rationale for such an operationalist approach—more on this in a moment.

Finally and relatedly, recent historical scholarship has indicated that Hempel's 1959 essay, based on his address to the American Psychopathological Association, did in fact not have the direct influence on DSM-III or the related ICD-10 that has been widely suggested in the literature. In multiple papers Fulford, writing with several different co-authors (see citations below), has argued that the operationalism ultimately adopted by the American Psychiatric Association (APA), characterized by the attempt to exclusively use theory-free atomized behavioral facts for the purposes of diagnosis, was not a *direct* result of Hempel's influence but rather a *perversion* of Hempel's 1959 talk by the psychiatrist Sir Aubrey Lewis (perhaps among others). While Hempel made clear in his talk that an operationalized vocabulary was only important in the service of theoretical advances and urged the continued investigation of psychiatric laws (psychodynamic or otherwise), it was Lewis who argued that psychiatric nosology should limit itself to the first, descriptive step. While Fulford et al. may overemphasize the importance of Lewis (as opposed to other figures like Stengel and Kendell) it is worth noting that Hempel himself urged the grounding of claims about etiology in an operationalized vocabulary, rather than the exclusion of etiological theories altogether from psychiatry.

This modification of the historical record is germane because it makes clear that the shift towards operation was *not* motivated by an admiration for the logical positivist program in philosophy of science—as Fulford et al. note, if this were the case, Hempel's emphasis on a second, theoretical stage of scientific progress would also have been incorporated by the APA. Rather, Lewis selectively isolated logical empiricism's descriptivist project because, as an important member of the World Health Organization's revision task force for the ICD-8, his primary concern was with international statistical and diagnostic projects—for which an observational basis for diagnosis was deemed essential (Fulford 2006; Fulford and Sartorius 2009) see also (Kendler et al. 2010). This history only helps Parnas and Bovet's case, in so far as Fulford et al.'s research reveals that the operationalist stance of the DSM was originally deemed appropriate only for the international statistical setting, rather than the demands of clinical intervention or psychiatric research. As the authors observe in a footnote, Lewis advocated for different classification systems for different purposes, so he himself recognized the restricted applicability of operationalism.

24.2 **Bridgman and Einstein**

We agree with our authors that it is worth evaluating how the form of operationalism cited in the psychiatric literature differs from the philosophical meaning of the term.[1] Bridgman in particular may have some useful lessons for contemporary philosophers of psychiatry. Parnas and Bovet note that Bridgman himself focused on one of Einstein's *annus mirabilis* papers of 1905, "Zur Elektrodynamik bewegter Körper," which detailed his special theory of relativity. In that revolutionary paper, Einstein began by locating the hidden problem that had so plagued the

---

[1] In so doing, the authors dismiss Hempel's more permissive account of operationalism, which allows for observation of an object to count as an operation, claiming, "this modification empties the concept of 'operation' of all its epistemological or scientific meaning." We believe this to be too strong. As Fulford et al. 2006 (p. 337) note, Hempel indicates that by observations he means something akin to measurements, rather than interpretations—his example is the characteristic physical features of endomorphy which, unlike many *DSM* criteria, do not demand inference to the presence of mental states by the observer. *DSM* criteria that depend on assessing mental states from outward behavior would thus not be covered under Hempel's use of the term.

optics and electrodynamics of bodies in motion (Jammer 2006; Schaffner 1974) in the concept of time and the synchronization of clocks in motion. Influenced by the earlier work of the philosopher-physicist Ernst Mach on operational definitions of inertial mass and temperature (Mach 1960, 1896), Einstein provided an operational definition of time at two points distant in bodies at rest and relative motion. Using this definition, Einstein was then able to recast electrodynamics and optics, and revolutionize science. Bridgman generalized—perhaps overgeneralized—this lesson, along the lines that Parnas and Bovet outline in their chapter.

Bridgman's analysis of the role of an operational definition seems critically wrong to us, since a close historical analysis of Einstein's 1905 relativity article and the available historical documents show that the operational definition is heavily laden with theory, and needs to assume the relativistic "light postulate" in order to have any empirical content. This interpretation is, interestingly, essentially Hempel's view about operationalism and scientific theory as detailed in papers written in the 1950s.

For support of this theory-laden view of Einstein's definition of simultaneity, we can refer to Jammer's close analysis of the available historical documents, which indicate that Einstein's operational definition was in fact deeply anchored in the theories of electrodynamics, light and mechanics (Jammer 2006). Jammer writes the following, which is worth quoting *in extenso*:

> After having studied Heinrich Hertz's reformulation of Maxwell's electrodynamics Einstein wrote in August 1899 to Mileva that he was becoming more and more convinced that the electrodynamics of moving bodies, as currently presented, is not correct, and that it should be possible to present it in a simpler way. All his attempts to construct such a theory on the basis of the relativity principle and the principle of the invariance of the velocity of light were thwarted by the apparently irreconcilable conflict between the light principle and the rule of the addition of velocities as used in mechanics. In an impromptu talk on the creation of the theory of relativity, delivered at Kyoto University on 14 December 1922, Einstein reportedly gave the following account:

> Why do these two concepts contradict each other? I realized that this difficulty was really hard to resolve. I spent almost a year in vain trying to modify the idea of Lorentz in the hope of resolving this problem. By chance a friend of mine [Michelo Besso] in Bern helped me out. It was a beautiful day when I visited him with this problem. I started the conversation with him in the following way: "Recently I have been working on a difficult problem. Today I come here to battle against that problem with you." We discussed every aspect of this problem. Then suddenly I understood where the key to this problem lay. Next day I came back to him and said to him, without even saying hello, "Thank you. I've completely solved the problem. An analysis of the concept of time was my solution." Time cannot be absolutely defined, and there is an inseparable relation between time and signal velocity. With this new concept I could resolve all the difficulties completely for the first time. Within five weeks the special theory of relativity was completed. (Jammer 2006, pp. 106–107)

The reference to "signal velocity" in Einstein's 1922 reflection quoted earlier is to the "light postulate." Jammer writes separately "Einstein [...] arrived at the important conclusion that distant simultaneity is a relativistic concept and that, almost paradoxically, its relativity is a consequence of the invariance of the velocity of light (i.e., of the postulate of the constancy of the velocity of light [Einstein's light postulate])" (Jammer, p. 118). We view this is as an extraordinary repudiation of the view that relativity theory is a triumph of pure operationalism.

24.3 Hempel and Kuhn

As Parnas and Bovet note, Bridgman himself expressed concerns about the overextension of his operationalist philosophy. Hempel, too, wrote critically of the possibility of replacing theoretical analyses with observational and/or operationalist statements. Even in the early 1950s, probably under the partial influence of W.V. Quine's famous "Two Dogmas of Empiricism," Hempel had moved to a view that based science on large theoretical systems, laying the groundwork for the Kuhnian revolution of the 1960s and 1970s in philosophy of science (see Hempel 1950s references cited earlier). In point of fact, in his later years Hempel agreed much more with Kuhn's radical approach to science than is commonly realized. On this point Fetzer writes that:

> [B]y the end of his career, Hempel had become one of the most astute and devastating critics of the logical positivist/logical empiricist program. He was almost certainly influenced in that direction at least partly by his association with Thomas Kuhn when both taught at Princeton. Kuhn proposed and argued that the logical/formalist view and program of the logical positivists (the members and descendants of the Vienna Circle) should be replaced by a view grounded in the history, sociology, and psychology of science, and Hempel, while never fully embracing Kuhn's view, seems to have moved a large distance toward it." (New World Encyclopedia 2014)[2]

24.4 Defining Psychiatric Terms

Parnas and Bovet note other historical forces that influenced the development and acceptance of operationalism in psychiatry, including the decline of psychoanalysis and reactions to the antipsychiatry of the 1970s, though space does not permit additional comments on those aspects of the history. What does seem worth commenting on, however, is a discussion of the epistemological alternative that Parnas and Bovet summarize in those sections of their article. Our authors pose the question: "Are, then, the diagnostic *criteria* 'operational' in any remotely significant, epistemological sense?" (p. 199). Their "answer to this question is a clear-cut *no*." They elaborate: "The operational definition, as a *measurement rule whose execution links the concept with its referent in reality* in a clear-cut, unambiguous way (e.g., like the notion of 'harder' in mineralogy, vide supra) is simply *inapplicable*, and therefore *unapplied*, to the vast majority of psychiatric terms." (p. 199). Further, they write: "psychiatric terms are impossible to define unequivocally as

---

[2] Fetzer's suggestion about Hempel and Kuhn is also supported by one of our (KFS's) own recollections of discussions with Hempel during his 5 years in Pittsburgh in the 1980s.

simple atomic entities but nearly always require an embeddedness in a conceptual/theoretical and ostensive context (e.g., with prototypical examples and discussions of their limits)" (p. 199) here providing some additional references to Parnas and colleagues' earlier articles.

We strongly agree with Parnas and Bovet's view here, and it interestingly mirrors our analysis of the key Einstein example, as illuminated by Jammer's account summarized earlier. As Parnas has convincingly argued in a series of articles on the importance of a phenomenological treatment of consciousness in psychiatric nosology, psychopathological signs and symptoms should not be viewed atomically, but rather as part of the complex semantic structures of the individual's life—encompassing not only their mental states but their broader social and environmental milieu (see Parnas [2008, 2011] and Parnas et al. (2005) for introductions and a list of related references.) As the authors note in their valuable discussion of prototypes, the DSM's purportedly operational definitions, and its concomitant reliance on structured diagnostic interviews, have led to a poverty of psychiatric description that has grave implications for clinical training and practice. This theoretical embeddedness view also resonates with Hempel's later views referenced above, though perhaps not with the potted version sometimes attributed to Hempel (but better attributed to the likes of Lewis).

24.5 Reduction, Emergence, and RDoC

There is, however, more to say about the even conceptually deeper "epistemological considerations" sections of Parnas and Bovet's article. Their perspective here is strongly anti-reductionistic, opposed to the medical-scientific approach exemplified by Kendell's statement that "the only reason most mental disorders are still defined by their clinical syndromes is that the human brain is infinitely *more complex machine* [… than] the heart, kidney, or liver" (p. 202). Their thesis in these pages is that:

> Kendell's equation of nephrology with psychiatry (*pace* complexity) is a prevalent, alas unquestioned, category mistake. In this reductionistic model, mental disorders are seen as signaling natural kind-like "brain disorders" and the individual symptoms/signs are considered to be meaningless causal referents, pointing to specific, dysfunctional neural networks.

It is worth noting that in criticizing reductionism in psychiatry, the authors are addressing a distinct, though related, target from their original adversary, operationalism. While operationalism and reductionism promote some shared values, they are distinct positions in the philosophy of psychiatry and have distinct histories. On the most superficial level, the behaviorist slant of twentieth-century psychiatric operationalism is opposed to the theorized unobservables that often play a role in reductionist accounts of psychopathology. But the authors are justified in asserting that the search for discrete and atomic signs and symptoms led both to reductionism and to an exclusion of phenomenological approaches that emphasize the overall Gestalt of the patient.

Parnas and Bovet seem to be particularly concerned about attempts to explain psychopathology using basic scientific knowledge about the brain. One target is the National Institute of Mental Health's new Research Domain Criteria (RDoC) framework that focuses on circuits, albeit also allowing higher (and lower) units of analysis to define the psychiatric object (National Institute of Mental Health n.d.). For Parnas and Bovet, such a potentially reductionistic analysis is in fact a serious "category mistake," (p. 202)—one which fails to appreciate the "distinctiveness of the ontology and epistemology of human consciousness." Such distinctiveness has both historical antecedents, as in Jaspers' work and the phenomenological philosophical tradition, as well present advocates as in current debates about the "explanatory gap" and the "hard problem" in philosophy of mind (Chalmers 1996; Levine 1983). Note too that the target here moves from a critique of operationalist approaches to psychiatric nosology to a more general criticism of reductive approaches to psychiatric explanation. The RDoC, for example, is precisely *not* interested in diagnosis (at least at present); its target is the use of the DSM in classifications of research proposals, rather than in patients, and it aims to foster new *theoretical* accounts of etiology.

While we share Parnas and Bovet's anxiety about the neurocentrism of the NIMH's approach, in our view there is more than a whiff of substance dualism in their views (though we do not think that such dualism is an inevitable implication of anti-reductionism). Calling naturalistic approaches to mental illness a category mistake is reminiscent of Thomas Szasz's claim that mental illness is a contradiction in terms, since if something is "mental" it cannot be embodied, and therefore cannot be diseased. If one claims that psychiatric objects would, even in an ideal world (that is, not just given the limits on human knowledge) be inexplicable in terms of the brain and its interactions with its environment, what ontology other than substance dualism could one claim allegiance to? In regards to the relationship between mind and brain we would rather take a position once developed by Herbert Simon (1981), and defended in the philosophical literature by writers such as William Wimsatt (1974) as well as by one of us (Schaffner 1993, 2006), that can be called "pragmatic holism" or "pragmatic emergence." On this view, as Simon wrote:

> Roughly, by a complex system I mean one made up of a large number of parts that interact in a non-simple way. In such systems, the whole is more than the sum of the parts, not in an ultimate, metaphysical sense, but in the important pragmatic sense that, given the properties of the parts and the laws of their interaction, it is not a trivial matter to infer the properties of the whole. In the face of complexity, an in-principle reductionist may be at the same time a pragmatic holist. (Simon 1981, p. 195)

This pragmatic holism or emergence view also resonates well with epistemological pluralism and a multilevel, "dappled" view of the world (Cartwright 1999; Kendler 2012). While neuroscientific and neurocognitive approaches might not be the most efficacious (and are certainly not the only) modes of explanation in psychiatry, they cannot be, at this point, ruled out, especially considering modest evidence of their success in explaining aspects of psychopathology. Therefore, *pace* Parnas and Bovet, pragmatic emergence cannot endorse, and in fact due to its inclusiveness will work against, the exclusion of brain-based explanations of the psychiatric object. While we join the authors in condemning the atomizing and oversimplifying effects of operationalism (*sensu* Lewis), we do not follow them in painting all reductionism with the same brush.

References

Bridgman, P.W. (1927). *The Logic of Modern Physics*. New York: The Macmillan Company.

Cartwright, N. (1999). *The Dappled World: A Study of the Boundaries of Science*. Cambridge: Cambridge University Press.

Chalmers, D.J. (1996). *The Conscious Mind: In Search of a Fundamental Theory*. Philosophy of Mind Series. New York: Oxford University Press.

Chang, H. (2009). Operationalism. In E.N. Zalta (ed.) *The Stanford Encyclopedia of Philosophy*. [Online] Available at: <http://plato.stanford.edu/entries/operationalism/>.

Fulford, K.W.M. (2006). *Oxford Textbook of Philosophy and Psychiatry*. Oxford: Oxford University Press.

Fulford, K.W.M and Sartorius, N. (2009). The secret history of ICD and the hidden future of DSM. In M.R. Broome and L. Bortolotti (eds.) *Psychiatry as Cognitive Neuroscience; Philosophical Perspectives*, pp. 29–48. Oxford: Oxford University Press.

Hempel, C.G. (1965a). Empiricist criteria of cognitive significance. In *Aspects of Scientific Explanation, and Other Essays in the Philosophy of Science*, pp. 101–122. New York: Free Press.

Hempel, C.G. (1965b). Fundamental of taxonomy. In *Aspects of Scientific Explanation, and Other Essays in the Philosophy of Science*, pp. 137–154. New York: Free Press.

Hempel, C.G. (1965c). A logical appraisal of operationalism. In *Aspects of Scientific Explanation, and Other Essays in the Philosophy of Science*, pp. 123–133. New York: Free Press.

Jammer, M. (2006). *Concepts of Simultaneity: From Antiquity to Einstein and Beyond*. Baltimore, MD: Johns Hopkins University Press.

Kendell, R.E. (1975). *The Role of Diagnosis in Psychiatry*. Oxford: Blackwell Scientific Publications.

Kendler, K.S. (2012). The dappled nature of causes of psychiatric illness: replacing the organic-functional/hardware-software dichotomy with empirically based pluralism. *Molecular Psychiatry*, 17(4), 377–388.

Kendler, K.S., Muñoz, R.A., and Murphy, G. (2010). The development of the Feighner criteria: a historical perspective. *American Journal of Psychiatry*, 167(2), 134–142.

Levine, J. (1983). Materialism and qualia: the explanatory gap. *Pacific Philosophical Quarterly*, 64, 354–361.

Mach, E. (1896). *Die Principien der Wärmelehre: historisch-kritisch Entwickel*. Leipzig: Barth.

Mach, E. (1960). *The Science of Mechanics: A Critical and Historical Account of its Development* (6th ed.). LaSalle, IL: Open Court Pub. Co.

National Institute of Mental Health. (n.d.). *Research Domain Criteria (RDoC)*. [Online] Available at: <http://www.nimh.nih.gov/research-priorities/rdoc/index.shtml>.

New World Encyclopedia. (2014). *Carl Gustav Hempel*. [Online] Available at: <http://www.newworldencyclopedia.org/entry/Carl_Gustav_Hempel>.

Parnas, J. (2008). Varieties of "phenomenology": on description, understanding, and explanation in psychiatry. In K.S. Kendler and J. Parnas (eds.) *Philosophical Issues in Psychiatry*, pp. 239–278. Baltimore, MD: Johns Hopkins University Press.

Parnas, J. (2011). A disappearing heritage: the clinical core of schizophrenia. *Schizophrenia Bulletin*, 37(6), 1121–1130.

Parnas, J., Moller, P. Kircher, T. Thalbitzer, J. Jansson, L. Handest, P., et al. (2005). EASE: Examination of Anomalous Self-Experience. *Psychopathology*, 38(5), 236–258.

Schaffner, K.F. (1974). Einstein versus Lorentz: research programmes and the logic of comparative theory evaluation. *British Journal for the Philosophy of Science*, 25, 45–78.

Schaffner, K.F. (1993). *Discovery and Explanation in Biology and Medicine*. Chicago, IL: University of Chicago Press.

Schaffner, K.F. (2006). Reduction: the Cheshire cat problem and a return to roots. *Synthese*, 151(3), 377–402.

Simon, H. (1981). *The Sciences of the Artificial*. Cambridge, MA: MIT Press.

Stengel, E. (1959). Classification of mental disorders. *Bulletin of the World Health Organization*, 21, 601–663.

Wimsatt, W.K. (1974). Complexity and organization. In K.F. Schaffner and R.S. Cohen (eds.) *PSA-1972: Proceedings of the 1972 Biennial Meeting Philosophy of Science Association*, pp. 67–86. Dordrecht: Reidel.

Section 9
The evolution of genetic explanation in psychiatry

Chapter 25

Introduction to "The nature of nature"

Kenneth S. Kendler

It is a challenging task to introduce briefly this rich and far-reaching chapter. Turkheimer illuminates a major issue within psychiatric and behavioral genetics that has both substantive scientific content but also important conceptual and philosophical substrates. The logical entry point into this chapter is the question: "What have we learned about the nature of the underlying genetic contributions to psychiatric illness?" Turkheimer reviews the acrimonious "nature–nurture" debates of the last generation (that were more heated in psychology—with the especially emotionally charged issue of IQ—than in psychiatry) and declares that battle over. Nature has "won." However, the victory may be less revolutionary than some of its advocates thought. By "won," he means that it is now accepted by all serious researchers across the disciplinary spectra in psychiatry that genetic risk factors contribute meaningfully to all psychiatric disorders that have been studied. The parallel could be said for psychologists and all of the key traits that they study such as intelligence, personality, aggression, etc. But what exactly does this teach us? Empirically, this means that twin and adoption studies have, with substantial consistency, shown that every psychiatric disorder investigated is heritable with estimates typically falling in the range of 25–80%. None are zero. So, a radical environmentalist agenda for psychiatry is scientifically unsupportable. It will not be possible to construct anything close to a complete etiologic picture of a psychiatric disorder without including genetic risk factors.

But these findings can be viewed from a more conceptual perspective from which they may be less surprising and informative. Indeed, you could argue that they might be derived from first principles with no need for empirical verification. If we reject Cartesian dualism, then it follows that psychiatric illnesses have to be, in some way, instantiated in brains. We also know that brains arise from genetic blueprints interacting with environmental experiences in a complex developmental process. You cannot build brains without genes. So, if we agree that psychiatric disorders centrally involve brains and genes are critical to the construction of brains, is it at all surprising that we find that genes have something important to do with psychiatric disorders? Not really.

However, reality is not quite as simple as I have just argued. Genetics actually involves the study of individual differences, not just average overall effects. So, what I am really claiming is less obvious (and hence we might actually need all those twin and adoption studies after all). That is, the differences in how brains are constructed are a result, at least in part, of the differences in genetic blueprints between people. Given that we have long accepted that the differences between people in noses and height are partly a result of differences in their genes (i.e., "You have your uncle's nose"), it would take some special pleading to argue that brains are different. And, the last step then becomes, those differences in the way brains are made play an important role in differences in the risk for psychiatric disorders.

Given the victory of "nature" in these nature–nurture wars, Turkheimer then asks, "So what is next?" The field of psychiatric genetics has in effect already answered that question. Efforts to use increasingly sophisticated and inexpensive genotyping methods (and a deluge of varying statistical tools) to attempt to first localize and then identify individual genetic variants that impact on risk for psychiatric disorders has been gaining steam for at least 20 years. So, the current molecular psychiatric geneticist would have a ready answer for Turkheimer, "Find the damn genes!" Implicit in their approach—and sometimes it is made explicit—is that the existence of these genes can be assumed because of the results of twin (and adoption) studies. "We know they are there. We just have to find them."

Turkheimer says, in effect, "Hold on!" In what I would regard as the core of this chapter, he makes the critical observation that *"genetic variation does not imply genetic mechanism."* That is, showing from twin studies that genetic factors impact on disease liability is *not* the same thing as showing a biological disease mechanism involving an identifiable set of specific genes. The equation of these two kinds of genetic insights has been assumed by many in our field. Turkheimer would argue, with much force, that this equation represents a "level" or "category" mistake.

But we need to stop here for a conceptual clarification that I am not sure Turkheimer fully cashes out. Here are two possible claims:

C1. Results of heritability from twin and adoptions studies for complex psychiatric disorders (or psychological traits) do not guarantee that the individual risk variants will be identified using molecular methods.

C2. Results of heritability from twin and adoptions studies for complex psychiatric disorders (or psychological traits) do not guarantee that any individual risk variants which will be identified using molecular methods will form any coherent biological story.

I think that C2 is much more defensible that C1. I would argue, C1 is merely a problem of statistical power and Turkheimer (in a personal communication) agrees. If twin studies identify risk genes in aggregate, eventually—if those studies are true—with large enough sample sizes some individual variants will be identified. C2 is asking a far deeper and more interesting question.

I would agree that it is theoretically possible for some trait to be substantively heritable (Turkheimer used the example of "divorce") and yet for the individual genetic variants that make up that genetic "signal" to be so scattered across the genome and across biological systems that there is no coherent mechanism to be detected. As Turkheimer himself has argued, this is conceptually very similar to the idea that the "environment" could make a major contribution to the etiology of a disorder without revealing any useful environmental disease predisposing "mechanism." That environment could represent environmental processes that we could clarify and even prevent, like birth defects, toxin exposures, or some pathogenic aspects of parenting. But the environment could be hidden in the stochastic core of development and/or the numberless idiosyncratic aspects of human experience that we could never hope to understand let alone to intervene. That is, it could be "environmental" but contain no "actionable" mechanism that we could ever prevent.

So, on a logical basis, as Turkheimer has noted, we can divide what we might call a weak and strong role for genetics in the etiology of psychiatric illness. The question of the hour is: What is the likelihood that for some psychiatric or behavioral traits we care about, all we will ever find is the "weak" role—that is, variation but no mechanism? Turkheimer argues that this has already been shown for human personality. Many twin and adoption studies show personality to be heritable but current efforts to identify specific genetic variants, including those with quite large sample sizes, have turned up very little for their labors.

This is a subject I have treated at some length elsewhere (Kendler 2013). Here my intuitions—informed by some effort at studying over the years of what we have learned about the genetic substrate of other complex human disorders (admittedly not nearly as "complex" as psychiatric disorders)—differ from Turkheimer's. I am more optimistic that we will find at least moderately coherent biological systems underlying heritability estimates for most of our disorders. We will not likely have to wait long before the rapid advance of science will settle this issue. To be clear, it is not black and white. As I have argued previously (Kendler 2013), the extreme position that broadly equates variation and mechanism would postulate that all the small-effect variants contributing to psychiatric disorders are part of one global coherent biological pathway to illness. That is quite unlikely. But small patchy sets of variants that contribute to some "subphenotypes" are much more probable. Using Turkheimer's example of divorce, we might find genes that contribute to the mechanism of irritability, impulsivity, or alcohol dependence, each of which could increase the chances of divorce. Furthermore, the answer is likely to differ across different disorders. Genetic risk factors for some disorders might have higher mechanistic coherence than for other disorders.

The historical changes that have occurred in the nature–nurture debate in psychiatry are rich subject matters for the kind of analyses that are the focus of this volume. We have seen stunning "internal" developments in the areas of statistical methods that have pushed the science forward. Even more dramatic have been the technological developments that have enabled genotyping to be done so much more quickly and cheaply. We have seen a change in the organization of science with the Psychiatry Genomics Consortium playing a central role in building a more collective model that has enabled the sample sizes for analysis to grow to the size (tens of thousands) needed to produce reliable variant discovery. But the questions of the role of genetic factors in human behavior touch quite close to home and raise a host of "external" social-cultural and legal questions, for example, about heritability and responsibility, and the possibility that risk variants for psychiatric disorders could or should be tested for in utero. We might consider Turkheimer's chapter as a beginning look at this area rich for further philosophical-historical analysis.

Reference

Kendler, K.S. (2013). What psychiatric genetics has taught us about the nature of psychiatric illness and what is left to learn. *Molecular Psychiatry*, 18(10), 1058–1066.

Chapter 26

The nature of nature

Eric Turkheimer

> When we speak of genetic transmission, we are addressing the real problem of how far differences in the genotype and differences in the environment contribute to the development of such a character [...] If genetic differences make a contribution it is important to try to find out what we can about their nature.
>
> (Gottesman and Shields 1972, p. 10)

26.1 Introduction

Medicine is applied science, and the history of medicine tells a story about the emergence of medical practice from prescientific medieval beliefs into the bright light of modern science, especially modern biology. Vitalism and spiritualism are no more, and although "alternative" forms of medicine persist they are increasingly isolated from the scientific mainstream. Psychiatry is a branch of medicine, and for many good reasons, psychiatry has always wished to follow its sister disciplines into the light of science. The natural way to do this, it has always seemed, is to follow the other disciplines and become a form of applied biology, or what is now called clinical neuroscience (Insel and Quirion 2005), but that task has proved to be difficult to accomplish. The reason, I will suggest here, is that psychiatry is as much applied psychology as it is applied biology. Although some of the origins from which psychiatry is forever trying to lift itself are indeed prescientific, others are scientific in intent but behavioral in content, and psychology has not experienced the same decisive scientific success as biology during the last 150 years.

So to the extent the historical task of psychiatry has been to establish its scientific bona fides, biology usually appears superior to psychology as a means of doing so. As a result, psychiatry has felt a constant intellectual pressure in the direction of biology, a need to demonstrate that mental illnesses are biological, and therefore that psychiatry's clinical practitioners are applied biologists—real physicians. This chapter will explore one aspect of that historical trend, involving the role of genetics in determining of the biological status of psychiatric entities. In particular, after some historical introduction, the account will focus on a crucial moment in the history of both genetics and psychiatry: the end of the twentieth century, when long-established knowledge of the genetics of behavior based on quantitative studies of families was being supplemented and challenged by the explosion of DNA-based science that followed from the completion of the Human Genome Project. It was a time of great optimism, a feeling that the scientific millennium had arrived with the chronological one, but as we now know the story turned out to be much more complex than anyone anticipated. But to understand that moment we have to begin more than a century earlier, with the beginnings of modern genetics, modern psychiatry, and modern psychology, all in the person of Francis Galton.

26.2 **Nineteenth Century: The Galtonian Paradigm**

Questions of nature and nurture, famously, originated with Charles Darwin's cousin, Sir Francis Galton, who borrowed the phrase from Prospero's description of Caliban:

> A devil, a born devil, on whose nature Nurture can never stick; on whom my pains, Humanely taken, all, all lost, quite lost. And as with age his body uglier grows, So his mind cankers. I will plague them all, Even to roaring. (Shakespeare, *The Tempest*, Act IV Scene I)

Galton (1875), like so many who came after him, liked the sound of the phrase "nature-nurture":

> The phrase 'nature and nurture' is a convenient jingle of words, for it separates under two distinct heads the innumerable elements of which personality is composed. Nature is all that a man brings with himself into the world; nurture is every influence without that affects him after his birth. (p. 9)

Questions of nature and nurture scratch a deep itch in the human psyche. Although most discussions of nature and nurture eventually turn into deconstructions, it is worth considering seriously for a moment how strong our nature–nurture intuitions are. Children are not given lessons to learn how to run or to speak their native language: they just learn it, and even our nagging awareness that children raised swaddled and isolated might not learn to do either does not dissuade us from thinking of language and locomotion as "inborn," "innate," or (in the modern era), "hard-wired." But no one, or almost no one, emerges full-blown as a virtuoso oboe player or champion pole-vaulter: those we do have to take lessons for. We say they are learned, the result of specialized and systematic exposures. Dogs bark, but they don't roll over unless you teach them how.

Galton's intuition about nature and nurture went one step beyond the classification of abilities into the inborn and learned, however. It is not only running in general that feels like it is inborn, it is also the fact that some people can run faster than others. Humans differ on even the most universal of behavioral characteristics, and it seems—still referring only to widely held intuitions, perhaps misguided but worth taking seriously for a while—that some of those differences are more the result of nature and others the result of nurture. Few of us would contend that we might have been concert musicians or Olympic champions if only we had the training,[1] but getting to Carnegie Hall is at least to some extent a

---

[1] As Billy Martin put it, "Well, you got your mules and you got your racehorses, and you can kick a mule in the ass all you want, and he's still not gonna be a racehorse."

matter of practice. Spelling out the intuition in this way has already clarified one important conclusion: nothing is purely the result of either nature or nurture. Olympic sprinters have to train, great oboe players have some hard-to-define quality called musical talent, and even the ordinary among us can improve ourselves with practice.

Reading Galton 150 years later is an experience in simultaneously appreciating the breadth of his genius and the opacity of the blinders placed on him by the common prejudices of his era. In his famous studies of "eminence," he examined the familial clustering of men (again, accepting without question that there was no place else to look) of great accomplishment in Victorian society. Along the way he invented much of what we recognize as modern social science, starting with a compulsion to quantify what he studied, including the correlation coefficient and at least a portion of the twin method.

It comes as no surprise today that Galton's men of eminence were, indeed, clustered in families; what is remarkable is the extent to which Galton was willing to accept this clustering as evidence of "nature." Although Galton labored mightily to develop methods to differentiate nature and nurture, from a modern perspective it is clear that Galton was so firmly rooted in the pre-genetic, rigidly stratified socioeconomic confines of the nineteenth century that he could not fully appreciate the magnitude of the fundamental problem. It is more obvious today that clustering of human beings in families is the result of both genetic relatedness (which Galton recognized as "nature") and environmental relatedness of various kinds, including especially social class, the elephant in the room throughout Galton's studies.

Galton was, however, not so thoroughly naïve. As pointed out in Rende et al.'s (1990) excellent history of the early development of the twin method by Galton and others, in a 1876 article entitled "The History of Twins, As A Criterion Of The Relative Powers of Nature And Nurture," Galton considered the role of the environment in familial clustering and differentiation. Galton had some premonition of the existence of identical and fraternal twins, but did not have the scientific tools to fill it out. As a result he did not use the twin method in what we now think of in the "classical" way, via comparison of the similarity of monozygotic and dizygotic twins. Instead he analyzed the developmental tendency of twin pairs to become more alike or different over time, an idea with strikingly modern resonances of its own (Beam and Turkheimer 2013).

26.3 Twentieth Century: Twin Method

The development of the classical twin method as we know it today awaited genetic advances by Weinberg at the turn of the twentieth century, leading to an explosion of twin studies in the 1920s, mostly on the subject of human intelligence (Rende et al. 1990). The classical twin method is based on the existence of two distinct types of twins: monozygotic (MZ), who share 100% of their DNA sequence (within an order of approximation; epigenetics and other aspects of contemporary genomics have complicated this simple picture somewhat), and dizygotic (DZ) who are essentially ordinary siblings, sharing on average 50% of the DNA sequence, but who happen to share a womb and be born at nearly the same time.

The conceptual, genetic, and statistical details of the twin method have been described and debated many times already, and I will do so as briefly as possible here, with a goal of neither supporting nor undermining its many genetic and scientific assumptions. There are two sources of resemblance in twin models: a broadly genetic source, labeled A for additive and one environmental source, labeled C for common. I will have more to say about both of these, but for now it is simply an observation that members of twin pairs resemble each other because they share DNA on the one hand (A) and share a rearing environment on the other (C). The genetic source of resemblance is twice as large for MZ pairs than it is for DZ pairs, the family environmental source is the same for both of them. The third term, labeled E (for environment, though it is actually one of two environmental terms in the model), is not a source of resemblance: in fact it represents all the environmental factors that make siblings and twins raised in the same family different from each other. Given a sample of identical and fraternal twins that varies in some outcome, one can use these relationships to partition the variation in outcome into independent sources of variation attributable to A, C, and E. Before reviewing how such twin studies have come out for commonly studied forms of psychopathology, it is necessary to describe some details that are crucial to understanding the results.

The name additive that is given to the genetic term in the twin model is very important. What is being added in such models are the tiny effects of many individual genetic loci. A major task of genetics during the first half of the twentieth century was the unification of Mendelian genetics, in which characteristics like smooth and wrinkled peas "segregated" in known ratios according to laws of discrete genetic transmission, with quantitative genetics, in which continuously distributed characteristics like height are transmitted from parents to children but do not segregate into types. Twin designs are very much an example of the latter. The integration is accomplished by assuming a very large number of segregating genes of small effect, which, when summed (thus the A) produce a quasi-continuous, bell-shaped curve according to the binomial theorem.

An additional complication of quantitative models in psychiatric genetics is that for better or for worse, psychiatric outcomes have historically been represented as classifications rather than as continua. This adds one more layer to models of familial resemblance: variation in many discrete genetic loci is combined with whatever environmental risk can be identified to create a latent continuous distribution of liability to disorder with a threshold: individuals with liability scores greater than the threshold develop the disorder. The quasi-categorical character of psychiatric disorder also means that twin similarities are usually expressed as concordances (percentage of pairs with one affected individual in which the other is also affected) rather than as the correlation coefficients developed by Galton for the analysis of continuous traits like height and ability.

Also in the category of fortunately or unfortunately is the fact that twin and family studies result in an index, called a heritability coefficient, that varies from zero to one, expressing the proportion of variance in outcome that is accounted for by variance in genotype. The heritability coefficient is one of the most reified, vilified, and generally misunderstood parameters in the history of science, and its strengths and weaknesses do not need to be rehashed here. The current author has addressed the issues quite recently (Turkheimer and Harden 2014); more (Visscher et al. 2008) and less (Charney 2012) sanguine views are also available.

In any event, in the 1920s the twin method evolved from the early sketches provided by Galton to the "classical" method in which the similarities of identical and fraternal twins were compared and modeled. Although the slow and shifting development of reliable diagnostic systems and the relatively smaller sample sizes imposed by the rarity of psychiatric disorder may have resulted in somewhat more variable results than were obtained for more easily measured normal characteristics like intelligence, from an historical bird's-eye view the results were unanimous. Psychopathology is heritable, in all its forms, in the simple sense that MZ twin concordances are consistently higher than DZ twin concordances; there is little evidence for systematic environmental effects originating in families; but there is persistent evidence of unsystematic environmental variability within families, which is simply a way of saying that identical twins raised together are substantially less than perfectly similar for any form of psychopathology

The discovery that all major forms of psychopathology were substantially heritable was, at the time, a source of some degree of triumphalism among psychiatric geneticists (Seymour Kety, 1974, replying to Thomas Szasz' (1960) *Myth of Mental Illness*, famously quipped, "If schizophrenia is a myth, it is a myth with strong genetic component"). The ubiquity of genetic variance and the defeat of traditional family environmentalism led to a widely held point of view that major psychopathology had turned out to be "genetic," and that it would therefore only be a matter of time before the scientific details were filled in, as they had been for Huntington's disease once the autosomal dominant mutation that is its basis was finally discovered, a century after the clinical syndrome was first systematically described. Schwarz, for example, in the 1991 *Review of Psychiatry*, put it as follows:

> Even as the epidemiologic [i.e., twin and family] studies continued, it was clear to the field that if there was a genetic etiology to schizophrenia, it would act through a biological mechanism. Therefore, studies aimed at understanding the biological pathophysiology of schizophrenia take on a new importance for genetic hypotheses, especially if the factor being studied is likely to be under somewhat simple genetic control (e.g., an enzyme level of neurotransmitter receptor density). (p. 85)

It was common at the time to go as far as to declare that schizophrenia is a "brain disease" (Heinrichs 1993; Henn and Nasrallah 1982; Johnson 1989). Chua and McKenna (1995), for example, stated:

> In recent years, the hypothesis that schizophrenia is a biological brain disease has spectacularly gained the upper hand. The origins of this paradigm shift can be traced

directly to two incontrovertible findings: first, the hereditary contribution to the disorder and, secondly, the antipsychotic effect of neuroleptic drugs. (p. 563)

To be fair, Chua and McKenna expressed at least a modicum of skepticism about the idea. What they shared with every other theorist who introduced the idea, however, is that they didn't stop to analyze exactly what it meant for something to be a brain disease, or the role that genetic variance might properly play in the determination.

At the time, findings of genetic variance in psychopathology also sparked considerable resistance and controversy. From a contemporary perspective it may be difficult to remember that 50 years ago, the goal of behavior genetic studies of psychiatric illness was not so much to uncover the biological etiology of psychopathology, but simply to "unravel" (as was commonly said) genetic from environmental sources of etiology. The prevailing criticisms of the day were psychoanalytic and family environmental, holding that family dynamics were the most important determinant of psychopathology, including for schizophrenia (Lidz and Blatt 1983). Although twin-study-based behavior genetics still has its critics, are there any surviving "environmentalists" as regards psychopathology? In the middle of the twentieth century, the behavioral sciences were dominated by two great schools of thought that were, in different ways, deeply environmental in outlook: psychoanalysis and behaviorism. There are, of course, still psychoanalysts and behaviorists, but modern Freudians and Beckians don't bother to deny the importance of genetic factors in mental illness; it is considered a given, an etiological background against which any treatment modality does its work.

The environmentalists—the Laingians, the Szaszians, the humanists, the Sullivanians—may have been routed, but there were nevertheless worrisome signs that the Galtonian victory of nature over nurture in psychopathology still faced difficult obstacles. The first was the very ubiquity of heritability. It wasn't as though some mental disorders had been shown to be thoroughly genetic while others were thoroughly environmental. All psychopathology is substantially heritable, and none of it is perfectly so. It is true that psychopathology has produced a more reproducible gradient of heritability than other areas of behavior, with schizophrenia and bipolar disorder showing heritabilities close to 0.8 in meta-analyses (Sullivan et al. 2003), and major affective disorder, anxiety disorders, and substance abuse disorders more in the range of 0.4–0.6 (Sullivan et al. 2000, 2001), similar to normal individual differences like personality and intelligence. The biological or psychological implications of these heritability differences remain unclear, however (Turkheimer 2011). There is no well-documented theory of the heritability of complex behavior showing why some behaviors are more heritable than others, and it is not as simple as expecting that more highly heritable syndromes will yield more easily to genetic explanation, as cancer genetics has demonstrated (Risch 2001). (Much of this difficulty is based on foundational difficulties in the concept of heritability itself. See Turkheimer and Harden (2014) for a review.)

Even more potentially troubling, the ubiquity of heritability turned out to extend beyond the bounds of major psychopathology. Following from Galton, differences in human intelligence were found to be heritable; so were differences in normal personality. Moreover, differences in human traits that seem well beyond the usual extent of biological explanation are heritable. Political attitudes are heritable (Hatemi et al. 2009), religiosity is heritable (Waller et al. 1990), how much television people watch is heritable (Plomin et al. 1990). And, in an example this author has pursued theoretically and empirically for the last 20 years, divorce is heritable (D'Onofrio et al. 2007). The heritability of divorce has implications for too-easy inferential leaps from quantitative genetics to genetic and biological explanation.

A third difficulty in the transition from quantitative genetic to mechanistic accounts of psychopathology is that as it became more and more possible to identify actual genes that caused psychopathology, it became increasingly clear that it was going to be very difficult to do so. It is commonplace to locate the beginnings of the search for DNA related to psychopathology with the completion of the Human Genome Project, but more limited searches for linkage with genetic markers have been possible for much longer than that, and the troublesome patterns that have come to characterize much modern genomic research—early reports of large effects greeted with great enthusiasm, followed by disappointment in replication and meta-analysis—plagued the field from the beginning. In a passage entitled, "The Pond is Empty," Crow (2008), recalled:

> Many in linkage research thought that success was inevitable—one would "drain the pond dry" and there would be the genes! However, the reality is that in spite of a plethora of well-hyped findings no linkage claim has proven robust. In each case an apparent finding in a modest-sized population of families that was then used to "identify" a candidate gene has not been found linked in more systematic and larger studies. (p. 1682)

In fact, the absence of genes of large effect for psychopathology should not have come as a surprise. As I have already described, the additive action of many genes of small effect is an *assumption* of routine quantitative genetics. When comparisons of polygenic and of single-gene or "oligogenic" (specifying a handful of genes of intermediate effect against a polygenic background) models were actually conducted, they invariably favored the polygenic theories. Thoughtful psychopathologists of the era were troubled by the prospect: what kind of biological mechanism could be invoked if genetic effects were so completely distributed across the genome? Faraone and Tsuang (1985) put it as follows:

> The mode of inheritance has substantial implications for etiological research and clinical practice. A conclusive demonstration that a single major locus is involved in schizophrenia would hold the promise that a relatively direct biochemical pathway accounts for the psychophysiology of the disorder. If a multifactorial polygenic model describes the mode of transmission, the search for a simple biochemical pathway is likely to be less fruitful. (p. 44)

A final indication that the victory of nature over nurture was not complete is that the opposition never conceded. In fact, the growing biogenetic consensus of the time was paralleled, then as now, by an anti-hereditarian opposition that dismissed the entire quantitative genetic enterprise as ill-conceived. The most comprehensive early attack on the foundations of behavior genetics is a book entitled *Not in Our Genes*, by Lewontin et al. (1984). In the first pages of the book, the authors were clear about the twin foundations of behavior genetics they wished to undermine. The first is reductionism:

> The first is *reductionism*—the name given to a set of general methods and modes of explanation both of the world of physical objects and human societies. Broadly, reductionists try to explain the properties of complex wholes—molecules, say, or societies—in terms of the units of which those molecules or societies are composed. (p. 5, emphasis in original)

The second is determinism:

> The second stance is related to the first; indeed, it is in some senses a special case of reductionism. It is that of *biological determinism*. Biological determinists ask, in essence, why are individuals as they are? Why do they do what they do? And they answer that human lives and actions are inevitable consequences of the biochemical properties of the cells that make up the individual; and these characteristics are in turn uniquely determined by the constituents of the genes possessed by each individual. (p. 6, emphasis in original)

Lewontin et al. were correct in identifying reductionism and determinism—as opposed to heritability—as the important theoretical issues underlying nature and nurture. In their concluding chapter, they endorsed a view of biological systems according to which complexity of biological determination is the source of what we perceive as our psychological freedom from biology:

> What characterizes human development and actions is that they are the consequence of an immense array of interacting and intersecting causes. Our actions are not at random or independent with respect to the totality of those causes as an intersecting system, for we are material beings in a causal world. But to the extent that they are free, our actions are independent of any one or even a small subset of those multiple paths of causation: that is the precise meaning of freedom in a causal world. When, on the contrary, our actions are predominantly constrained by a single cause ... we are no longer free. (p. 289)

Although the authors of *Not in our Genes* recognized that heritability per se has an oblique relationship to their legitimate concerns about reductionism and determinism, they never gave up the attack on its empirical validity. Heritability, however, is precisely a means for computing genetic effects summed over a large "subset of those multiple paths of causation." In the kind of complex hierarchical biological model endorsed in *Not in Our Genes*, heritability is not a problem to be explained away; rather, it is inevitability, an assumption of the model.

Lewontin et al.'s analysis of the genetics of schizophrenia is particularly telling: Although they laid the groundwork for a compelling argument that the nonzero heritability of schizophrenia does not commit us to a biological "cause" of schizophrenia, any more than the heritability of divorce must lead to a neuroscience of marital status, they never make the case. Instead, they fall back on the traditional anti-hereditarian strategy of sniping at the methodology of twin and adoption studies, apparently hoping to convince the reader that a methodologically correct study (which, of course, is never actually conducted) would show the heritability of schizophrenia to be negligible. Finally, having convinced themselves that their stance against determinism commits them to radical environmentalism, they end the chapter with an endorsement of the views of Michel Foucault and R.D. Laing.

We can see in this progression the same confusions that plague traditional behavior genetics and biological psychiatry, precisely the confusions that Lewontin et al. set out to avoid: confounding of determinism and heritability, and commitment to a dichotomous view of the role of biology in behavior. Setting out to bring down reductionism, they end up in a futile attack on the empirical status of heritability; and once they have rejected reductionist models of schizophrenia, all they have at their disposal is the opposite extreme, the discredited Laingian contention that schizophrenia is no more than a lifestyle, and a heroic one at that.

26.4 Twenty-First Century: The Nature Debate

In Turkheimer (2000) I wrote that "The nature–nurture debate is over" (p. 160). The debating hasn't actually stopped, of course, and in that sense my declaration was premature, but that isn't really what I meant. Although there was obviously no particular date when it occurred, at some point around the turn of this century, the Galtonian nature–nurture project reached its logical conclusion: there is genetic variance in everything, psychopathology included; there is also environmental variance in everything; and most important, genetic variation does not imply genetic mechanism. The nature–nurture community in general, and the psychopathology community in particular (because questions of mechanism are especially important for psychopathology) have been trying to recover from this last conclusion ever since. The nature–nurture debate has not so much ended as it has been transformed into a debate about the meaning of the "nature" term in Galton's "convenient jingle." Call it the nature debate.

Establishing what the nature debate is about necessitates beginning with the obvious. Not all genetically influenced characteristics are etiologically alike. Figures 26.1 and 26.2 illustrate the relationship between genetic structure and behavior for two "syndromes" that are observable at the level of behavior. Figure 26.1 represents Huntington's disease. A clinical neuropsychologist might observe that a subset of patients in a neurological clinic display a characteristic pattern of disparate symptoms. Among other symptoms, these patients experience rapid cognitive decline in midlife, and a particular form of motor disturbance. Indeed, these clinical characteristics are what were observed by Huntington, well before the genetic basis of the disorder was known. Huntington's disease is "genetic" in two senses. The first is the Galtonian sense, according to which differences in the expression of Huntington's status are correlated with genotype and therefore cluster in families, but that is the less important part of what we mean when we say Huntington's is genetic. Once the genetic nature of the disorder was known, our understanding of its etiology was changed. In particular, explanations at the

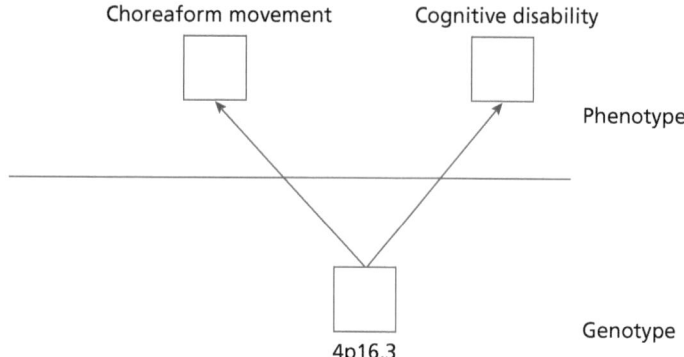

Fig. 26.1 The genetic structure of Huntington's disease is the explanation of the phenotypic structure. Choreiform movements occur in the presence of early dementia because the dominant gene explains both of them.

level of behavior—why people with particular kinds of motor disorders might be motivated to experience cognitive decline, or vice versa—became pointless. Both are caused by a single dominant gene. Differences in Huntington's status contain genetic variance, and Huntington's disease is explained by a genetic mechanism: these are two different things.

Figure 26.2 displays a similar set of circumstances for divorce. A social worker might observe a "syndrome" in which two kinds of activities co-occur in some individuals: they argue a lot with their partners, and spend time in court hearings. These two behaviors co-occur because the individuals in question are divorced, and the heritability of marital status ensures that genes are correlated with the likelihood that a person will have these experiences. Like Huntington's, differences in marital status are correlated with differences in genotype. But in the case of divorce, we have not discovered a gene responsible for the relationship, or a well-specified mechanism linking the genetic and behavioral levels of explanation; presumably we don't expect to discover one. Nevertheless, the heritability of divorce ensures that as married people descend into conflict with their spouses and head into court, their genes will come along for the ride. Nature, in the Galtonian, genetic epidemiological sense, contributes to both Huntington's disease and divorce, but the nature of Huntington's disease is different to the nature of divorce. The difference between Huntington's disease and divorce is not that the former involves genetics and the latter does not; it is that the former is *defined* by genetics whereas the latter is *defined* by behavior.

A conventional account of the difference between Huntington's disease and divorce would emphasize that Huntington's is the result of a single major locus whereas divorce is polygenic, and that is of course true. One way to understand the problem faced by modern complex genomics is to say that we are still searching for coherent ways to specify genetic etiologies of the radically polygenic causal architectures that have turned out to be the norm for behavior. This problem has faced the field of psychiatric genetics from its earliest days. Gottesman and

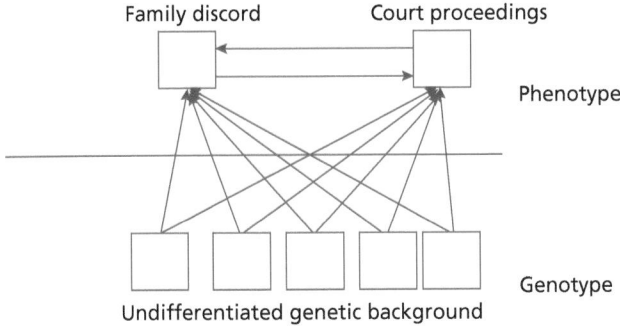

Fig. 26.2 Although divorce proceedings are associated with genetic variation, the structure of divorce-related activities is not apparent at a genetic level of analysis.

Shields (1972), in their classic theoretical and empirical account of the genetics of schizophrenia, were the first to insist on a polygenic model of inheritance, but they remained troubled by the relation between variation and etiology. In particular, they struggled with the Meehlian concept of "specific genetic etiology." I have argued for some time that "specific genetic etiology" is exactly what we are talking about: Huntington's disease has a specific genetic etiology, and divorce does not. Gottesman and Shields were convinced that their polygenic model of the transmission of schizophrenia was compatible with a specific genetic etiology, but Meehl (1972) himself was not. In his lengthy (and generally admiring) afterword to the volume, he wrote:

> One understands fairly clearly what it means to conjecture that a "big-effect monogene" is the specific etiology of a disease [...] But once we have excluded that simple situation, the very meaning of the phrase "specific etiology" begins to "fuzz up," and I wish the authors had said more about how they conceive it. (p. 376)

It is an extraordinary fact that 50 years later, biological and genetic psychiatry still lacks a coherent theory of mechanism that allows us to distinguish between the explanatory mechanisms underlying Huntington's disease and divorce. There are, in my view, only three broad possibilities for how a theory of specific etiology of polygenic characteristics might work. The first two are the perpetually embattled doppelgangers that have dominated the discussion for a long time: reductionist hereditarianism on the one side, and radical anti-hereditarianism on the other.

The hereditarian view, which is not often spoken out loud but is, I suspect, held in the breach by many working behavioral and psychiatric geneticists, is that despite our intuitions to the contrary, it *is* only a matter of time before things like divorce succumb to mechanistic genetic analysis. The unstated assumption of reviews of the biological nature of psychopathology is that anything detectably syndromal, and certainly anything both syndromal and heritable, must have a genetic mechanism to explain it. This assumption is often adopted out of either explanatory desperation (if there is no genetic mechanism, how can science proceed?) or oversimplified materialism (see, for example, Guze's famous question,

"Can psychiatry be too biological?" and my affirmative reply (Turkheimer 1998)). The second possibility, following *Not in Our Genes*, is a long antihereditarian tradition holding that the Galtonian, quantitative genetic empirical work showing marital status to be heritable is methodologically flawed and biologically oversimplified, and that the failure to identify genetic mechanisms of complex behavior is simply a reflection of those mistakes. These arguments have survived, virtually unchanged, into the genomic era (e.g., Joseph 2004).

The perpetual opposition between the reductionists and the antireductionists is potentiated by a common assumption that there are only two choices: something is either a brain disease or a lifestyle. If mechanistic genetic explanation cannot be brought to bear on psychopathology, the reductionists envision their field undone by naïve dualism, or at best, relegated to murky methodological domains of social science. The antireductionists envision a dehumanized world in which all human suffering, up to and including marital status, has been reduced to deterministic genetic effects. But fortunately for all concerned, it is actually glaringly obvious that most forms of psychopathology are neither brain diseases nor lifestyles. What is lacking is a sensible theory that offers some middle ground. The remainder of this chapter will begin to outline such a theory.

The third option, that of developing a meaningful theory of biological and psychological explanation in psychiatry, will require giving up on the first two possibilities in a way that the poles of the old nature–nurture argument have never been able to do. Has there ever been a heritable syndrome for which the biogeneticists have finally said, "You know what? This syndrome may have some genetic variance like everything else, but it doesn't have a genetic mechanism. We are going to have to leave this one to the psychologists." Conversely, has there ever been a syndrome for which the anti-hereditarian community has, finally, conceded that despite omnipresent environmental variation, psychological explanation isn't leading anywhere? The first task of any meaningful theory of biogenetic and psychological explanation is to distinguish them; no theory is plausibly independent of its mindless or brainless prejudices (Lipowski 1989) unless it can offer a meaningful example of a syndrome that does *not* fit the author's preferred explanatory modality.

One appealing possibility is to endorse a catholic scientific approach that welcomes top-down and bottom-up science for all behavior. Individual differences in personality may not have a genetic mechanism, but understanding of biology and genetics is certainly not irrelevant to personality. Schizophrenia may, when all is said and done, be well described as a brain disease with a genetic etiology, but schizophrenia is still experienced psychologically by individuals (e.g., Sullivan 1962). There are also contemporary genetic methodologies that go some distance in the direction of "unfuzzing" Meehl's concern with the meaning of specific etiology for complex disorders (Jia et al. 2010), although they are yet to produce decisive results.

In general, it is difficult to disagree with a causally pluralistic approach to science (Kendler 2012), but two caveats must be borne in mind. First, in accordance with the theme of this volume, there are powerful historical forces pushing psychiatry in the direction of biological explanation. No human behavior is viewed as too complex for biological explanation nowadays, but the psychology of schizophrenia is a relic. Sullivan (1962) seems inconceivable today, although Sullivan was hardly naïve about biology and genetics. Pluralism is a two-way street. Second, it is too easy to conclude that since all behavior comprises some kind of complex hierarchy of psychological, biological, neuronal, and genetic processes, it is necessarily the case that all behavior has the same causal structure and can be studied in the same way. Divorce *is* different from Huntington's chorea, and it needs to be studied differently, particularly along a dimension running from the biological to the psychological. Pluralism is not absolute.

My own account of the relationship between genetic versus environmental variation on the one hand and biological versus psychological explanation on the other is in its early stages. In Turkheimer et al. (2014) we suggest that the hallmark of genetic variation that does not play a specific mechanistic role is that the multivariate structure of the genetic variability is indistinguishable from the structure of the phenotype. We build the case that human personality is the first well-documented example of a domain of behavior that is demonstrably heritable in the Galtonian sense but has nevertheless resisted all forms of genetic explanation for so long that the time has arrived to declare it "phenotypic."

For example, our fundamental understanding of phenotypic differences in human personality has been developed with factor analysis. Large matrices of personality responses are analyzed with the goal of identifying the minimum number of latent dimensions that account for their multivariate structure. These exercises have led to the Five Factor Model of personality, which has become the almost universally accepted standard in the field. If one has access to genetically informative personality data on a matrix of personality items, it is possible to conduct factor analysis separately on the genetic, shared environmental, and nonshared environmental matrices. This possibility leads to an interesting question: if the phenotypic variance in personality can be described in terms of the Five Factor Model, what about the genetic variance? Perhaps if we factor analyze the genetic variation separately from the environmental, we can learn something about the genetic etiology of personality that contributes to the observable phenotype. But despite many attempts, the answer is that when we factor analyze the genetic variance–covariance matrix, we get—the Five Factor Model. There is usually not enough shared environmental variance to conduct a meaningful factor analysis, but if we factor analyze the nonshared environmental variance, we get—the Five Factor Model again. John Loehlin, at the end of a 30-year program of research on the topic, concluded, "the primary organization of personality is at the level of the phenotype" (Loehlin and Martin 2013, p. 766).

Space does not permit a full adumbration of all of the ways in which the genetics of human personality look like phenotypic human personality, described at a different level of analysis. Several findings are worth noting briefly. First, attempts to specify the molecular genetics of personality, initially with linkage and candidate gene studies, and more recently with genome-wide association studies, have been singularly unsuccessful. As one would expect based on a radically polygenic, phenotypically driven model, there are associations to be found between personality and individual genes, and if sample sizes become large enough we will "detect" them at whatever level of statistical significance we like, but that is irrelevant to the question at hand. A rejection of the phenotypic null model requires discovery of genetic-level structures that display meaningful differences from phenotypic structure, in the way that (in the extreme case) the highly structured familial segregation of Huntington's differentiates it from other forms of dementia or chorea.

By the same token, the failure to develop a biologically interesting molecular genetics of personality should not be taken of evidence that the original impression of genetic *variation* in personality was incorrect. The two findings are compatible; in fact they are both specific predictions of a radically polygenic phenotype-driven model. Finally, characterization of the phenotypic hypothesis as "null" is important. Null hypotheses can't be proven, in the sense that it is not possible to prove that a mechanistically meaningful personality gene will never be found. This is one of the reasons that dreams of biological explanation die so hard. All I can do is predict that in the long run personality will be seen to be phenotypic, make the case that things certainly look that way so far, and remind those who continue to expect a biological explanation to emerge that the burden of proof is ultimately on them.

The most comprehensive account of a post nature–nurture model of psychiatric explanation is found in Kendler (2013). Kendler begins with the universal heritability of "human traits and disorders," which he accepts as evidence that, "because genetic effects must be expressed through biological processes, these findings suggest that psychiatric disorders are 'biological.'" Later, however, Kendler is appropriately skeptical about this "weak" claim of biological explanation, because, as he correctly recognizes, in its most general sense the epithet "biological" refers to little more than the obvious facts that behavior begins, one way or another, in the brain, and differences in behavior begin, one way or another, in the genome.

Kendler's further analysis depends on the concept of biological coherence: "by coherence, I mean the genes whose altered expression or structure is indexed by the detected common or rare genetic variants or [copy number variations] tell a sensible biological story" (Kendler 2013, p. 1061). He describes four "scenarios" with different degrees of coherence. (It would seem that four per se, or really breaking coherence down into categories at all, is more a matter of explanatory convenience than anything else. The four scenarios are basically no coherence, two levels of middling coherence, and high coherence.)

When all the analysis is complete, I expect that Kendler's appeal to coherence and my phenotypic null hypothesis will wind up pointing in more or less the same direction. In the meantime, however, I will express one concern: how exactly is coherence to be detected? Kendler's examples come exclusively from consensually recognized medical disorders: Crohn's disease, Parkinson's diseases, multiple sclerosis, and Alzheimer's disease. These examples are ultimately too easy: no one has ever mistaken Alzheimer's disease for a lifestyle. The judges of coherence seem to be the working geneticists who study the syndromes, and they—unsurprisingly—are unanimous in concluding that the genetics of their respective disorders are headed in a coherent direction. Scientists always think this way, and I for one will be more convinced that the coherence criterion is going to work when someone identifies a meaningful domain of behavior where coherence doesn't seem to obtain. Kendler does not offer a suggestion.

In the consideration of the (no coherence) Scenario 1, Kendler concludes, "I consider Scenario 1 to be improbable. Although psychiatric disorders are likely etiological heterogeneous, and some of the coherence may be emergent at levels in the mind–brain system too high for us to now study, the chances that no meaningfully connectivity between variants will emerge seems low" (2013, pp. 1064–1065). For the record, it doesn't seem so low to me, given the history of biological psychiatry up to this point, and an exhaustive review of the personality literature has convinced me that Scenario 1 is already here for normal personality. Once again, any attempt at a theory of biological explanation in psychiatry has to set a marker on the left edge of the domain, identifying something that is *not* biological, if it wants to be taken at its word about things that are.

26.5 Conclusion: The Meaning of Nature

When one starts to enumerate the great theoretical questions in the history of psychiatry, it is striking how many of them depend crucially on the nature question and questions of mechanism, and how few of them hang on Galtonian concerns with untangling genes and environment:

- Diagnostic realism and natural kinds versus social construction.
- The organic–functional distinction.
- Mental illness as "myth" and medical reality.
- Disease models of addiction.
- Treatment with pharmaceuticals as opposed to talk therapy.
- Considerations of moral responsibility in the legal system.
- The possibility of objective biological diagnosis of psychopathology.

Galton's pleasing jingle of nature and nurture has become so familiar that it is easy to forget that nature in this sense, as what is inherited as opposed to inculcated, is not even its oldest or most common meaning in connection to human behavior. Neither is it the most profound. The other meaning of nature, as in the phrase *human nature*, owes less to Galton, and more to another late nineteenth-century interpreter of complex human biology, Freud. To ask about human nature, at the species level, is to wonder whether humans in general are universally endowed or burdened with desires or capacities that are beyond their willful control. At the individual level, to speak of a person's nature is to consider the possibility that some personal desires are not to be explained in terms of conscious intentions and observable life narratives, but instead by inner mechanisms of which a person may be only dimly aware. The relation between these levels—the expression of primitive species-typical desires (biology) in the presumably civilized minds (psychology) of modern individuals—is the central concern of Freudianism.

Nature versus nurture in the Galtonian, genetic epidemiological sense has little to do with the determination of human nature at either the species or the individual level, and questions of human nature remain undecided once the Galtonian questions have been answered. Another important usage of the word nature is important in this context. One of the attractions of natural explanations of human behavior is that they offer a route to natural science, a way out of the gloomy methodological swamp of the behavioral sciences. Freud was not immune to this temptation. In the famous opening to his never-completed "Project for a Scientific Psychology," he wrote:

> The intention is to furnish a psychology that shall be a natural science: that is, to represent psychical processes as quantitatively determinate states of specifiable material particles, thus making these psychical processes perspicuous and free of contradiction. (Freud 1895/1953–1974, p. 295)

In the contrast between Freud and the unexamined materialism of modern biological psychiatry we can see both horns of the dilemma that has plagued psychiatry from the start: indulge a high-level, humanistic model of causation and explanation, paying a price in methodological rigor, or indulge an exclusively reductionist view grounded in the natural sciences, paying a price in psychological relevance. Galtonian questions of nature and nurture are not irrelevant to this dilemma so much as orthogonal to it. Natural scientific explanations of human behavior must recognize that genetic variability does not guarantee the success of bottom-up explanation, or risk losing their relevance to human suffering as it is actually experienced. Psychological theories must remain compatible with genetic variation, or risk losing their relevance to the world of empirical science.

References

Beam, C.R. and Turkheimer, E. (2013). Phenotype–environment correlations in longitudinal twin models. *Development and Psychopathology*, 25(1), 7–16.

Charney, E. (2012). Behavior genetics and postgenomics. *Behavioral and Brain Sciences*, 35(5), 331–358.

Chua, S.E. and McKenna, P.J. (1995). Schizophrenia—a brain disease? A critical review of structural and functional cerebral abnormality in the disorder. *The British Journal of Psychiatry*, 166(5), 563–582.

Crow, T.J. (2008). The emperors of the schizophrenia polygene have no clothes. *Psychological Medicine*, 38(12), 1681–1685.

D'Onofrio, B.M., Turkheimer, E., Emery, R.E., Harden, K.P., Slutske, W.S., Heath, A.C., et al. (2007). A genetically informed study of the intergenerational transmission of marital instability. *Journal of Marriage and Family*, 69(3), 793–809.

Faraone, S.V. and Tsuang, M.T. (1985). Quantitative models of the genetic transmission of schizophrenia. *Psychological Bulletin*, 98(1), 41–66.

Freud, S. (1953–1974). Project for a scientific psychology. In J. Strachey (ed. and trans.) *The Standard Edition of the Complete Psychological Works of Sigmund Freud* (24 vols.), pp. 281–391. London: Hogarth Press. (Work originally published in 1895.)

Galton, F. (1875). *English Men of Science: Their Nature and Nurture*. London: D. Appleton.

Galton, F. (1876). The history of twins, as a criterion of the relative powers of nature and nurture. *The Journal of the Anthropological Institute of Great Britain and Ireland*, 5, 391–406.

Gottesman, I.I. and Shields, J. (1972). *Schizophrenia and Genetics: A Twin Study Vantage Point*. New York: Academic Press.

Guze, S.B. (1989). Biological psychiatry: is there any other kind? *Psychological Medicine*, 19(2), 315–323.

Hatemi, P.K., Funk, C.L., Medland, S.E., Maes, H.M., Silberg, J.L., Martin, N.G., et al. (2009). Genetic and environmental transmission of political attitudes over a life time. *Journal of Politics*, 71(3), 1141–1156.

Heinrichs, R.W. (1993). Schizophrenia and the brain: conditions for a neuropsychology of madness. *American Psychologist*, 48(3), 221–233.

Henn, F.A. and Nasrallah, H.A. (1982). *Schizophrenia as a Brain Disease*. Oxford: Oxford University Press.

Insel, T.R. and Quirion, R. (2005). Psychiatry as a clinical neuroscience discipline. *Journal of the American Medical Association*, 294(17), 2221–2224.

Jia, P., Wang, L., Meltzer, H.Y., and Zhao, Z. (2010). Common variants conferring risk of schizophrenia: a pathway analysis of GWAS data. *Schizophrenia Research*, 122(1–3), 38–42.

Johnson, D.L. (1989). Schizophrenia as a brain disease: implications for psychologists and families. *American Psychologist*, 44(3), 553–555.

Joseph, J. (2004). *The Gene Illusion: Genetic Research in Psychiatry and Psychology under the Microscope*. New York: Algora Publishing.

Kendler, K.S. (2012). The dappled nature of causes of psychiatric illness: replacing the organic–functional/hardware–software dichotomy with empirically based pluralism. *Molecular Psychiatry*, 17(4), 377–388.

Kendler, K.S. (2013). What psychiatric genetics has taught us about the nature of psychiatric illness and what is left to learn. *Molecular Psychiatry*, 18, 1058–1066.

Kety, S. (1974). From rationalization to reason. *American Journal of Psychiatry*, 131, 957–963.

Lewontin, R.C., Rose, S., and Kamin, L.J. (1984). *Not in Our Genes: Biology, Ideology and Human Nature*. New York: Pantheon Books.

Lidz, T. and Blatt, S. (1983). Critique of the Danish-American studies of the biological and adoptive relatives of adoptees who became schizophrenic. *American Journal of Psychiatry*, 140(4), 426–435.

Lipowski, Z.J. (1989). Psychiatry: mindless or brainless, both or neither? *Canadian Journal of Psychiatry*, 34(3), 249–254.

Loehlin, J.C. and Martin, N.G. (2013). General and supplementary factors of personality in genetic and environmental correlation matrices. *Personality and Individual Differences*, 54(6), 761–766.

Meehl, P.E. (1972). A critical afterword. In I.I. Gottesman and J. Shields *Schizophrenia and Genetics*, pp. 367–416. New York: Academic Press.

Plomin, R., Corley, R., DeFries, J.C., and Fulker, D.W. (1990). Individual differences in television viewing in early childhood: nature as well as nurture. *Psychological Science*, 1(6), 371–377.

Rende, R.D., Plomin, R., and Vandenberg, S.G. (1990). Who discovered the twin method? *Behavior genetics*, 20(2), 277–285.

Risch, N. (2001). The genetic epidemiology of cancer interpreting family and twin studies and their implications for molecular genetic approaches. *Cancer Epidemiology Biomarkers and Prevention*, 10(7), 733–741.

Schwarz, S.C. (1991) Genetics of schizophrenia: a status report. In A. Tasman and S.M. Goldfinger (eds.) *American Psychiatric Press Review of Psychiatry, Volume* 10, pp. 79–97. Washington, DC: American Psychiatric Press.

Sullivan, H.S. (1962). *Schizophrenia as a Human Process*. New York: W.W. Norton.

Sullivan, P.F., Kendler, K.S., and Neale, M.C. (2003). Schizophrenia as a complex trait: evidence from a meta-analysis of twin studies. *Archives of General Psychiatry*, 60(12), 1187–1192.

Sullivan, P.F., Neale, M.C., and Kendler, K.S. (2000). Genetic epidemiology of major depression: review and meta-analysis. *American Journal of Psychiatry*, 157(10), 1552–1562.

Szasz, T.S. (1960). The myth of mental illness. *American Psychologist*, 15(2), 113–118.

Turkheimer, E. (1998). Heritability and biological explanation. *Psychological Review*, 105(4), 782–791.

Turkheimer, E. (2000). Three laws of behavior genetics and what they mean. *Current Directions in Psychological Science*, 9(5), 160–164.

Turkheimer, E. (2011). Genetics and human agency (Commentary on Dar-Nimrod and Heine, 2011). *Psychological Bulletin*, 137, 825–828.

Turkheimer, E. and Harden, K.P. (2014). Behavior genetic research methods: Testing quasi-causal hypotheses using multivariate twin data. In H.T. Reis and C.M. Judd (eds.) *Handbook of Research Methods in Personality and Social Psychology* (2nd ed.), pp. 159–187. Cambridge: Cambridge University Press.

Turkheimer, E., Horn, E.H. and Pettersson, E. (2014). A phenotypic null hypothesis for the genetics of personality. *Annual Review of Psychology*, 65, 515–540.

Visscher, P.M., Hill, W.G., and Wray, N.R. (2008). Heritability in the genomics era—concepts and misconceptions. *Nature Reviews Genetics*, 9(4), 255–266.

Waller, N.G., Kojetin, B.A., Bouchard, T.J., Lykken, D.T., and Tellegen, A. (1990). Genetic and environmental influences on religious interests, attitudes, and values: a study of twins reared apart and together. *Psychological Science*, 1(2), 138–142.

Chapter 27
Is it time for a "Copenhagen interpretation" in behavioral genetics?

Peter Zachar

27.1 Introduction

Reductionism in the psychiatric and psychological sciences refers to explaining phenomena at higher levels of analysis with reference to causal mechanisms at lower levels. For example, accounting for the co-occurrence of coughing, fever, and fatigue with respect to the mechanisms of a viral infection is a reductionist explanation. Causal explanations of this sort are important achievements of scientific medicine.

So why does reductionism have such a negative connotation for many in psychiatry and psychology? To some extent it is because of claims such as the following:

> The lesson of the history of psychiatry is that progress is inevitable and irrevocable from psychology to neurology, from mind to brain, never the other way around. Every medical advance leads to the list of diseases which may cause mental derangement. (Macalpine and Hunter 1974, pp. 256–257)

This claim is incorrect. Many important advances in our understanding of schizophrenia, depression, and autism have resulted from an increase of information at higher levels of analysis involving facts about conditioning, attention, emotion, memory, and personality.

The disagreement that many people have with such claims is not only with their inaccuracies. The philosophically important disagreement with "ruthless" reductionism is the implied metaphysics which holds that what occurs at the level of the brain is *really real* as opposed to the "fictional" mental referents of abstract psychological concepts.

Science is replete with metaphysical assumptions that have influenced the various positions advocated for in what Turkheimer (Chapter 26, this volume) calls "the nature debate." Drawing both on Turkheimer's chapter and on his larger body of work, in what follows I will examine why some behavioral geneticists are questioning the metaphysics of a previous generation (Turkheimer, 1998, 2012, Turkheimer, Pettersson and Horn, 2014). To better understand this development, I will compare this skepticism to another rejection of a metaphysics in the early days of quantum physics by scientists working at the University of Copenhagen.

Although the Copenhagen interpretation will be described later in the chapter, for now let me summarize the main idea: because the information needed to develop precise causal models is unmeasurable at the subatomic level, some physicists asserted that the nineteenth-century notion of causality as both completely determined and necessary was a metaphysical elaboration that was superfluous and should be discarded in quantum physics.

27.2 *Fin de siècle* Psychiatry and Genetics (Nineteenth/Twentieth Century)

The metaphysics of genetic reductionism was part of the intellectual landscape of the seventeenth century, but its more proper origin lay in the *fin de siècle* period of the late nineteenth century and early twentieth century.

According to Gregory (2008), the most widely accepted theory of biological growth in the early modern era was preformationism. The preformationist thinker Nicholas Malebranche declared that all the living beings that will ever be born were preformed by God and encased in embryos. As this theory was advanced by subsequent thinkers, growth into the adult form was not considered to be guided by the deity directly but consisted in the unfolding of these nascent structures according to natural laws. By the end of the next century, after Laplace's determinism had gained acceptance in the scientific community, the concept of preformation entailed that both positive and negative traits are destined. The major issue of dispute was whether the preformed structures reside in the egg or the sperm.

The contrast theory to preformationism was called epigenesis. Advocated by both Aristotle and Harvey, epigenesis referred to a process in which form *developed* out of an unformed mass. In the embryology of the seventeenth and eighteenth centuries, preformation was the preferred scientific theory because it was more mechanical in nature. Epigenesis was considered too spooky. By the middle of the nineteenth century, however, with the introduction of cell biology by thinkers such as Virchow and von Baer, organisms were seen to develop through a mechanical process of cell division and specialization, and epigenesis became the preferred scientific theory (Magner 2002).

Although thinkers in the nineteenth century were concerned about heredity, it was largely a topic in embryology. The science of heredity came into being with classical (or Mendelian) genetics, which was founded by de Vries, Correns, and Bateson in the early 1900s. In classical genetics, an organism was construed as a mosaic of segregated traits that are each genetically encoded. Such Mendelian traits are inherited from parents and passed down to offspring.

Interestingly, the formal discipline named "psychiatry" appeared about the same time as did genetics. Its emergence consisted in a lumping of the more functional, neurotic disorders of neurologists with the insanities treated by the asylum doctors into a single domain. Despite this emphasis on functional conditions, many academic psychiatrists maintained a commitment to an organic model of mental disorders as diseases of the brain.

In pondering *hereditary insanity*, the academic psychiatrists found it appealing to combine the new genetic ideas with late nineteenth-century degeneration theory. Degeneration referred to a regressive developmental process involving a reversion to an ancestral form. As degeneration theory spread, it was conceptualized in terms of Lamarckian soft inheritance and was considered just as likely to result from exposures to bad environments (Chamberlin and Gilman 1985). With the Mendelian emphasis on hard inheritance, in the early twentieth century the causes of degeneration were moved inside the body.

Inspired by the new genetics, insanity came to be seen as the manifestation of a causally potent, hereditary taint—ultimately residing in the genes. Those who specialized in embryology criticized the new genetics by claiming that it represented a resurrection of preformationist assumptions that ignored the constitutive role of development. According to Kendler (2005), this preformationist causal metaphysics became an implicit background assumption for twentieth-century psychiatric genetics, leading many researchers to minimize developmental processes and instead seek things like a discrete gene for schizophrenia or a gene for autism.

27.3 *Fin de siècle* Psychiatry and Genetics (Twentieth/Twenty-First Century)

So what has happened in 100 years? One thing that is the same in comparison to the beginning of the last century is that the scientific understanding of heredity still plausibly offers one of the best models for thinking about the nature of psychiatric disorders. As Turkheimer's chapter suggests, however, several of the metaphysical assumptions of the early geneticists are in the process of being rejected in favor of a more empirically constrained understanding. This ongoing process also represents a rejection of a metaphysical picture that many scientists (who are not behavioral geneticists) still find attractive, and even indispensable.

In the science of the last century genes were thought of as physical entities that causally determined psychological traits. In contrast, behavioral geneticists such as Turkheimer (1998) argue that whatever we take to be "a gene," it is usually a probability *enhancer*, not a *maker* of traits. Furthermore, the relationships that genes have with psychological traits lack the immediate proximity of an underlying physical substrate.

When purveying major events in the history of science, the phrase *fin de siècle* calls to mind a nearly century-old story about what happened to Laplace's determinism in the early twentieth century. In quantum physics, the concepts of position and momentum are borrowed from the macro-world (such as the solar system) to understand the micro-world (such as an electron). Due to the small size of electrons compared to the wavelength of light, it is not possible to measure the position and momentum of an electron simultaneously with certainty. Making a precise measurement about position means that our uncertainty about its momentum must be large. If we attempt to be more precise in the measurement of an electron's momentum, our uncertainty about its position increases correspondingly.

There is no getting outside of measurement for quantum events. According to the Copenhagen interpretation, to assert that an electron simultaneously possesses a precise position and a precise momentum independently of being measured is a metaphysical assumption. Such an assumption, it was thought, muddles the scientific issues. Our notion of what electrons are like should be based on what we can know about them, not based on a conceptual and semantic framework used to understand a very different level of reality.

One famous philosophical implication of the Copenhagen interpretation was the undermining of Laplacian determinism. According to Laplace, if an omniscient being could know the current position and momentum of all the matter in the universe for a single slice of time, that being could predict the entire future of the universe and could retrodict the entire history of the universe. If simultaneous position and momentum cannot be precisely known, Laplace's deterministic universe can be seen as resting on a metaphysical assumption that muddles the scientific issues.

Based on this brief summary of quantum uncertainty, let us explore three features of a Copenhagen interpretation that are relevant to understanding recent developments in behavioral genetics. The first is that the meanings of concepts are embedded in the experimental practices in which they are used. The second feature is that the names we use to describe our quantifications are not always interpretable in terms of familiar semantics. The third feature refers to the metaphysical notion of "a cause." If the fundamental causal set-up is different than assumed, then our understanding of the relationship between the putative cause and the outcome may have to be altered.

27.3.1 Concepts as Experimental Practices

What many readers likely find interesting about the debate in physics is the notion that position and momentum are concepts that are inseparable from measurement. From this, advocates of Copenhagen-like interpretations infer that when the measurement practices change, there may also be slight changes in the meaning of related concepts (Bridgman 1927; Chang 2004).

Similar empiricist considerations are also relevant to understanding the concept of a gene. In biology, what the concept of a gene refers to differs depending on whether what is being sought is a unit of mutation, of recombination, or of function (Falk 2000; Fogle 2000). In some experiments a gene refers to a long section of DNA. In others it refers to a transcript of messenger RNA with the "intron" sections transcribed from DNA edited out. In linkage studies "candidate genes" are genetic markers on chromosomes. In genome-wide association studies a "gene" is effectively reduced to what makes an allele different, often a single alteration in a base pair (or single nucleotide polymorphism—SNP).

RNA transcripts are not SNPs. The changes in meaning that are contingent on the measurement of a transcript and then of a SNP are fairly obvious but the noticing of these changes is sometimes ignored—despite the fact that researchers readily accommodate themselves to local meanings. When this failure to notice occurs, it is likely related to a reliance on an essentialist metaphysics according to which a gene refers to a single, universal kind of thing with an inherent nature. A Copenhagen interpretation, focusing as it does on the constructive aspects of measurement, could serve as a prophylactic against essentialism about the gene.

27.3.2 Statistical Indices are not always Interpretable in Terms of a Familiar Semantics

Another advantage of a Copenhagen interpretation would be to see that some of our concepts refer primarily to measurements and not to previously developed, semantically inspired concepts. The concept of heritability is a good example. Behavioral geneticists are constantly informing people that high heritability is not synonymous for *highly inherited* (versus acquired in development). For instance, being an oxygen breather has a heritability of zero because it does not vary in the population, but it is highly inherited. The concept of heritability refers to a statistical index, not to a pre-existing semantic concept like "inherited." Although to some extent this problem is primarily due to a sloppy use of the term "heritability" by some scientists, people in general would be less surprised at finding out that depression, extroversion, religiously, and time watching television are all heritable to the same extent (about 0.50) if they did not think of heritability in familiar semantic terms.

Turkheimer (2012) further suggests that both "additive genetic effects" and "nonshared environment effects" are also better understood, not as expressions of a familiar semantics, but as mathematical abstractions/measurements. For example, he and his colleagues note that nonshared environment is a name for a quantitative estimate of "whatever makes identical twins raised together different." Many different things can lead identical twins to vary. When we lump all those particulars under a single name like nonshared environment, we should not assume that the name refers to a homogeneous entity.

27.3.3 The Nature of Cause

The features of a Copenhagen interpretation just explored are understandably controversial for being too instrumental and too operationalist. A less controversial feature of a Copenhagen interpretation in behavioral genetics would be what it says about the concept of a cause.

Laplacian determinism assumed that all matter has a simultaneous position and momentum, but the quantum revolution argued that at the fundamental level such information is empirically unknowable. Einstein, as many are aware, asserted that information about simultaneous position and momentum was potentially empirically knowable, but he never said that it was currently knowable (Fine 1986).

The genetic determinism of the past century assumed that scientists could specify mechanistically the relationship between the information contained in genes (or in a group of genes) and the production of psychological traits. Consider, however, the following statement from Eric Turkheimer et al. (personal communication, May 6, 2013):

> A psychologically determined complex human trait is influenced by the combined action of a very large number of genetic loci, and the fact that a process is circumscribed and definable at a behavioral level of analysis does not imply that it will be systematic at a genetic level as well. Although quantitative genetics allows us to compute gross sums over these undifferentiated genetic effects and thus to compute statistical estimates of their joint effect, the effects of individual genes will be tiny to the point of being undetectable and, more strongly, unspecifiable.

In behavioral genetics, different metaphysical assumptions are put into doubt, but like in physics these are assumptions about the causal set up. As Kendler (2005) notes, much work in behavioral genetics seeks to find genes for schizophrenia, or anger, or extroversion. He terms this the *gene for X* research program. The basic idea of "gene for" research programs is that once the relevant genes are identified, they will represent the starting point for discovering the underlying biological mechanisms for the target psychological states. The problem with this set-up is that it assumed that much of the causal information would be contained in a single gene, or if polygenic would still constitute a well-demarcated package that would allow the discovery of genetically controlled mechanisms in general. Both Turkheimer (2012) and Kendler (2005) argue that the actual causal set-up is very different than assumed. The relevant genes are copious, their effects are not solely additive, which genes are significant shift from study to study, and each gene can explain only a small part of the variance.

A key philosophical issue here is the metaphysical concept of cause. As Turkheimer and his colleagues note, the "genetic effect" is a statement about a population of genes, not about single genes. In this sense, looking for a gene that causes schizophrenia is like looking for the voter who caused Barrack Obama to become the President of the United States. It is a type of category mistake.

Gene–trait and voter–victor relationships are probably not best understood using the metaphysics of causal reductionism. For instance, the concept of a cause includes the notion that the outcome would be different if the cause was absent (Lewis 1983). If, however, our identified person had not voted, Obama would still have won the election. We can also intervene on a cause and alter the outcome (Woodward 2008). If an intervention had caused our person to change his/her mind and vote for another candidate, Obama still would have won. The relationship between polygenes and phenotypes is similar to that between voters and winning candidates. For most constructs of interest in psychiatry and psychology, the effect of a single gene is not necessary for the outcome to occur, nor is it sufficient for it to occur. The causal factor is an aggregate in the form of a mathematical abstraction.[1]

---

[1] The concept of cause is obscure enough to accommodate construing single genes and singles voters as causes when they are part of larger casual packages, even if they are causes in a minimal sense.

Behavioral genetics is even more causally complicated than elections because a candidate is a concrete particular. Psychological states such as anger and extroversion are abstract concepts that refer to amalgamations.

Let us explore this issue further by considering basic emotions. Essentialist theories like that of Ekman and Friesen (1975) construe basic emotions as possessing a definite and inherent nature that is the result of a single causal mechanism called an "affect program." Examples of basic emotions are anger and fear.

In contrast, nonessentialist theories construe a basic emotion such as anger to be a moving target made up of a dynamic and shifting combination of subjective feelings, cognitions, facial expressions, physiognomy (body language), and behavioral tendencies (Ortony and Turner 1990; Russell 2003; Zachar 2006). According to nonessentialists, anger can be decomposed in many ways (e.g., furrowed brows, glares, and yelling), and each of the decompositions might be easier to explain causally than the global construct of anger. The features associated with anger may also be reshuffled to create a family of higher-order constructs such as annoyance, ire, wrath, fury, and rage.

To the extent that a construct such as anger is not a concrete particular but a moving target with shifting features and boundaries, any causal sketch of that construct will also be subject to ongoing modifications. Of course we can (and should) fix the construct by idealizing it into something less complex, thereby stabilizing the causal sketch. This is a necessary scientific practice and is what Meehl (1986) calls "malignant" only if we do not realize that both the causal sketch and the construct to be explained are open concepts.

Although Kendler (Chapter 39, this volume) is more hopeful than Turkheimer (Chapter 27, this volume) that a decomposition and reduction strategy might lead to some progress in the discovery of underlying mechanisms of phenomena grouped under abstract names like negative affect and depression, neither of them is very confident that these idealizations will be best described as "genetic."

27.4 Conclusions

I am mindful that comparing quantum physics and behavioral genetics primarily because at a certain point in both of their histories a 100-year-old metaphysics (Laplace and Mendel respectively) was subject to rejection is a tenuous rationale. Also, in each case the key concepts involve technical aspects of measurement that fall outside my own area of expertise. Nevertheless, a historical and philosophical comparison may still be *historically* and *philosophically* informative. With that in mind let me push the comparison further.

Arthur Fine (1986) argues that Einstein adhered to the metaphysical skepticism and instrumentalism of empiricists such as Hume, Mach, and Poincaré when he was developing his theories of relativity. This instrumentalism, suggests Fine, liberated Einstein from the metaphysical assumptions of Newton and Maxwell. Only later did Einstein abandon instrumentalism in favor of scientific (causal) realism. Furthermore, after the debate between Einstein and those who followed Bohr and Heisenberg's Copenhagen interpretation was made public, some young physicists who were interested in joining Einstein's attempt to save Laplacean determinism were dissuaded from doing so by their supervisors because those supervisors believed that such a research program was a scientific dead end.

The strength of empiricism is that its adherents are often more able to see metaphysical elaborations as metaphysical. In the case of behavioral genetics, the ontology of genetic reductionism and the causal models used to think about genetic determinism are the kind of metaphysical elaborations that empiricists tend to notice. If these metaphysical elaborations are used to design research programs that are also scientific dead ends as Turkheimer, Kendler, and many of their colleagues are beginning to suggest, then perhaps the time has come for a Copenhagen interpretation in behavioral genetics.

Acknowledgments

Randy Russell, Rosine Hall, Robyn Bluhm, Bob Krueger, and Ginger Hoffman made helpful comments on an earlier version of this chapter.

References

Bridgman, P.W. (1927). *The Logic of Modern Physics*. New York: Macmillan.

Chamberlin, J.E. and Gilman, S.L. (eds.) (1985). *Degeneration: The Dark Side of Progress*. New York: Columbia University Press.

Chang, H. (2004). *Inventing Temperature: Measurement and Scientific Progress*. New York: Oxford University Press.

Ekman, P. and Friesen, W.V. (1975). *Unmasking the Face*. Englewood Cliffs, NJ: Prentice Hall.

Falk, R. (2000). The gene—a concept in transition. In P.J. Beurton, R. Falk and H.-J. Rheinberger (eds.) *The Concept of the Gene in Development and Evolution*, pp. 317–348. Cambridge: Cambridge University Press.

Fine, A. (1986). *The Shaky Game: Einstein, Realism, and the Quantum Theory*. Chicago, IL: University of Chicago Press.

Fogle, T. (2000). The dissolution of protein coding genes in molecular biology. In P.J. Beurton, R. Falk and H.-J. Rheinberger (eds.) *The Concept of the Gene in Development and Evolution*, pp. 3–25. Cambridge: Cambridge University Press.

Gregory, F. (2008). *Natural Science in Western History*. Boston, MA: Houghton Mifflin Company.

Kendler, K.S. (2005). 'A gene for': the nature of gene action in psychiatric disorders. *American Journal of Psychiatry*, 162(7), 1243–1252.

Lewis, D. (1983). *Philosophical Papers* (Vol. 2). Oxford: Oxford University Press.

Macalpine, I. and Hunter, R. (1974). The pathology of the past. *Times Literary Supplement*, March 15, 256–257.

Magner, L.N. (2002). *A History of the Life Sciences* (3rd ed.). New York: CRC Press.

Meehl, P.E. (1986). Diagnostic taxa as open concepts: metatheoretical and statistical questions about reliability and construct validity in the grand strategy of nosological revision. In T. Millon and G.L. Klerman (eds.) *Contemporary Directions in Psychopathology: Toward the DSM-IV*, pp. 215–231. New York: Guilford Press.

Ortony, A. and Turner, T.J. (1990). What's basic about basic emotions? *Psychological Review*, 97(3), 315–331.

Russell, J.A. (2003). Core affect and the psychological construction of emotion. *Psychological Review*, 110(1), 145–172.

Turkheimer, E. (1998). Heritability and biological explanation. *Psychological Review*, 105(4), 782–791.

Turkheimer, E. (2012). Genome wide association studies of behavior are social science. In K.S. Plaisance and T.A.C. Reydon (eds.) *Philosophy of Behavioral Biology* (Vol. 28), pp. 43–64. New York: Springer Science + Business Media.

Turkheimer, E., Pettersson, E., and Horn, E.E. (2014). A phenotypic null hypothesis for the genetics of personality. *Annual Review of Psychology*, 65, 515–540.

Woodward, J. (2008). Cause and explanation in psychiatry: an interventionist perspective. In K.S. Kendler and J. Parnas (eds.) *Philosophical Issues in Psychiatry: Explanation, Phenomenology, and Nosology*, pp. 136–184. Baltimore, MD: Johns Hopkins University Press.

Zachar, P. (2006). The classification of emotion and scientific realism. *Journal of Theoretical and Philosophical Psychology*, 26(1–2), 120–138

Section 10
Psychiatry and evolution

Chapter 28

Introduction to "What can evolution tell us about the healthy mind?"

Josef Parnas

Pathogenetic hypotheses and theories of modern psychiatry changed or became regularly modified over the course of the last 150 years, not only due to the developments within psychiatry itself but also due to developments in other disciplines. The appearance of an evolutionary approach to mental illness, the so-called evolutionary psychiatry, is an example of such a change that was initiated in the scientific domain external to the field of psychiatry itself, namely the evolutionary theory of biology. This is of course not to say that evolutionary thought was completely absent in psychiatry prior to the articulation of evolutionary psychiatry; Hughlings Jackson's theory of mental pathology as a product of "dissolution" (a kind of "reverse" evolution) is one familiar to most readers. Interestingly, the impact from evolutionary biology on psychiatry is itself a subject to quick changes because the notions of gene, genome, and genetic transmission have all undergone rapid scientific developments.

Chapter 29, written by John Dupré, a leading figure in contemporary philosophy of biology, addresses the epistemological and scientific status of evolutionary psychiatry (an offshoot of evolutionary psychology). After the arrival of sociobiology in the second half of the twentieth century, the evolutionary approach quickly found its way into psychiatry.

Evolutionary psychology and psychiatry are seen by Dupré partly as products of what he calls a "scientific imperialism," that is, a situation in which a theory, successful in one particular domain (e.g., biology), exports its concepts, perspectives, and domination to other domains (e.g., psychology and psychiatry), even though when such transfer is not be entirely justified or even applicable in the extended, target domain. Evolutionary theory is regarded by some psychiatrists as a paradigm for understanding the human mind and its pathologies. In other words, psychiatry, an essentially pragmatic discipline with unclear contours and mixed theoretical perspectives, needs to embrace an evolutionary approach as a unifying framework, conferring on psychiatry a status of "real" science (see also E. Bovet, Chapter 14 and Kendler Chapter 32, this volume).

Evolutionary psychiatry considers a psychopathological phenomenon as an abnormal expression of a mental disposition or function, both assumed to have developed and to have become genetically fixed during the Pleistocene. Mental pathology, simply stated, is a misfit between our ancient behavioral heritage and the context of modern societies. In order to address, for example, emotional disorders, we need to know what emotions are and that requires knowledge of their evolutionarily derived functions.

It occurs to me that it is a quite heavy theoretical and empirical task to define or individuate what a given "function" or "motivation" is, especially if the purpose is to arrive at a concept similar to that of a "natural kind." Second, behavior does not leave a fossil record (apart from cultural artefacts). Finally, it seems to me that requiring knowledge of the phylogenesis of a given function in order to understand it, is an exaggeration.

Jerry Fodor, an astute philosopher of cognition, once proposed the following thought experiment: We all assume that the function of the heart is to pump blood and that the heart must have evolved to do that. Imagine then that recent and very solid fossil discoveries contradict this second assumption, namely that the evolution of the heart actually happened in the assumed way. Would this new and dramatic fossil record stop us from continuing to consider the heart as having the function of pumping blood? Surely not; in fact, we are already in the phase of constructing mechanical heart-like devices (pumps) in order to reduce the need of heart transplants.

Dupré's chapter offers a systematic and critical assessment of the theoretical and empirical problems of evolutionary psychiatry, ending with a brief presentation of the dynamic systems theory. This latter approach will in all likelihood become an important tool for psychopathological theory and empirical research in the future. The chapter also provides a very relevant reference list for a reader eager to expand their knowledge of recent developments in this area.

Chapter 29

What can evolution tell us about the healthy mind?

John Dupré

29.1 Introduction

Change in science is commonly thought of as being endogenously driven. The internal logic of a body of scientific theory suggests lines of experimental or theoretical investigation, and unanticipated results of such investigations prompt more or less major modifications to the theory. But there are also exogenous sources of change from quite distinct and sometimes distant successful theories, which offer new ways of looking at a domain or findings that must be reconciled with a distinct domain. New ways of doing chemistry grew out of the acceptance of quantum mechanics, for example, and geological views about the rates of geological change had to be reconciled with new technologies for radioactive dating.

Generally this kind of cross-fertilization between scientific research programs should be seen as beneficial. But in some cases it can be less benign. It is a natural tendency for a successful research program to attempt to apply itself as widely as possible, and sometimes this can lead to attempts to colonize areas of inquiry for which it is poorly equipped. I have described this process, in its worst manifestations, as scientific imperialism (Dupré 1994). The power and generality of the central idea of natural selection has made it a particularly attractive base for such imperialism; *loci classici* are the notorious aspirations to colonize the humanities and social sciences in E.O. Wilson's *Sociobiology* (1975), or Daniel Dennett's conception of natural selection as a universal acid (Dennett 1995), capable of dissolving a vast array of problems.

It is hardly surprising that attempts have been made to expand the scope of evolutionary theory to the domain of human behavior, a project initiated by Darwin himself in *The Descent of Man*. Given that we evolved, and that therefore our behavior evolved, such attempts are surely sensible. Nevertheless, the processes through which our behavior evolved may be very different from those responsible for most of biological evolution; and biological evolution itself may involve a wider range of processes than are typically given much weight. So there are good reasons why these expansionist projects may prove unsuccessful. One project of this kind that has been particularly prominent for the last 30 years is the evolutionary psychology associated especially with Leda Cosmides and John Tooby (see, e.g., Barkow et al. 1992). It is also, according to several philosophers, including myself (Dupré 2001), a deeply ill-conceived project.

Some fields of investigation seem particularly liable to invite contributions from outside, whether beneficial or malignly imperialistic. It is unsurprising that psychiatry should be such a field, both because it lacks a dominant paradigm equipped to repel invaders, and because the complexity of the phenomena it addresses will very likely benefit from being considered from multiple perspectives. As chapters in the present volume illustrate, fields including genetics, neurophysiology, and evolution have volunteered to reform psychiatric thinking. All of these may well have significant contributions to make, though almost certainly less extensive contributions than their more enthusiastic advocates suppose. This chapter will explore the claims of evolutionary psychiatry, derived directly from the school of evolutionary psychology mentioned earlier, to hold the key to a proper understanding of the diseases of the mind. The chapter will outline the deficiencies of some of the arguments offered in favor of this reforming movement. More generally, it is hoped, it will provide a cautionary tale to deter excessive enthusiasm in assessing such offers of radical reform from distant intellectual arenas.

29.2 Evolution and the Human Mind

I introduce the substantive discussion of this chapter with some platitudes. First, we evolved: our distant ancestors were much simpler organisms, and at some point in the very distant past there are ancestors that we share with all other terrestrial organisms. I do not make any assumptions about the process of evolution, for example, on the role of natural selection or the extent to which natural selection guarantees optimal outcomes. It does follow from the fact that we evolved, however, that our capacities to develop healthy or unhealthy minds are products of our evolutionary history.

What does not follow from any of the above is that evolutionary theory will be useful in understanding either what constitutes a healthy mind or why, and under what circumstances, our minds sometimes become unhealthy. There are at least two reasons for this. First, our concepts of health and disease are partly normative concepts. This is most obviously the case for psychological health. In some historical periods, homosexuality, for instance, was taken to be a disease; moral reflection and political action have subsequently overturned this categorization. This is not to deny that there is an organic basis for many mental disorders or traits (homosexuality might in principle turn out to have a systematic neurological cause), nor that some organic conditions can produce conditions that would be drastically debilitating in any imaginable society. It is rather a reminder that in attempting to understand a psychiatric disorder we should always be prepared to ask why this condition is judged pathological. In some cases, no doubt, the answer will be obvious.

The normativity of at least some kinds of psychopathology is hardly controversial. Continuing the previous illustration, it was not that long ago that homosexuality was considered both a disease and a crime. It was then hazardous to be homosexual—leading to disastrous outcomes such as incarceration—and even today it exposes people to dangers from social discrimination and the violence of homophobic gangs. This observation points to the second problem I want to stress for evolutionary approaches to the pathological: pathology is a relation between an organism and an environment not, in general, an intrinsic feature of an organism. Although, as noted above, there are conditions that would very probably be considered pathological in just about any imaginable society, these constitute a limiting case rather than the paradigm. There is a sense in which homosexuality really is a pathology in a homophobic society: it is a dangerous and unhealthy behavioral disposition, though the danger derives not from any inherent features of the trait, but from the behavior it may precipitate in others.

We might also consider the suggestion deriving from Foucault that homosexuals, as a class of people with a particular distinguishing characteristic, are a social construct. Where once homosexual acts were just a behavior that many or most people engaged in on occasion, they were gradually interpreted as the symptoms identifying a special kind of person, or a pathology afflicting an unfortunate or sinful minority. While not forgetting that there are people with massive cognitive deficits that impair their functioning in any imaginable society, psychiatry is often concerned with more subtle mismatches between individual behavior and social norms. Much psychopathology can be, to a greater or lesser extent, partly constructed by these norms. This is nicely illustrated by Ian Hacking's discussion (Chapter 38, this volume) of the conditions under which (some) autistic people can lead worthwhile lives. My point here is not to promote general skepticism about psychopathology but only to recall the quite familiar difficulty of saying what it is, what its various manifestations are, and what are the conditions, internal and external to the patient, that make these manifestations pathological. This is important for understanding the difficulties with evolutionary approaches to the subject that will be the main topic of this chapter.

29.3 Is Evolution the Key to Understanding Human Behavior?

While evolutionary theory has had extraordinary successes in explaining biological phenomena, it is quite another matter to use it to predict, to tell us what organisms must be like ahead of our empirical discovery that they are or are not like that. Advocates of an evolutionary approach to psychiatry do not merely point to a well-understood phenomenon, say, schizophrenia, and explain how it came about. Given the limitations of our understanding of the mind it is inevitable that a general theory of its origin and function will reshape the categories in which we think about the mental. Evolutionary theorists indeed do propose that reflection on the evolutionary origins of our psychopathologies will help us to understand what these are, and even whether they are pathological. What they propose is, therefore, often more like prediction than explanation.

There are several grounds for skepticism about this general project. Evolution is an extremely complex process, the upshot of processes of many different kinds, and the nature and importance of these is by no means fully understood (Dupré 2012, chapter 9; Gould and Lewontin 1979). Moreover, if there is one feature that most clearly distinguishes human behavior, it is its plasticity. Of course, this plasticity evolved. But what is part of the normal scope of this evolved plasticity, and what lies beyond it in the realm of the abnormal or pathological, becomes a difficult, perhaps even incoherent, question. At any rate, behavioral plasticity makes it easy to understand how the realm of the normal may be an evolving function of the social environment as much or more than an intrinsic feature of the individual. With these concerns in mind, I turn to the claims made by advocates of evolutionary psychiatry for the relevance of their approach. Perhaps the best known such advocate is Randolph Nesse.

29.4 Nesse on the Proper Functioning of the Emotions

The evolutionary approach to psychiatric issues is well illustrated by Nesse's treatment of emotional disorders (Nesse and Jackson 2006). Nesse and Jackson's starting point is that we need evolutionary insight to understand why the emotions exist at all and hence what their proper functions are. Only from this perspective can we provide a proper taxonomy of emotions, realizing, for example, that sadness, depression, or anxiety may have different evolutionarily derived functions. Identification of these functions, in turn, can show us that some distressing emotions are normal given their occurrence in circumstances for which they are appropriate. This realization will enable the avoidance of false positives that can lead to inappropriate attempts to treat normal, functional emotional states. More generally, the evolutionary perspective is required if we are to analyze the motivational structure of an individual's life.

I offer no opinion on whether Nesse and Jackson's evolutionary reflections may have provided valuable insights into emotional disorders. Nevertheless, the path by which they have reached them is problematic. First, as already noted, inferring how something evolved presupposes knowing what it is that evolved. It is not now possible, and very probably never will be possible, to infer what features an organism must have from reflection on its evolutionary history. So whether sadness, depression, and anxiety are importantly different states is a question for empirical investigation of contemporary humans, not for theoretical evolutionary speculation.

A second difficulty is the omnipresence of exaptation, the adaptation of traits evolved to serve one function to entirely different uses. The fact that lungs evolved from structures that served to keep our fishy ancestors afloat doesn't imply that our present lungs are really flotation devices. This is a general problem with evolutionary accounts of function, which has led philosophers to the 'recent history' account of function, the idea that function is what currently maintains or has recently maintained a trait in a population (Godfrey-Smith 1994). The plasticity of human behavior makes it plausible that exaptation could happen on a very short timescale, so that identifying what evolutionary psychologists refer to as the "environment of evolutionary adaptation" (see further discussion later in this chapter) becomes an extremely difficult task.

Given these problems, it is no surprise that the possibility of inferring the functional organization of individuals from evolutionary reflection is typically grounded in simplistic and increasingly outdated ideas about evolution. Here are two indicative quotes from Nesse (2008):

> Biologists have known for decades that selection is much stronger at the level of the individual, so benefits to groups are rarely substantial. (p. S24)
>
> There is no single normal genome, there are just genes, some of which have been more successful than others in making bodies that survive to reproduce. (p. S26)

Both of these statements are highly contentious. While group selection became very unfashionable in the 1970s and 1980s, especially under the influence of Williams (1966) and the very successful popularization of Williams's views by Dawkins (1976), more recently the issue has become far more open (Sober and Wilson 1998). Notoriously, group selection has recently been strongly endorsed by E.O. Wilson (2012), the founder of sociobiology (Wilson 1975), the intellectual ancestor of evolutionary psychology. Needless to say, perhaps, the question of group selection is of central relevance to human behavior, much of which is undoubtedly directed at developing and maintaining cohesion and cooperation within groups, whether or not that is the evolutionary explanation of its existence.

The status of genes is also a matter of intense debate among philosophers of biology (Stotz and Griffiths 2013). An uncontentious point is that the behavior of genes, whatever exactly these are, is always dependent on many aspects of their cellular context, including other features of the genome. Arguably the genome is a much less theoretically problematic entity than the gene (Barnes and Dupré 2008). Certainly there is no normal genome if that is taken to mean some precise sequence of nucleotides; but there is a great deal more to a genome than a sequence of nucleotides. And in fact equally, there surely are abnormal, or at least pathological, genomes, for example, trisomies such as that which results in Down syndrome. There are invariably pathological genes, for example, the extended trinucleotide repeat that causes Huntington's disease, though this might equally well be seen as a genomic pathology. Most potentially harmful genes are only abnormal, however, in the sense of having harmful effects, in specific genomic contexts. As is a familiar finding from classical genetics, many recessive deleterious genes, genes that are harmful in the homozygous state, may be beneficial as heterozygotes.

My point here is not to develop an argument in favor of one position or other on these controversial and difficult questions, but to point out that evolutionary theory is in a dynamic and rapidly changing state, and that to take it as a firm body of established principles from which conclusions can be drawn in other equally difficult and contentious domains, is highly problematic (Dupré 2012, chapter 9).

29.5 Evolutionary Psychology and Evolutionary Psychiatry

Many attempts to apply evolutionary thinking to psychiatry follow closely the program of evolutionary psychology often referred to as the Santa Barbara School, associated especially with Leda Cosmides and John Tooby (Barkow et al. 1992; Buss 1999). Because there is an uncontroversial sense in which there must in principle be some legitimate study of Evolutionary Psychology—since humans evolved, their psychology must have evolved—it has become common to refer to the specific approach of the Santa Barbara School as Evolutionary Psychology, a convention I shall follow here after. Unfortunately Evolutionary Psychology suffers from serious deficiencies, including the general problems sketched in section 29.4 (Buller 2005; Dupré 2001). In this section I shall briefly describe Evolutionary Psychology, and the evolutionary psychiatry that derives from it, and point toward some of their failings. This will lead, in the section 29.5, to some suggestions about a more adequate way of thinking about human nature and, thus, its possible pathologies.

Representative applications of Evolutionary Psychology to psychiatry include a general treatment by Anthony Stevens and John Price (2000) and a more specific treatment of depression by Keedwell (2008). In briefest outline, these works take psychopathology to consist of a misfit between a universal evolved human nature and the actual (social) conditions of an individual. The contribution from Evolutionary Psychology is that human nature is to be discerned by reflection on a particular phase of evolutionary history, the Pleistocene, approximately the 2 million years preceding the Holocene, roughly the last 11,000 years. During this period, according to Evolutionary Psychologists, humans evolved a large number of specialized mental modules designed to deal with the problems posed by the natural and social environment of that time period.

Here is how Stevens and Price describe our general predicament:

> From a biological point of view, the ultimate purpose of our existence is the perpetuation of our genes. The transmission of our genes to the next generation is the *ultimate cause* of our behaviour. The archetypal propensities with which we are endowed are adapted to enable us to survive long enough in the environment in which we evolved ("the environment of evolutionary adaptedness") to give our genes a fair chance of transmission to our offspring. (Stevens and Price, p. 11; emphasis in original)

And here is why this leads to psychological disorder:

> cultural development now occurs too quickly for genes to adapt, resulting in a split between our genes and our lifestyles; this mismatch ... can bring about illness ... the brain is a physical structure ... and one that has been under genetic control. (Keedwell, pp. 6–7)

I, and others, have offered extensive criticism of the general picture assumed in these quotes, and I won't try to rehearse these in any detail here (Buller 2005; Dupré 2001). One central point is that, as is standard in Evolutionary Psychology, development is not highlighted—emphasis is on dispositions that develop similarly in the Stone Age and a modern city, that is, are genetically determined independent of any external developmental contingencies. Stevens and Price elaborate this in terms of Jungian *archetypes* and though these are no doubt controversial, I don't think their peculiarities are essential to the argument beyond proposing developmental trajectories that are evolutionarily selected and genetically determined.

Of course both Evolutionary Psychologists and their psychiatric followers universally deny that their doctrines embody genetic determinism. And of course this is quite correct if determinism is taken to deny any interaction between goals, drives, needs, etc. and the environment. But the basic goals are given: "psychopathology results when the environment fails ... to meet one (or more) archetypal need(s) in the developing individual" (Stevens and Price 2000, p. 34). At the very least these archetypal needs are seen as developmentally deeply entrenched and hard to deflect.

29.6 Against Atavism

The views I have been describing see human behavioral dispositions as *atavistic*. Though of course we may often manage to adjust our behavior to the exigencies of modern life, the dispositions from which we begin are designed for the very different conditions of the Stone Age. I have criticized this idea in some detail elsewhere (Dupré 2012, chapter 14), and I shall not rehearse the arguments in detail here. The key point is that the thesis of atavism is based on assumptions about the rate of evolution. Evolution is understood as involving random changes in genomes and selection of any that prove to be beneficial, and this is taken to be far too slow a process to result in significant changes in the short time period since the Pleistocene. But this is a quite inadequate account of human evolution. Changes in human behavior can be brought about, and passed on to descendants, by a variety of processes, notably cultural and epigenetic, that can operate on much shorter timescales. In the following sections I shall give some indications of how this can work, and how it wholly undermines the program of Evolutionary Psychology and its offspring in psychiatry.

29.7 Genetic versus Cultural Causes of Human Behavior

Notoriously, there is a good deal of mudslinging in debates over human nature, with opposing camps hurling accusations of genetic and cultural determinism. We can begin to move beyond these stark oppositions by noting a fundamental point about scientific explanation. In contrast with the grand theories espoused by an earlier generation, contemporary philosophers of science see explanation, at least in the social and biological sciences, as deriving from various kinds of models (Bailer-Jones 2009; Morgan and Morrison 2000). All models provide only partial representations of the real systems that are their targets. Certain features are highlighted and others ignored. This enables the understanding of important tendencies or capacities of real systems, but in the open real-world contexts in which living systems reside, scientific models cannot provide universally reliable predictions.

Given this basic point we might conclude that both genetic "determinist" and cultural "determinist" models were perfectly legitimate scientific tools. Up to a point this is correct. However, first, advocates of models of both kinds are sometimes inclined to what I have called scientific imperialism, the view that their favorite tools are far more widely applicable than they really are (Dupré 1994). (If you have a hammer, everything looks like a nail.) Second, and more important, in human development biological and cultural factors are almost invariably so deeply intertwined that a one-sided model is almost inevitably misleading. But finally, as I shall argue shortly, there are good reasons for paying more attention to cultural models.

One area where the atavistic perspective described in the preceding section might seem especially attractive is that of phobias. The dangers posed today by snakes and spiders are trivial compared to, say, cars or electric outlets. Yet the former are much more frequent subjects of phobia. It is hard to resist the conclusion that some atavistic predispositions are at work here. On the other hand there are also distinctively modern phobias, such as going to school or to the dentist, or of contracting AIDS. According to Stevens and Price (2000, pp. 103–104.) "[these] are contemporary versions of going off the home range, getting hurt, or of getting infected." Perhaps. But this is then looking a disturbingly Procrustean or even Panglossian program. (If you have a hammer…)

Surely a better way to understand this case is to see an interaction of biological, evolved tendencies with environmental factors that can lead to a wide variety of more or less pathological outcomes. Learning what to be afraid of is, presumably, an important part of development, and one that undoubtedly depends on both biological capacities and environmental inputs (learning of various kinds). Sometimes this fear is disproportionate, and sometimes it is directed at largely inappropriate objects, perhaps for reasons of phylogenetic inertia. There are no dangerous spiders where I live, but perhaps they were a serious threat to many generations of my ancestors.

A more complex example will show why generally we should be more interested in cultural determinants of behavior. Stevens and Price divide the fundamental goals of human life shaped by our Stone Age history into those concerned with rank and with attachment. Rank, or status, provides access to resources of all kinds, but especially mates. Attachment, cooperative relations with other humans, provides allies and again mates. They remark that "The commitment of social scientists to … cultural relativity and behavioral plasticity … has meant that the universal importance attributed to rank and status in human societies has been largely overlooked" (2000, p. 25). Knowing a few social scientists, I found this comment extraordinary. I'm inclined to say, rather, that the commitment of Evolutionary Psychologists to natural selection and reproductive success has meant that the universal importance attributed to rank and status by social scientists has been largely overlooked. Status is a (or the) fundamental organizing concept for much of social science.

There is an important point here beyond the mudslinging. While it may be true and important that a generalized drive to achieve high status can be found in the great majority of humans, the implications that this has in any particular human society are enormously more complex and interesting than the identification of such an allegedly general drive. And the implications in a particular complex modern society are quite different from those in a particular hunter-gatherer society. It is perhaps because of this that social scientists have been interested in the diversity of social contexts more than the possible universality of very basic human goals. No one is likely to deny that sex is a very widespread human goal, but it does not follow, nor is it true, that the implications of this are the same in Los Angeles, Teheran, and Beijing.

At any rate, the division of labor provides a foundation for all human societies, is a central feature that distinguishes one society from another, and provides a range of crucial differentiations within any society by giving rise to multiple, often cross-cutting status groups. Occupational status groups determined by the division of labor are cross-cut by countless other status groupings: race, gender, class, caste; nerds, geeks, skinheads, *Guardian* readers. As, for example, Bourdieu (1984) has elegantly demonstrated, status is also acquired and confirmed by a multitude of matters of taste and style. The fact that people seek status, at least within a more or less narrow group to which they belong, is a necessary background to the interest in considering these various sources of status. But if one in interested in how people actually behave there is no substitute for mapping the complex and intersecting paths to multiple different kinds of status in particular societies. In the present context it is surely these that must be understood if we are to discern the frustrations that the attempt to follow these winding paths can engender, and which can, in extreme cases, lead to mental illness. Social scientists are surely right to resist the reduction of this complexity to the quest for reproductive success.

29.8 Developmental Systems Theory

A much more useful approach to evolution, especially human evolution, than the neo-Darwinism implicit in the evolutionary psychiatry I have been criticizing is provided by developmental systems theory (DST) (Gray and Griffiths 1994; Oyama et al. 2001). DST sees evolution not as a sequence of statically defined things (adult organisms or genomes) but as a series of cycles of development, which also involve the assembly of the resources necessary for the next cycle. These resources certainly include genes, but also features of the "environment," from multiple features of cellular chemistry and structure beyond the mere sequence of nucleotides in the genome, to nests, dams, or hospitals. In the human case, a central aspect of the developmental niche is technology.

The emphasis on technology fits nicely with an important topic in recent evolutionary theory, niche construction (Odling-Smee et al. 2003). Emphasizing a feature of evolutionary thinking that was classically elaborated in Darwin's work on earthworms (Darwin 1881), the concept of niche construction captures the way that organisms do not merely evolve to adapt to a pre-existing environment, but also shape the environment to fit with their evolved needs. A glance at contemporary human environments makes the relevance of this point obvious. Indeed, few humans could survive at all outside the elaborate contexts that they have constructed for themselves. And this is not merely a matter of constructing environments suited to the thriving of humans as they have come to be. Within the perspective of DST it is clear that technology, by changing the conditions under which humans can develop, can itself provide real changes in human evolution. I would argue that technologies from clean water and drainage to rapid transport, computers, or cell phones provide just such potential agents of evolutionary change.

One other widely discussed feature of human evolution is the importance of cultural transmission. Most of human behavior is learned from parents, peers, teachers, or other role models. Innovations in behavior, often connected to new technologies, can spread rapidly through human populations, sometimes within the time frame of a single generation. It is sometimes objected that such changes should not count as evolutionary because of their potential impermanence. But I can see no force to this point. There is no theoretical reason why rapid transport, say, should not remain a feature of human existence for another million years nor, for that matter, why we should not be wiped out by familiar biological forces next week. Generally, the attempt to find something conceptually unique about genetic transmission seems increasingly unpromising, an observation that is in fact central to the widespread acceptance of DST by philosophers of biology.

The rejection of the privileged status of genetic transmission, finally, completely undermines the standard Evolutionary Psychological argument for privileging the conditions of the Pleistocene in understanding human evolution. The human environment has changed massively and dramatically in the last 11,000 years, the Holocene, as has the variety of human behavior. At some level of abstraction there are no doubt neural structures that have remained pretty much the same over this period, many of which date from far earlier periods than the Pleistocene. Similarly, much basic metabolic chemistry has remained largely unchanged for much of the history of life, but no one supposes that this is the right level of abstraction to understand general morphology or physiology. It is worth mentioning that as well as genetic and cultural transmission, there has recently been an explosion of interest in epigenetic transmission, heritable changes to the genome that do not involve changes to nucleotide sequence (Jablonka and Lamb 1995, 2005). The diversity of kinds of change and modes of transmission that can be involved in human evolution makes the Evolutionary Psychologists' obsession with genetic evolution in the Pleistocene entirely without defensible rationale.

29.9 Human Nature as a Process

Evolutionary Psychology offers us a theory of a universal human nature. Even if this particular approach is misguided, there remains a widespread intuition that there must be some such human nature, and that discovering what this is must be the key to understanding the deviations from it that constitute psychopathology. The intuition is expressed by William James (1890, emphasis in original):

> Why do we smile, when pleased, and not scowl? Why are we unable to talk to a crowd as we talk to a single friend? Why does a particular maiden turn our wits so upside-down? The common man can only say, *Of course* we smile, *of course* our heart palpitates at the sight of the crowd, *of course* we love the maiden, that beautiful soul clad in that perfect form, so palpably and flagrantly made for all eternity to be loved!

The 'of course' in this quote, I take it, points to the idea that this is just what people are like, something that is just obvious to all of us, even the common man. These are commonplace remarks about human nature. Such an appeal to human nature seems plausible because certain abstractions across human behavior seem both intuitively and evolutionarily inescapable: expression of emotions (an element of sociality), interest in (usually) the opposite sex, etc. But once again, the problem is with the level of abstraction. To know how real people will actually behave, we need to know more specific facts about a particular cultural context or a particular individual. *When* we smile, or *which* maidens turn our wits upside down, etc., can vary greatly and change rapidly. The most distinctive thing about human "nature" is its flexibility. And the specific, local level at which behavior is underdetermined is crucial for understanding human evolution. The level at which behavior is underdetermined by biologically inherited factors provides the material for cultural evolution, and cultural evolution can produce profound changes in the developmental niche. Through such processes changes in behavior can be firmly entrenched in human lineages.

According to Cosmides and Tooby, "Our modern skulls house a stone age mind," (Cosmides and Tooby 1997). But this is just wrong. For one thing, according to many contemporary philosophers from followers of Wittgenstein to various kinds of externalists and adherents of extended mind theses, our skulls don't house minds of any kind. The most that can be said with any confidence is that our skulls house a partly Stone Age brain. I say "partly," first, because much of the brain has a history that goes back far beyond the Stone Age. This evolutionarily ancient structure may be said to provide the physiological basis for the modern mind, and maybe even for Stone Age (or much earlier) dispositions, provided these are described in a sufficiently broad and abstract way. But the modern mind is codetermined by the context, especially social, in which it develops. And this context, and the minds that have developed within it, have changed at a far greater rate than genetic evolution alone could allow.

Human nature is generally understood as a common property of all humans. But there are also the particular natures of individual humans. I suggest that one way of thinking more clearly about both these topics is to understand them as processes. It is uncontroversial, of course, that whatever universal human nature there may be at any time is always evolving, and hence is a developing process not a static thing. My argument here has been that many theorists, including some evolutionary psychiatrists, have entirely misconstrued the rate of change of this process. To whatever extent there is, nonetheless, a universal human nature at a time, what it contributes to individual humans is just one of a number of developmental resources. Individual human nature is then a process of development in which these resources interact with a wide range of environmental conditions and contingencies to produce the particular nature—habits, dispositions, etc.—of the individual human. This nature is itself subject to continuous change and development over the life course. Except in cases of extreme dysfunction, trying to understand this process in terms of something as static as gene sequence is bound to fail. The clearest empirical observation about evolved human nature, to repeat, is its perhaps unique flexibility.

I must leave it to psychiatrists themselves to decide whether this perspective is helpful in understanding mental illness. It is uncontentious that mental illness is a developmental outcome, so it seems likely that a clearer view of the nature of human development is the best resource for a proper conceptual grasp of the causes and character of psychopathology. At the very least, it should be clear that reflection on Stone Age life is an unpromising path for gaining insights into psychiatry. Much more generally, we should be extremely wary of inferring from the fact that a theoretical perspective can in principle be applied to a domain of inquiry that it will be useful to do so. It is undoubtedly true that our minds evolved. But whether the models of evolutionary process that have proved useful in understanding many aspects of the history of life will be illuminating in understanding this particular and perhaps unique episode in the history of life is another matter. And indeed much experience to date suggests that such a strategy will provide more confusion than illumination.

Acknowledgments

This chapter has benefitted greatly from the thoughtful comments of Kenneth Kendler and Josef Parnas. The research leading to these results has received funding from the European Research Council under the European Union's Seventh Framework Programme (FP7/2007-2013)/ERC grant agreement no. 324186.

References

Bailer-Jones, D. (2009). *Scientific Models in Philosophy of Science*. Pittsburgh, PA: University of Pittsburgh Press.

Barkow, J., Cosmides, L., and Tooby, J. (eds.) (1992). *The Adapted Mind*. New York: Oxford University Press.

Barnes, B. and Dupré, J. (2008). *Genomes and What to Make of Them*. Chicago, IL: University of Chicago Press.

Bourdieu, P. (1984). *Distinction: A Social Critique of the Judgement of Taste*. (R. Nice, trans.) Cambridge, MA: Harvard University Press.

Buller, D. (2005). *Adapting Minds: Evolutionary Psychology and the Persistent Quest for Human Nature*. Cambridge, MA: MIT Press.

Buss, D. (1999). *Evolutionary Psychology: The New Science of the Mind*. New York: Doubleday.

Cosmides, L. and Tooby, J. (1997). *Evolutionary Psychology: A Primer*. [Online] Available at: <http://www.cep.ucsb.edu/primer.html>.

Darwin, C. (1881). *The Formation of Vegetable Mould, through the Action of Worms, with Observations on their Habits*. New York: D. Appleton.

Dawkins, R. (1976). *The Selfish Gene*. Oxford: Oxford University Press.

Dennett, D. (1995). *Darwin's Dangerous Idea: Evolution and the Meanings of Life*. New York: Simon and Schuster.

Dupré, J. (1994). On scientific imperialism. *Philosophy of Science Association Proceedings*, 2, 374–381.

Dupré, J. (2001). *Human Nature and the Limits of Science*. Oxford: Oxford University Press.

Dupré, J. (2012). *Processes of Life: Essays in the Philosophy of Biology.* Oxford: Oxford University Press.

Godfrey-Smith, P. (1994). A modern history theory of functions. *Noûs,* 28, 344–362

Gould, S.J. and Lewontin, R.C. (1979). The spandrels of San Marco and the Panglossian program: a critique of the adaptationist program. *Proceedings of the Royal Society of London,* 250, 281–288.

Griffiths, P. and Stotz, K. (2013). *Genetics and Philosophy: An Introduction.* New York: Cambridge University Press.

Griffiths, P.E. and Gray, R.D. (1994). Developmental systems and evolutionary explanation. *Journal of Philosophy,* 91, 277–304.

Jablonka, E. and Lamb, M.J. (1995). *Epigenetic Inheritance and Evolution: The Lamarckian Dimension.* New York: Oxford University Press.

Jablonka, E. and Lamb, M.J. (2005). *Evolution in Four Dimensions: Genetic, Epigenetic, Behavioral, and Symbolic Variation in the History of Life.* Cambridge, MA: MIT Press.

Keedwell, P. (2008). *How Sadness Survived: The Evolutionary Basis of Depression.* Oxford: Radcliffe Publishing.

Morgan, M. and Morrison, M. (1999). *Models as Mediators: Perspectives on Natural and Social Science.* Cambridge: Cambridge University Press.

Nesse, R.M. (2008). Evolution: medicine's most basic science. *The Lancet,* 372, S21–S27.

Nesse, R.M. and Jackson, E.D. (2006). Evolution: psychiatric nosology's missing biological foundation. *Clinical Neuropsychiatry,* 3, 121–131.

Odling-Smee, F.J., Laland, K.N., and Feldman, M.W. (2003). *Niche Construction: The Neglected Process in Evolution.* Princeton, NJ: Princeton University Press.

Oyama, S., Griffiths, P.E., and Gray, R.D. (eds.) (2001). *Cycles of Contingency: Developmental Systems and Evolution.* Cambridge, MA: MIT Press.

Sober, E. and Wilson, D.S. (1998). *Unto Others: The Evolution and Psychology of Unselfish Behavior.* Cambridge, MA: Harvard University Press.

Stevens, A. and Price, J. (2000). *Evolutionary Psychiatry: A New Beginning* (2nd ed.). Hove: Routledge.

Williams, G.C. (1966). *Adaptation and Natural Selection.* Princeton, NJ: Princeton University Press.

Wilson, E.O. (1975). *Sociobiology: The New Synthesis.* Cambridge, MA: Harvard University Press.

Wilson, E.O. (2012). *The Social Conquest of Earth.* New York: Norton.

Chapter 30

What can history and social studies of sciences teach us about evolutionary psychiatry?

Emilie Bovet

30.1 Introduction

I am far from being an expert in evolutionary psychiatry, but Chapter 29 by John Dupré gave me the opportunity to think about the issues we can address to this field through the two perspectives that I favor in my research: epistemological history of psychiatry and social studies of sciences. It also seems to me that these two perspectives are very complementary to the philosophy of sciences in adopting a critical stance toward evolutionary psychiatry.

30.2 In Search of Scientific Legitimacy

Even if I share Dupré's skepticism about the arguments put forward by evolutionary psychiatry, my goal is not to deconstruct these arguments one by one. I'll rather try to provide some clues to think about how such a discipline can emerge and be strengthened in the field of psychiatry.

We can first mention briefly the paradox of psychiatry as a scientific discipline. Among medical and scientific disciplines, psychiatry is often considered as a "separate" one since it tries to treat pathologies whose etiologies are unknown and where diagnosis can vary depending on theoretical and therapeutic approaches. There is indeed no way to act on the pathology except through drugs and various forms of psychotherapy. Clinicians in psychiatry are thus always forced to do a sort of therapeutic "trial and error" to alleviate mental suffering. The immense diversity of the psychiatric field, both at a practical and at a theoretical level, tends sometimes to discredit psychiatry toward other scientific communities whose theories and therapeutic tools do not represent a source of such strong disagreements.

The whole question of the status of psychiatry as a "scientific" discipline appears tangentially. Psychiatry is indeed generally considered as the "orphan child" in medical sciences, and this complex is not only apparent in the current literature in the field. It also appears throughout the decades in all the issues concerning the training of clinicians in psychiatry, such as: Does specialization in psychiatry have to be part of the training in medicine? Should psychiatry be definitely integrated with neurology? Is psychoanalysis really scientific? We can thus easily understand that psychiatry is struggling to find its place at a time when the practice of evidence-based medicine is increasing.

Psychiatry has always been in search of scientific legitimacy and we find in its history many attempts to anchor it in a more scientific field, by searching for explanations which link mental suffering to brain or somatic disturbances. Identifying the attempts of psychiatry to strengthen its scientific status is part of my work as a historian. Indeed, most of the recent books on biological psychiatry or on psychiatric neurosciences put forward their own narrative and often forget to mention that the interest of psychiatry in biology and brain is far from being new. This kind of narrative actually gives the impression that psychiatry had finally become scientific at the end of the twentieth century. However, there have been many schema and theories which claimed that psychiatry was part of biology and which finally attempted to give some explanatory dimension to mental illness. Although the hope of finding an explanation for the etiology of mental disorders has mostly not been achieved, it has always motivated the psychiatric hypotheses which focused on the biological part of the pathology.

I think that evolutionary psychiatry is one example of these numerous attempts to make psychiatry more "explainable," to give it a more scientific status. In this respect, it is interesting to read the first paragraphs of Stevens and Price's book (2000), mentioned by Dupré, which underline the paradoxical situation of every clinician in psychiatry: according to Stevens and Price, the psychiatrist is a doctor, whose primary tasks are to examine, diagnose, and treat. They say that "a psychiatric examination, like any medical examination, is designed to elicit signs and symptoms and to establish the history and course of a diagnosable disease" (Stevens and Price 2000, p. 3). They add that if psychiatrists persuade themselves that they are dealing with clinical entities which possess a known origin, a definable course, and a definite cure, it is largely an illusion.

This kind of introduction is often found in books which try to stress the necessity of strengthening the links between psychiatry and biology. This strategy also allows the reader to think that he or she is faced with a revolutionary step which will change the way of conceiving psychiatry. Moreover, we cannot forget that Stevens and Price's book, like many studies on evolutionary psychiatry, was first published during the 1990s, the decade of the brain. Evolutionary psychiatry takes then part in the rise of psychiatric neurosciences, and the promises made by Stevens and Price about the future of psychiatry also concern a strong bond between psychiatry and neurosciences.

However, a closer look at the emergence of evolutionary psychiatry reveals that this discipline is actually not so unprecedented as it pretends to be. This is where the use of history may be relevant. Indeed, even if their purposes were not described in the same words, psychiatrists from the first part of the twentieth century were already concerned with the Darwinian perspective. We can, for example, quote some French or Swiss psychiatrists such as Henri Ey, Jean Delay, or Hans Steck who shared a strong interest in a neo-Jacksonian model of mental pathology. They were thus persuaded that our nervous system was hierarchical; it could indeed be compared to a pyramid with different levels: at the base are the most archaic and automatic levels, which remain almost unchanged from birth to death, while the upper levels keep evolving and are less firmly organized than the lower ones. If the Jacksonian conception of the nervous system and mental pathology cannot be qualified as "evolutionist," it is striking to see how the psychiatrists who support this model have referred to evolution in their attempts to understand the emergence of mental pathology. The French psychiatrist Henri Ey, for example, often used the terms "regression" or phylogenetic archaism to qualify the pathological behaviors; mental pathology could thus correspond to a primitive state of evolution. That is why the idea prevailed that people falling into madness show the same characteristics as "primitive" people, as he calls them. A huge literature can thus be found from this period on the comparison between mentally ill people, "primitive" people, and animals. Most of this literature also refers to ethnology and anthropology, which at that time were mostly used to justify colonization, by studying the "archaic behaviors" of colonized populations. The diencephalic hypothesis of mental pathology (see E. Bovet, Chapter 14, this volume) certainly pertains to a conception which neglects the cultural aspects of the patient's life. The aim is really to find a common point in each brain to explain the emergence of mental pathology. This part of the brain is supposed to regulate instinct and emotions, which are the most primitive reactions in human behavior. That is why studies on the diencephalon are performed as much on humans as on animals, in order to confirm that this part of the brain can be universally considered as the seat of primitive instincts that have not really evolved since the beginning of humanity and which we share with animals. Paul MacLean, who published a lot of studies on the diencephalon and is also one of the promoters of the limbic system theory, claimed himself to be an evolutionist neurophysiologist and wrote some texts on this subject, insisting on the fact that each human brain still has a strong animal heritage. It is still today very common to hear that we react with our reptilian brain, mainly to explain an emotion like fear or a reaction like running away when we face a danger. If I cannot go into the issue of normativity, which Dupré evokes in his chapter, it is essential for me to consider the strong normative dimension of theories such as those focusing on the diencephalon or other parts of the brain in psychiatry, because they allow psychiatrists to define pathological behaviors by anchoring them in a somatic (or cerebral) dysfunction.

It seems to me that referring to history can help to relativize the revolutionary discourse put forward by the supporters of evolutionary psychiatry. Indeed, I consider that the success of evolutionary psychiatry was clearly linked with the rise of psychological neurosciences and was useful to its promotion. It should be pertinent to wonder why these neurosciences, when they put forward their promises, forget to mention that long before the "decade of the brain," psychiatry had tried to explain the link between the development of the brain and the emergence of mental pathology through a perspective which relied on the theory of evolution.

30.3 Which Evolution for Evolutionary Psychiatry?

As a social scientist interested by the social studies of science and medicine, I always find it useful to think about the political and institutional repercussions which can be provoked by this kind of discipline. It seems that today, evolutionary psychiatry from the 1990s has progressively been replaced by less deterministic approaches, mentioned by Dupré, such as those which mobilize epigenetic or cerebral plasticity. The references to epigenetic plasticity, as well as the references to cerebral plasticity, are very practical because they underline a constant interaction between genetics, brain, and environment. At first sight, these new theories seem closer to social sciences than evolutionary psychiatry, because they take into account cultural and environmental aspects of development. However, when it comes to simplifying these kinds of theories, evolutionist perspectives are really not so far away. It is indeed striking to see how the notion of attachment which prevails in evolutionary psychiatry, remains one of the main notions in the field of social neurosciences. This notion is also related to many others, such as nurture, fidelity, protection, pair-bounding or monogamy ... all the new trends of social neurosciences which, however, draw on theories of evolution to explain most of our behaviors.

Living in a town famous worldwide for its teams and research projects in the field of neurosciences, I would give as an example a local and current problem concerning theories about the expression of violence. There are indeed a lot of studies conducted with animals in behavioral genetics laboratories at the Lausanne Polytechnical University. Most of these studies put forward an epigenetic explanation of violent behaviors, in which the "environment" is considered as central to explain the emergence of violence. It remains that these studies rarely mention the complex environments in which human beings evolve: most of the time, the environment evoked in behavioral genetics refers either to the device of the experiment or to the natural environment of the animal in which the researchers seek to identify the origin of violent behavior. In a large interdisciplinary conference called "Understanding Violence" organized in 2009 by the Lausanne Polytechnical University, I assisted in a lot of meetings where human beings were compared to animals in the expression of violence, and where evolutionist theories prevailed. At the conclusion of one of the meetings, an internationally famous researcher in behavioral genetics claimed that beards in human males were related to the lion's mane, which could explain a lot of similarities in the way both act. If epigenetic and cerebral plasticity are supposed to provide theories more complex than genetic determinism, it seems that this complexity disappears when it comes to drawing easy conclusions to understand where violence comes from. In this context, evolutionist theories continue to be mobilized to explain violence in humans, especially men's domestic violence against women. Today in the French-speaking part of Switzerland, the tendency to organize political conferences on violence focusing on the genetic and hereditary dispositions to this behavior is clearly increasing. There is almost no more discussion on the social construction of violence, as if this theory was too obsolete and militant to be taken into account. In the long term, one might fear a reduction in budgets for organizations which don't share the theoretical basis of social neurosciences.

It thus seems that we have to analyze how evolutionary psychiatry is itself evolving today in order to adapt itself to new kinds of theories which are less deterministic than before. It is also a big issue for social scientists to keep a critical distance toward theories which don't oppose cultural and environmental development with genetic dispositions. We are indeed currently facing a new step in the way of conceiving the interaction between culture, environment, brain, and genetics, and it is important that theories coming from the social sciences do not end up being totally confounded with theories coming from the social neurosciences.

Reference

Stevens, A. and Price, J. (2000). *Evolutionary Psychiatry: A New Beginning* (2nd ed.). Hove: Routledge.

Part III
Specific disorders from a historical perspective

Section 11
Schizophrenia and the dopamine hypothesis

Chapter 31

Introduction to "Dopamine hypothesis of schizophrenia: an updated perspective"

Josef Parnas

In Chapter 32, we are offered a thoughtful historical and conceptual analysis of the most influential etiological theory of schizophrenia, that is, the dopamine hypothesis of schizophrenia (DHS). Kenneth Kendler is a perfectly suitable candidate for venturing on such a critical enterprise, given his long track record of research in psychopathology, epidemiology, and genetics, combined with an interest in and study of conceptual and philosophical dimensions of science.

The chapter starts with the history surrounding the first articulations of the DHS, followed by a summary of findings from a previously published review (Kendler and Schaffner 2011), an update of empirical findings since 2008, and a thorough weighing of empirical evidence and nonempirical influences on the changing formulations and status of the DHS.

As it will become clear from reading this dispassionate text, a critical examination of the DHS is a quite sensitive undertaking, perhaps bordering on blasphemy. For this reason, it is not strange that Kendler and Schaffner's (2011) first paper on the DHS only succeeded in appearing in *Philosophy, Psychiatry, & Psychology* (a highly specialized journal for a philosophically minded audience) rather than in a general psychiatric journal with a high impact factor.

Kendler's chapter is an excellent example of an analysis of the historical vicissitudes of an important, unifying etiological theory of schizophrenia, its attractiveness as a simple explanatory model, its professional appeal through a medicalization of psychiatry to the status of "real science," its unsurpassed adaptability in the face of negative findings, and of a host of nonempirical factors contributing to its persistence. For the unlikely reader, who mistakenly considers the scientific activity as an exclusively unselfish pursuit of truth, the reading of this chapter may be discomforting.

I will end the introduction with two personal comments. A few days ago, I had a conversation with a 26-year-old woman with schizophrenia, who told me that during a high-school class (when she was 16–17 years old), a "depression dawned on her," a depression that manifested itself by a realization that the very process of asking certain theoretical and scientific questions necessarily involved *not asking other*, potentially equally relevant questions, with deleterious consequences for humanity. She had a solipsistic sense of having a deeper access to reality than other people (including her ability to ask the unasked questions). Yet, what she expressed is a truly important philosophical issue with serious epistemological and metaphysical implications, namely the issue of "unconceived alternatives." In our particular context, a rigid and concerted pursuit of a dominating scientific path not only entails not asking other, potentially relevant questions but it restrains the very conceivability of the latter type of questioning. We can only imagine to what extent the domination of the "chemical imbalance" theory diverted resources and efforts, which might have been better used elsewhere. The second point relates to the widespread and unquestioned popularity of the DHS. My personal professional trajectory is very much influenced by Bleuler's, Minkowki's, Meehl's, Kety's, and others' concept of the schizophrenia spectrum of disorders—a view of schizotypy with its autistic features as the most elementary phenotype of the spectrum and expressive of a certain structural alteration of consciousness (subjectivity) (Parnas and Henriksen, in press). I always failed to grasp how an etiological theory, which from the beginning was only really designed to address the positive symptoms of schizophrenia, often considered as "secondary" attempts at coping or mal-adaptation, could achieve such a dogmatic credibility despite leaving out of its account the phenomenological core of the illness.

Reference

Parnas, J. and Henriksen, M.G. (n.d.). Disordered self in the schizophrenia spectrum: a clinical and research perspective. *Harvard Review of Psychiatry*. [Online] Available at: <http://journals.lww.com/hrpjournal/toc/9000/00000>.

Chapter 32

The dopamine hypothesis of schizophrenia: an updated perspective

Kenneth S. Kendler

32.1 Introduction

This chapter is best seen as a continuation and update of a prior detailed historical and philosophical analysis of the dopamine hypothesis of schizophrenia (DHS) that I completed with Kenneth Schaffner in 2008, although published several years later (Kendler and Schaffner 2011). This chapter has four major parts. First, I briefly summarize our prior findings. Second, I update the review with several relevant developments. Third, I review, utilizing the frameworks developed in this book by Longino (Chapter 2) and Solomon (Chapter 8) (Solomon 2001), the role of empirical and nonempirical factors that impacted on the DHS during its development and subsequent history. Finally, I try to contextualize the DHS story in light of the histories of etiologic controversies in other medical disorders and see if we can begin to determine what features of the DHS might be typical versus more unique.

32.2 A Brief History of the DHS

We should begin by asking why it is important to study the history of the DHS. This can be easily answered. In approximately the last quarter of the twentieth century (e.g., ~1975–2000), the DHS was arguably the most prominent etiologic theory in psychiatry, widely discussed, taught to all medical students and psychiatric residents, and routinely reviewed in major textbooks. It has stimulated a huge biomedical literature—with a current PubMed search on "dopamine" and "schizophrenia" yielding 7785 hits (May 2014). Understanding its origins and evolution should help clarify the nature of modern psychiatry. Furthermore, given the focus of this volume on the ways in which historical changes in psychiatry respond to empirical versus nonempirical forces, the DHS is likely to be a good "teaching case."

To understand the origins of the DHS, it is important to review briefly the scientific context of American psychiatry in the 1950s–1960s. Both the clinical and academic psychiatric worlds were dominated by psychoanalysis. A long period of therapeutic pessimism had come to an end by a very exciting series of developments in the late 1940s and 1950s that produced the first specific pharmacologic treatments for psychiatric illness—antipsychotic drugs for schizophrenia, lithium for bipolar illness, and antidepressants for major depression. The field of neuroscience was in an early growth spurt. Researchers spoke for the first time of being able to read "the chemical language of the brain." The National Institutes of Health was growing and beginning to widely fund research, thereby supporting the rise of research-oriented medical schools. A number of leaders of the field of psychiatry were uneasy. Psychoanalytically dominated psychiatry was widely perceived as distant from the rest of medicine. Its prestige, in many circles, was low and it seemed very difficult to link psychoanalysis to mainstream medicine, especially as it was becoming increasingly based in the biomedical sciences.

A few key scientific developments played a central role in the emergence of the DHS. In 1957, Montagu discovered dopamine (DA) in brain tissue (Montagu 1957) and 1960 saw the publication of dramatic results from Ehringer and Hornykiewicz of the lowered content of DA in postmortem brains of patients dying with Parkinson's disease (Ehringer and Hornykiewicz 1960). This opened up the possibility of linking a clinically complex neuropsychiatric disorder to dysfunction in a single neurotransmitter system. In 1960–1965, histofluorescence stains were developed whereby the cell bodies and the neuronal pathways for the monoamine neurotransmitters DA, norepinephrine, and serotonin could be traced in the brain (Dahlstrom and Fuxe 1964; Falck et al. 1982; Fuxe et al. 1966). The year 1963 saw the key discovery by Carlsson and Lindqvist that neuroleptic drugs effective in the treatment of schizophrenia increased DA turnover in rodent brain (that is, augmented the amount of DA being produced and degraded) (Carlsson and Lindqvist 1963). L-dopa, a precursor of DA, entered clinical practice in 1967, and the first large study reporting improvements in people with Parkinson's disease resulting from treatment with levodopa was published in 1968 (Kopin 1993). This suggested that effective therapy for neuropsychiatric disorders could be based on single neurotransmitter models.

The first hints about an emerging DHS were published from 1967 to 1973, always in the context of evidence that the effective antipsychotic drugs increased DA turnover. This view is well captured by this brief quote from one of the key early proponents of the DHS—Matthysse—in 1973:

> Suppose we now assume that the hypothesis of specific blockade of dopamine transmission by neuroleptic drugs is true [...]. Does the theory give us any clues to the neuropathological basis of schizophrenia? [...] From the blocking action of neuroleptics on dopamine synapses, it is a relatively small step to postulate over-activity of dopaminergic transmission in schizophrenia, whether generalized or confined to one nuclear group. (Matthysse 1973, p. 204)

Here are two more brief definitions of the DHS from other key early papers:

> [T]oo much dopamine is released at synapses in the central nervous system. (Matthysse and Lipinski 1975, p. 558)
>
> [S]chizophrenia may be related to a relative excess of DA-dependent neuronal activity. (Meltzer and Stahl 1976, p. 19)

The subsequent history of the DHS has two major themes. After an early key success—in which the potency of antipsychotic drugs was shown to be highly correlated with their ability to block DA receptors—the DHS failed considerably more tests than it succeeded at. We presented a "box-score" in our prior review (Kendler and Schaffner 2011, table 2) of eight predictions of the DHS examined in multiple studies. Six of them produced results contrary to predictions of the DHS, one was consistently positive, and one equivocal. The one positive finding was that, as predicted, the administration of amphetamine (a "dirty drug" which among other things indirectly stimulates DA receptors) consistently made individuals with schizophrenia worse. Prominent negative findings were the inability to detect increased levels of DA or key DA metabolites in cerebrospinal fluid or postmortem samples from individuals with schizophrenia. The one equivocal finding emerged from imaging studies of brain DA receptors with some evidence that receptor levels were elevated in schizophrenia (of that more later). We then reviewed results from eight DA-related genes, variants at which the DHS predicted would be involved in risk for schizophrenia. Results for one of these were equivocal, five were negative, and one was modestly positive.

The second theme in the history of the DHS was how poorly specified the theory was. It became, over time, protean, shifting to accommodate failures. It was the opposite of a clean "Popperian" refutable hypothesis. For example, should the abnormalities be seen in all major DA systems in the brain (there are, depending on how you count, four or five of them) or only some? If some, which ones? (Ironically, while most theorists focused on the mesolimbic and mesocortical DA tracts that subserve brain areas likely involved in schizophrenia, much of the subsequent work has been done on the nigrostriatal system which largely governs motor movements because it is so much more accessible for study.) Would the excess DA function result from too much DA or receptors that were too sensitive? If we looked for alterations in DA receptors, which ones (there are at least five)? Should we examine postsynaptic receptors or presynaptic receptors? What about the role of synthetic or degradative enzymes?

Of note, a major revision of the DHS was proposed by Davis and colleagues in 1991 (Davis et al. 1991). They moved away from a single global DHS into a theory with two subcomponents:

> The authors hypothesize that schizophrenia is characterized by abnormally low prefrontal dopamine activity (causing deficit symptoms) leading to excessive dopamine activity in mesolimbic dopamine neurons (causing positive symptoms). (Davis et al. 1991, p. 1474)

32.3 An Update on the DHS

Of the many research approaches to the testing of the DHS, only two have remained highly active since we completed our prior review in 2008—imaging and molecular genetics. In the area of imaging, an important meta-analytic review of positron emission tomography (PET) studies in schizophrenia was published by Howes and colleagues (Howes et al. 2012). They addressed evidence for in vivo altered brain DA function in schizophrenia in three possible ways: presynaptic DA function (DA synthesis capacity and release, and synaptic DA levels), DA transporter, and D2 and D3 postsynaptic receptor availability. For DA transporter availability, the meta-analysis was clearly negative—no difference between cases and controls. For the D2/D3 receptors (the major focus of prior work both in vivo and in postmortem studies), results were marginally positive for all studies but disappeared when drug-naïve patients were studied (which here is critical because antipsychotic drugs can elevate levels of brain DA receptors). Note that this research area had produced equivocal findings on our prior review and these authors are clearly skeptical about the small positive effects observed. The authors were skeptical about these findings and felt that they were likely negative. However, Howes et al. found significant evidence for elevated presynaptic DA function in schizophrenic patients, consistent with predictions of the original DHS. But the area studied was the basal ganglia and so these results were not actually consistent with the modified version of DHS by Davis et al. who predicted DA hyperactivity in mesolimbic pathways. One other meta-analysis of striatal DA transporter activity in drug-naïve schizophrenia patients was published by Chen and colleagues in 2013 with negative results (Chen et al. 2013).

By far the most important development in the genetics of schizophrenia since 2008 has been the success of genome-wide association studies (GWAS). This approach, for the first time, gives us an unbiased view of the association with schizophrenia risk of all variants across the genome. The most important paper published to date was by Ripke and colleagues (Ripke et al. 2011) in 2011. In samples of schizophrenic patients and controls in both the discovery and replicate samples of over 50,000, seven risk loci were identified. What is important for the current discussion is that none of those loci were in or near genes directly involved in any aspect of DA function. **While many more risk genes remain to be discovered, and further results are sure to be available before this book is published, these results clearly suggest that variants in DA-related genes are not going to be among the strongest identified for schizophrenia. Given the high heritability of schizophrenia (Sullivan et al. 2003), if abnormalities in DA systems were central to the pathophysiology for this disorder, this would not be the expected pattern of results.

One further development in the DHS since 2008 is noteworthy. In 2009, Howes and Kapur published an important review paper with the title "The dopamine hypothesis of schizophrenia: version III—the final common pathway" (Howes and Kapur 2009). I quote from their abstract (where they consider the Davis et al. paper noted above version II of the DHS):

> The dopamine hypothesis of schizophrenia has been one of the most enduring ideas in psychiatry. Initially, the emphasis was on a role of hyperdopaminergia in the etiology of schizophrenia (version I), but it was subsequently reconceptualized to specify subcortical hyperdopaminergia with prefrontal hypodopaminergia (version II). However, these hypotheses focused too narrowly on dopamine itself, conflated psychosis and schizophrenia, and predated advances in the genetics, molecular biology,

and imaging research in schizophrenia [...]. We selectively review these data to provide an overview of the 5 critical streams of new evidence [...] We synthesize this evidence into a new dopamine hypothesis of schizophrenia—version III: the final common pathway. This hypothesis seeks to be comprehensive in providing a framework that links risk factors [...] to increased presynaptic striatal dopaminergic function [...] Future drug development and research into etiopathogenesis should focus on identifying and manipulating the upstream factors that converge on the dopaminergic funnel point. (Howes and Kapur 2009, p. 549)

We see here another significant shift in the focus of the DHS. Most importantly, from being an etiologic theory—that excess DA function caused schizophrenia—Howes and Kapur view DA as a final common pathway (aka "funnel point") with the causal effects now a result of various "upstream factors." Also, we have greater biological specificity with a focus solely on one anatomical location—the striatum—and one kind of DA dysfunction—presynaptic. They note correctly that most (but not all) prior work on the DHS has focused on postsynaptic receptor alterations. This work was informed by reviews of the PET literature described earlier in this chapter. The authors in the body of the article also back away from the concept that DA can really explain schizophrenia at all and focus instead on the broader state of psychosis.

This brief updating on the last 5 years of the DHS suggests that our two main conclusions of our prior review still hold. Empirically, the performance of the DHS remains spotty. Some work, especially in the area of presynaptic functioning, appears consistent with the theory but other key findings, in D2/D3 receptors (a prior focus of much work) and genetic variants (ditto) have not been well verified. Finally, the protean nature of the theory has been well illustrated by yet another major revision.

32.4 Empirical and Nonempirical Forces Vectors influencing the DHS

In this section, I want to try to give my subjective weights to empirical and nonempirical factors impacting on the DHS following the broad approach taken by Solomon in her "decision vectors" (Solomon 2001). Two key issues quickly emerged in this effort. First, the factors involved in the early versus later phases of the DHS seemed quite different. So I decided to develop different ratings for these two stages that I labeled "proposal" and "persistence." Second, I had to decide at least roughly which of the major incarnations of the DHS I was going to try to treat in this exercise. I chose a rather nonspecific version of the "classical" DHS—that schizophrenia was largely the result of excess DA functioning somewhere in the brain.

Table 32.1 depicts my sense of the key empirical forces that impacted on the proposal and persistence of the DHS over its life course. The overwhelming empirical "push" for the proposal of the DHS was the evidence that antipsychotic drugs in large part worked through the blockade of dopamine receptors. This important influence carries a potentially major logical flaw—that of reasoning from treatment back to etiology. Medicine is full of examples where treatments work at biological levels remote from those involved in etiology. For example, fevers from pneumonia do not arise from aspirin deficiency. Heart failure is first treated by diuretic drugs which act in the kidney. Throughout the history of the DHS, there has been some conflation of the DHS and the "dopamine hypothesis of neuroleptic action." So I put an asterisk on the empirical support for the DHS provided this data, as it has this potentially deep conceptual weakness. The second less influential set of findings in the early days of the DHS was evidence from clinical studies that heavy use of amphetamines—which stimulate, among other things, DA receptors—could produce a schizophrenia-like psychosis (Connell 1958).

Neuroleptic blockade of DA receptors certainly also played a central role in the persistence of the DHS. Its influence became weaker as new "atypical" neuroleptics, especially clozapine, were studied where their clinical potency was not so strongly related to DA blockade. The other rows depicted in Table 32.1 tell briefly the story of the largely unsuccessful attempt to validate the DHS through more specific tests. For more details about these studies, see Kendler and Schaffner

Table 32.1 Empirical decision vectors for the proposal and persistence of the dopamine hypothesis of schizophrenia

Nature of evidence	Impact on proposal of DHS	Impact on the persistence of the DHS
Correlation of DA receptor blocking capacity with antipsychotic potency	+5[a]	+3[a]
Psychotogenic effects of DA agonist drugs	+2	+1
Failure to find excess DA metabolites in cerebrospinal fluid	0	−3
Failure of various neuroendocrine predictions	0	−1
Exacerbating of positive symptoms in patients by DA agonist drugs	0	+1
In vivo evidence for excess DA receptors in brain	0	−1
Absence of robust evidence for associated postmortem changes in DA level or turnover	0	−2
Failure to find robust evidence of genetic effects of DA variants	0	−3
Evidence for in vivo increased striatal presynaptic DA function	0	+1

[a] Potential major conceptual problem.

(2011). Two of these efforts produced weakly positive results (amphetamine making schizophrenia patients worse and those reviewed earlier reflecting increased in vivo presynaptic DA functioning in the striatum). The rest were consistently negative. I would conclude from this table that at its inception, the DHS had some plausible empirical support, although potentially flawed. However, over time, the weight of empirical evidence tipped against the validity of the DHS.

Evaluating a table like this requires some set of expectations about theory performance. How successful do we expect the predictions of our theories to be? My understanding is that the theory of general relatively has been consistently verified to very high precision. It has not failed a single major test. Contrast this to theories in the "soft" areas of psychology where a box score average on a literature review of 60% or 70% confirmation is seen as very good. What do we expect of the DHS? While the standards of physics are surely too high, I am not sure that even by the standards of soft psychology, the DHS is doing very well.

Table 32.2 summarizes the even more complex set of nonempirical factors that have influenced the proposal and persistence of the DHS. Here I would give preeminence to the strong desire within psychiatry as a whole but even more so among the nascent movement of biological psychiatry to show that psychiatry could connect itself with the exciting developments then ongoing in the neurosciences. Neurology—a sister field and competitor with psychiatry—had a tremendous success with Parkinson's disease, reducing a complex clinical syndrome down to a single specific neurotransmitter system. What could be better than psychiatry doing the same thing with schizophrenia? In its broad framing, the DHS was simple and powerful, rooting the etiology of this key devastating psychiatric syndrome with the latest neuroscience advances. Of course it would be appealing. Such an advance could reconnect psychiatry to biomedicine and usher in a period of dominance for the biological psychiatric paradigm and the associated decline in influence of psychoanalysis. One other factor favored the DHS in its early stages—the confounding of the DHS with the "dopamine hypothesis of neuroleptic action." Whether this surprisingly pervasive confusion should be considered empirical or nonempirical is unclear to me but I listed it as the latter.

Early on, there was opposition to the DHS by at least two important subgroups within psychiatry—the psychoanalysts and the social psychiatrists. Space constraints prevent any detailed discussion of this. Suffice it to say that the effectiveness of their opposition waned considerably over the years as the biological psychiatric paradigm (with the DHS as one of its "star" components) became increasingly dominant within American psychiatry.

In considering the nonempirical factors that impacted on the persistence of the DHS, I would emphasize three additional factors. First, as already noted and in Kendler and Schaffner (2011), the DHS was a shape-shifter over time and was very successful at absorbing negative findings. If results were not positive in the mesolimbic DA system, then look in the nigrostriatal system. If DA receptors were not altered, consider presynaptic DA functioning. If there was not too much DA, perhaps there was too little. This made definitive disproof of the DHS very difficult. Second, through most of its history, the DHS had no serious

Table 32.2 Nonempirical decision vectors for the proposal and persistence of the dopamine hypothesis of schizophrenia

Nature of evidence	Impact on proposal of DHS	Impact on the persistence of the DHS
Desire for "biological psychiatry" to develop plausible brain-based explanations of illness	+3	+5
Multiple versions of the hypothesis making definitive disproval very difficult	0	+4
Confusion about biology of treatment versus pathophysiology	+2	+3
Lack of viable competing hypotheses	0	+3
Role of pharmaceutical industry	0	+3
Opposition by psychoanalysts	−2	0
Opposition by social psychiatry	−2	0

competitors as theories for schizophrenia. Early on, several psychoanalytic theories were prominent but these had little traction with the major audience for the DHS. Other biological theories (methylation hypothesis, ideas about the possible roles of norepinephrine and serotonin, and more recently glutamate) were in the field, but they never coalesced into a powerful theory that could give the DHS a "run for its money." Third, the DHS was a boon for the pharmaceutical industry and made a great marketing tool. It allowed them to claim that their drugs "fixed" the essential abnormality in schizophrenia. Furthermore, the DHS was so influential that "big pharma" spent much more effort trying to find other DA blocking drugs for schizophrenia (whose efficacy provided further support for the DHS) rather than exploring with equal vigor other possible treatment approaches.

I would conclude from Table 32.2 that at its inception, the nonempirical factors in favor of and opposing the DHS were approximately balanced. This would be a situation that Solomon might consider fairly benign. But over time, the scales tipped considerably and an unhealthy situation developed that has helped explain the persistence of the DHS in the face of a weak empirical performance. I need to end this section with a personal anecdote. I reviewed some of the results from an early version of our chapter on the DHS at Psychiatry Grand Rounds in a biologically oriented department of psychiatry about 5 years ago. Toward the end of that section of my talk, several in the audience rose from their seats in vehement protest. They were indigent. How dare I attack this theory and I had not considered this finding or that finding. So there was empirical content to their attack on me. But the emotional tone was more striking. It was as if I had personally attacked them or a close family member.

32.5 Trying to put the DHS into a Broader Historical Context

I am at best an amateur medical historian. Nonetheless, I have read enough to provide what might be some helpful historical contextualization of the DHS story. I will tell three brief stories looking for potential parallels in debates about the etiology of medical disorders. The first comes from the excellent book by Worboys about the history of microbial theories of disease in Britain in the second half of the nineteenth century (Worboys 2000). Worboys documents the empirical struggles between two broad disease models for "infectious" disease: the old public health "miasma"-based model and the new microbial laboratory-based model. Of course, the later eventually wins out. But there are a range of nonempirical factors that enter into this story. Some (such as the opposition to the microbial theories because they were largely German in origin) have little bearing on the DHS. More relevant is the unsurprising observation of Worboys that, by and large, people working in the field used the science available to them to advance their own professional self-interests. If you were an older veterinarian responsible for inspecting cattle entering England, you did not want your overstretched public health budget eaten up by the costs of a new-fangled laboratory doing things you did not value or understand. On the other hand, if you were a young physician returning to England from a stint in one of the few German microbial laboratories, you saw an opportunity for professional advancement and increased status by advocating for the newer theories under the hope that you would be funded with a laboratory, attract students, become a professor, and so on. The obvious point here is that scientists often act in their own professional self-interest and this impacts on how they value certain sets of empirical findings. We should not be overly cynical and Worboys certainly documents evidence that some individuals truly changed their mind as the data in favor of the microbial causes of disease mounted and acted on those beliefs even if they did not serve their selfish professional interests. Lest the reader potentially feel smug about the eventual triumph of the microbial over the miasma theories ("at least the right side clearly won out here"), in fact nearly all the highly successful public health measures taken in Europe in the nineteenth century for clean water, disposal of sewage, and so on were motivated by the scientifically wrong miasma theories and not the correct microbial theories.

The second story is that of the etiology of peptic ulcer and the shift from an "excess acidity" model to a "*Helicobacter pylori*" disease model. Here I rely on the excellent recounting of this story by Thagard (2000). I would suggest four interesting parallels and contrasts between this story and that of the DHS. First, both stories involved a "re-telling" of the etiologic story of a disease from less specific to a more specific cause. Peptic ulcer disease was initially considered a multifactorial and potentially psychosomatic disease with a final common pathway in excess gastric acidity. It was a dramatic shift to consider it being an infectious disease with a far more specific etiology. Schizophrenia was a multifactorial syndrome with a range of postulated risk factors from psychodynamic to social to genetic. The DHS attempted to redefine it as a neurochemical disorder. Second, critical early empirical support for the *H. pylori* theory of ulcers came from the efficacy of antibiotics. So, the advocates of this theory used the same "back justification" from treatment to etiology as did those of DHS. But, the back justification in the ulcer story was on far firmer ground than in the DHS. In the case of antibiotics, treatment is typically specific and closely tied to etiology. Nothing parallel can be claimed for schizophrenia and DA blockade. Furthermore, in the ulcer story, they could examine subjects after antibiotic treatment and confirm that the *H. pylori* bacteria were gone, firming up their "treatment back to etiology" line of reasoning. Third, each theory could also be tested by trying to precipitate the disorder. In a famous episode, recounted by Thagard, one of the two early discoverers of the *H. pylori* story, Marshall, drank a beaker of *H. pylori* culture, became ill with nausea and vomiting, and showed on endoscopy 10 days later clear signs of gastritis and the presence of *H. pylori*. For the DHS, the prediction, eventually confirmed, was that high-dose DA stimulant drugs (amphetamines) could produce a model psychosis in a laboratory setting (Angrist et al. 1974; Griffiths et al. 1968). In the final loose parallel, there were two "subfields" in the peptic ulcer story as in the DHS. As might be expected, bacteriologists accepted this theory much more quickly than did gastroenterologists. The DHS achieved far more rapid acceptance within biological psychiatry circles than within more typical and especially psychodynamically oriented psychiatrists.

The final historical parallel to the DHS I want to review is the story of the clarification of the etiology of AIDS as recounted by Epstein (1996). Here the major debate was between the simple HIV theory and the more complex multifactorial "immune overload" hypothesis. This struggle occurred both within and outside science and involved a far greater and more energetic set of activists than were ever involved in the DHS. The stakes were high because tens of millions of dollars of research funding were to be disbursed. Epstein describes the state of the few retrovirus laboratories, including that of Gallo, before the intense interest in AIDS. Their funding was low. It was not clear whether this would be a fruitful area of research. Labs were considering shifting to other areas in virology. When early reports emerged about the possible role of retroviruses in the etiology of AIDS, would you expect these research groups to advocate for this line of research, as Gallo did strenuously? The answer here is obvious and again points to the ways in which empirical evidence and scientific self-interest interact in debates about the etiology of biomedical disorders. I end this section with the following poignant quote of Epstein's:

> In short, the commonly expressed preference of [...] biomedical researchers for simple, monocausal, microbial models may in an immediate sense have less to do with medicine's role in legitimating society than with doctors' and scientists' role in legitimating scientific medicine. (Epstein 1996, p. 58)

32.6 Conclusion

Since the completion of our prior review on the DHS in 2008, the basic pattern of this theory has been broadly stable. It has had some empirical success but more failures. It has maintained and perhaps enlarged its protean status. An admittedly somewhat subjective review of the empirical and nonempirical forces operating on the DHS suggests that at its inception, the nonempirical forces were relatively well balanced and the empirical forces—given the caveat of arguing from treatment to etiology—were somewhat favorably aligned. Over time, however, the empirical support for the DHS became weaker and its scientific quality declined as it morphed into what Lakatos might consider a degenerative research program (Lakatos 1970). At the same time, the nonempirical forces shifted more and more in favor the DHS producing what Solomon would consider an unhealthy situation. I would judge that the longevity of the DHS has more to do with nonempirical than empirical forces. Finally, a brief review of three other stories relating to the etiology of biomedical disorders—infectious diseases generally, peptic ulcers, and AIDS—suggest that in many of its themes the DHS is not unique. In their approach to advocacy for certain scientific positions, researchers are likely to consider both the nature of the data and what is in their own professional interests for advancement and increased status.

The story of the DHS provides one illustration of how empirical and nonempirical forces shaped a central etiologic theory of late twentieth-century psychiatry. It illustrates clearly that psychiatry does not, as a science, exist in the rarefied atmosphere postulated by the logical empiricists responding solely to empirical developments. Nonempirical forces, both within the field and from the outside, can impact on scientific developments. But empirical forces also played a strong role in our story. Looking forward, I predict that the DHS will end with a whimper, overtaken by further scientific advances in our understanding of the etiology of schizophrenia. One important lesson, however, is that the field of psychiatry needs better theories that are more specific and testable. There are hopeful signs that advances in molecular genetics, the neurosciences, and the fields of epidemiology can and will produce such theories and avoid undesirable situations where the persistence of major theories in our field are driven largely by nonempirical rather than empirical forces.

References

Angrist, B., Lee, H.K., and Gershon, S. (1974). The antagonism of amphetamine-induced symptomatology by a neuroleptic. *American Journal of Psychiatry*, 131(7), 817–819.

Carlsson, A. and Lindqvist, M. (1963). Effect of chlorpromazine or haloperidol on formation of 3-methoxytyramine and normetanephrine in mouse brain. *Acta Pharmacologica et Toxicologica*, 20, 140–144.

Chen, K.C., Yang, Y.K., Howes, O., Lee, I.H., Landau, S., Yeh, T.L., et al. (2013). Striatal dopamine transporter availability in drug-naive patients with schizophrenia: a case-control SPECT study with [(99m)Tc]-TRODAT-1 and a meta-analysis. *Schizophrenia Bulletin*, 39(2), 378–386.

Connell, P.H. (1958). *Amphetamine Psychosis*. Maudsley Monographs, No. 5. Institute of Psychiatry. London: Chapman and Hall, Ltd.

Dahlstrom, A. and Fuxe, K. (1964). Evidence for the existence of monoamine-containing neurons in the central nervous system. I. Demonstration of monoamines in the cell bodies of brain stem neurons. *Acta Physiologica Scandinavica. Supplementum*, 232, 1–55.

Davis, K.L., Kahn, R.S., Ko, G., and Davidson, M. (1991). Dopamine in schizophrenia: a review and reconceptualization. *American Journal of Psychiatry*, 148(11), 1474–1486.

Ehringer, H. and Hornykiewicz, O. (1960). Distribution of noradrenaline and dopamine (3-hydroxytyramine) in the human brain and their behavior in diseases of the extrapyramidal system. *Klinische Wochenschrift*, 38, 1236–1239.

Epstein, S. (1996). *Impure Science: Aids, Activism, and the Politics of Knowledge*. Berkeley and Los Angeles, CA: University of California Press.

Falck, B., Hillarp, N.A., Thieme, G., and Torp, A. (1982). Fluorescence of catechol amines and related compounds condensed with formaldehyde. *Brain Research Bulletin*, 9(1–6), xi–xv.

Fuxe, K., Hokfelt, T., Nilsson, O., and Reinius, S. (1966). A fluorescence and electron microscopic study on central monoamine nerve cells. *The Anatomical Record*, 155(1), 33–40.

Griffiths, J.J., Oates, J., and Cavanaugh, J. (1968). Paranoid episodes induced by drugs. *Journal of the American Medical Association*, 205, 39–46.

Howes, O.D., Kambeitz, J., Kim, E., Stahl, D., Slifstein, M., Abi-Dargham, A., *et al.* (2012). The nature of dopamine dysfunction in schizophrenia and what this means for treatment. *Archives of General Psychiatry*, 69(8), 776–786.

Howes, O.D. and Kapur, S. (2009). The dopamine hypothesis of schizophrenia: version III—the final common pathway. *Schizophrenia Bulletin*, 35(3), 549–562.

Kendler, K.S. and Schaffner, K.F. (2011). The dopamine hypothesis of schizophrenia: an historical and philosophical analysis. *Philosophy, Psychiatry, & Psychology*, 18(1), 41–63.

Kopin, I.J. (1993). Parkinson's disease: past, present, and future. *Neuropsychopharmacology*, 9(1), 1–12.

Lakatos, I. (1970). Falsification and the methodology of scientific research programmes. In I. Lakatos and A. Musgrave (eds.) *Criticism and the Growth of Knowledge*, pp. 91–97. London: Cambridge University Press.

Matthysse, S. (1973). Antipsychotic drug actions—a clue to the neuropathology of schizophrenia? *Federation Proceedings*, 32(2), 200–205.

Matthysse, S. and Lipinski, J. (1975). Biochemical aspects of schizophrenia. *Annual Review of Medicine*, 26, 551–565.

Meltzer, H.Y. and Stahl, S.M. (1976). The dopamine hypothesis of schizophrenia: a review. *Schizophrenia Bulletin*, 2(1), 19–76.

Montagu, K.A. (1957). Catechol compounds in rat tissues and in brains of different animals. *Nature*, 180(4579), 244–245.

Ripke, S., Sanders, A.R., Kendler, K.S., Levinson, D.F., Sklar, P., Holmans, P.A., *et al.* (2011). Genome-wide association study identifies five new schizophrenia loci. *Nature Genetics*, 43(10), 969–976.

Solomon, M. (2001). *Social Empiricism*. Cambridge, MA: MIT Press.

Sullivan, P.F., Kendler, K.S., and Neale, M.C. (2003). Schizophrenia as a complex trait: evidence from a meta-analysis of twin studies. *Archives of General Psychiatry*, 60(12), 1187–1192.

Thagard, P. (2000). *How Scientists Explain Disease*. Princeton, NJ: Princeton University Press.

Worboys, M. (2000). *Spreading Germs: Disease Theories and Medical Practice in Britain, 1865–1900*. New York: Cambridge University Press.

Chapter 33

Why is the dopamine hypothesis of schizophrenia the only game in town?

Miriam Solomon

33.1 Kendler's Analysis of Decision Vectors for the Dopamine Hypothesis of Schizophrenia

Kenneth Kendler and Kenneth Schaffner (2011) have written a fascinating history of the dopamine hypothesis of schizophrenia (DHS). My comments refer to this paper as well as to the 2013 analysis and update in this volume in Chapter 32. The DHS is particularly appropriate for historical and philosophical attention because it is still in progress. We do not know which theory or theories of schizophrenia—if any—will be fruitful. Historical and philosophical accounts are less likely to be distorted by hindsight (typically referred to as "Whiggism") in this situation than they are in cases in which we know the outcome. Moreover, because the questions are still live, we have the opportunity to put any normative recommendations into practice, making them more useful. In taking a look at this case, I will rely on Kendler and Schaffner's historical account, and Kendler's decision vector analysis, but take them a step further. I make use of epistemic tools from Helen Longino's work (Longino 1995) and my own (Solomon 2001).

A striking feature of the DHS is that it has been the central hypothesis available for some 40 years. It is also, as Kendler says, a protean theory, often modified to align with contrary data, yet without the continued empirical successes that would justify such ad hoc changes. The robust and early empirical successes of the DHS are that dopaminergic drugs can worsen or produce psychotic symptoms and that dopamine blockers have antipsychotic activity. The original simple theory that schizophrenia is due to "excess dopamine in the brain" has not been supported by other empirical measurements, such as examination of cerebrospinal fluid for dopamine metabolites. DHS was modified to postulate different imbalances of dopamine in different areas of the brain, with equivocal evidence. Most recently DHS has been modified to suggest that it is a "pathway" for schizophrenia—or at least for its psychotic symptoms—but not the basic cause (Howes and Kapur 2009).

Kendler lists and quantifies[1] the empirical and nonempirical decision vectors from the beginning of the DHS to the present. His assessment is that nonempirical decision vectors—such as pharmaceutical company interests, dominance of biological psychiatry, and lack of viable competing hypotheses—came to disproportionally favor the DHS. He suggests that the upshot is that this imbalance of nonempirical decision vectors got in the way of doing good science. The implication is that the DHS would have been abandoned long ago, if not for the imbalance of nonempirical decision vectors.[2]

33.2 Discussion of Kendler's Analysis

Kendler's analysis of empirical and nonempirical decision vectors is interesting and helpful. From what he says about the case, I agree that the nonempirical decision vectors have disproportionately favored the DHS and that they have grown in both magnitude and number over the last 40 years. Yet, unlike some other cases in the history of science and medicine—such as the cases of infectious disease, peptic ulcers, and AIDS that Kendler mentions—there has not been a viable alternative theory for some time. (At one time, psychoanalytic and social psychiatric theories of schizophrenia were offered. These were rapidly discredited in the early days of the DHS.) This is surprising, because the poor success rate of the DHS creates an opportunity for other hypotheses about schizophrenia to come forward. Why hasn't that happened?

To answer this question, we need to take a closer look at the nonempirical decision vectors supporting the DHS. Recall that nonempirical decision vectors include *any* causes of preference for aspects of theories other than their empirical success. They include traditionally described "external" or "social" factors such as cohesion with ideologies and interests but *also* include traditionally described "rational" or "cognitive" factors such as simplicity (a structural and/or psychological feature of theories) and conservatism (the smallest distance between accepted knowledge and a new theory). One of the nonempirical decision vectors listed by Kendler for the DHS is "Lack of viable competing hypotheses." Let's look more closely at it: *why* aren't there viable competing hypotheses? The answer to this question is the actual nonempirical decision vector. ("Lack of viable competing hypotheses" is an effect, not a cause, in this context. So technically "lack of viable competing hypotheses" is not a decision vector, although it is a placeholder for one or more.)

---

[1] In Solomon (2001) I did not quantify the decision vectors, because I do not have standard procedures for doing so. Kendler's quantitative assessments are his own judgments of the magnitude of decision vectors. However, analysis of the case does not crucially depend on these quantifications, and the same result is achieved when decision vectors are not quantified at all (as in an improper linear model).

[2] In social empiricism, the goal is not to eliminate nonempirical decision vectors but to balance them.

The DHS is, at root, a simple hypothesis (even though some of its recent forms are more complicated). Moreover, it is redolent of the ancient humoral theories, in which disease results from an imbalance—too much or too little—of some basic biological substance. Instead of having too much or too little black bile, yellow bile, phlegm, or blood, biological theories of mental illness theorize that we have too much or too little dopamine, serotonin, or norepinephrine. With this connection to ancient theories the DHS is also a conservative hypothesis, and indeed perhaps this is (at least in part) why it seems simple to us. Simplicity and conservatism are thought of as "rational" or "cognitive" factors for choice in traditional philosophy of science (see, e.g., Quine [1963]), but they are conceptualized as nonempirical decision vectors in social empiricism. The point is that they are, from a scientific and empiricist point of view, arbitrary constraints.

Their arbitrariness was beautifully revealed by Helen Longino in a piece in which she proposed an alternative set of feminist cognitive values (1995). These are complexity, novelty, ontological heterogeneity, mutuality of interaction, and responsiveness to human needs. Longino uses the word "value" rather broadly, to encompass all reasons and causes of choice. She argues that there is no epistemic justification for the traditional distinction between cognitive and noncognitive values (just as I argue that the category of nonempirical decision vectors comprises traditional cognitive as well social, ideological, and other factors).

If the values of simplicity and conservatism were not so pervasive in the psychiatry research community, perhaps we would see some alternatives to the DHS. Another way of putting this is to say that creative theorizing in the psychiatry research community is hampered by traditional ways of thinking about mental disorder. The DHS anchors theoretical speculations more than it should.

So I do not draw exactly the same conclusion as Kendler does. He concludes that the situation is due to scientists being affected by "both the nature of the data and what is in their own professional interests for advancement and increased status." But professional self-interest is just one of many different nonempirical decision vectors at play in evaluating the DHS, and it is not a particularly troubling nonempirical decision vector in this context. It is the nonempirical decision vectors of simplicity and conservatism, which limit the theoretical options, that are most responsible for the slow progress in understanding schizophrenia.

References

Howes, O.D. and Kapur, S. (2009). The dopamine hypothesis of schizophrenia: version III—the final common pathway. *Schizophrenia Bulletin*, 35(3), 549–562.

Kendler, K.S. and Schaffner, K.F. (2011). The dopamine hypothesis of schizophrenia: an historical and philosophical analysis. *Philosophy, Psychiatry, & Psychology*, 18(1), 41–63.

Longino, H.E. (1995). Gender, politics, and the theoretical virtues. *Synthese*, 104(3), 383–397.

Quine, W.V. (1963). *From a Logical Point of View; 9 Logico-Philosophical Essays* (2nd rev. ed.). New York: Harper & Row.

Solomon, M. (2001). *Social Empiricism*. Cambridge, MA: MIT Press.

Section 12
Conceptual status of depression today

Chapter 34

Introduction to "Depression in a biopsychosocioeconomic context"

Josef Parnas

The theme of Chapter 35 is the change in the concept of depression that has occurred during the last 30 years, since the introduction of the operational criteria for "major depression," and possible factors contributing to that change. The prevalence of depression has increased dramatically in the developed countries and a substantial, perhaps alarmingly high, percentage of the population in these countries is today treated with antidepressants, especially with selective serotonin reuptake inhibitor drugs. These changes are debated both within and outside psychiatry and are of substantial societal interest. The following factors, out of many, are emphasized as being at least partly responsible for this change. First, the very concept of depression underwent important modifications in the DSM-III diagnostic classifications. This process, broadening the notion of depression, was initiated by the construction of Feighner criteria and officially endorsed in the DSM-III/ICD-10. In the "operational" sense, depression may be defined as a condition that is present when a patient says yes to a certain number of questions from a specific checklist (frequently modelled upon the Hamilton Depression Scale) (see Parnas and P. Bovet, Chapter 23, this volume). Other factors, potentially contributing to this change, comprise increasing medicalization of human unhappiness and misery, a medicalization that has many roots but one of which is likely to be a result of marketing strategies of the pharmaceutical industry, unfortunately also endorsed by some of us with a strong reductionistic bent. Professor Sato's chapter can be read narrowly, as dealing specifically with the biosocial issues surrounding the changing concept of depression or more broadly, as an engaged voice of indignation with the current status of psychiatry and directed to all of us.

Chapter 35

Depression in a biopsychosocioeconomic context

Yuji Sato

There has been a tendency among intellectuals to prize and overprize objectivity and scientific method, even to the point where such objectivity becomes detachment [...] People engaged in psychological or physiological research are sometimes equally reluctant to admit their responsibility, though their experiments may lead to all kinds of astonishing transformations of human beings, and may give to certain individuals dangerous powers of conditioning people, of altering their responses. This is called detachment or objectivity of science.

(Isaiah Berlin, *The Role of the Inelligentsia*, 1968/2000)

35.1 Introduction

Disease concepts generally crystalize through gradual nosological demarcation of a distinct clinical entity based mainly on clinicopathological, epidemiological, and catamnestic data accumulated over a certain length of time. This process is carried out in medical academia by building a consensus through scientific organizations and accredited academic journals. Factors external to this academic process, such as accessibility to health care, dietary habits, and the economic status of a particular country in a given time period, can to some extent influence the clinical and epidemiological features of a disease, but such influences are seldom pivotal to the nosological definition of the disease concept per se. In contrast, psychiatric disorders are, due to the very nature of mental illness, often markedly influenced by sociocultural, political, and historical factors external to the normative academic process of nosological conceptualization. Therefore, conceptual historical analysis of psychiatric disorders is required, which invariably involves multidisciplinary viewpoints. Indeed, some mental illnesses are claimed to represent the dominant zeitgeist of the West in specific eras: hysteria in the late nineteenth century (Hollender 1972; Scull 2009), anxiety in the twentieth century (Lane 2007), and depression, perhaps, in the twenty-first century (Shorter 2009). These claims are generally metaphorical/literary and unsupported by epidemiological surveys, of course, as exemplified by the title of W.H. Auden's poem *The Age of Anxiety* (1948). Whether depression, however defined, does in fact represent the twenty-first-century zeitgeist is probably not for us to judge, but an attempt at a tentative historical overview and general analysis of the depression concept and its historical changes is surely a worthwhile undertaking. I must confess that research into depression per se is not particularly my forte. Nevertheless, this does not necessarily disqualify me from discussing the topic: lacking any significant vested interest in depression as a researcher myself may allow me to adopt a relatively neutral viewpoint, even though I do naturally have a clinical commitment to better understand depression in order to provide better treatment to my patients with the disease.

Ideally, an overview of the depression concept in the above sense should cover and analyze all the relevant factors as comprehensively and minutely as possible, but this is hardly feasible given the multifaceted nature of factors encompassing the wide range of relevant phenomena observed over several decades. Nevertheless, an overview of some kind is critical if we want to better understand the current conceptual status of depression, because the conceptual complexity of depression today cannot be fully elucidated by medical/nosological clarification alone. It seems to me that the depression concept consists of at least two major components: medical/nosological and nonmedical. Any overview will, therefore, present only a crude bird's-eye view of these two components across the relevant disciplines and cannot include a detailed analysis of each contributing factor within each component.

This chapter has two somewhat limited objectives: (1) to delineate the major medical and nonmedical components that form the depression concept today, and (2) to illustrate how these components interact in bringing about the current complex conceptual status of depression and the resultant practical issues that affect society at large, for example, confusions seen amongst practitioners as to how to understand, diagnose, and treat depression. Furthermore, as it is imperative that we all try to improve clinical practice after clarifying the confusing complexities of the depression concept, several possible remedial measures are proposed.

35.2 The Two Major Components of the Depression Concept at Large

35.2.1 Medical/Nosological Component

The philosophical and nosological issues concerning depression were discussed in depth (Maj 2012) at the second conference on philosophical issues in psychiatry (Kendler and Parnas 2012) and need not be repeated here, but for the present objective of gaining an overview of the current status of the depression concept, the kernel of the concept based on psychiatric nosology needs to be summarized.

I will provide a very quick summary, relying mainly on Berrios's seminal work (1996, pp. 289–331) (Figure 35.1).

The concept of melancholia has existed from time immemorial, but in the nineteenth century it was renamed depression, with a number of symptomatic features. From here Kraepelin developed and defined manic depressive illness (MDI) using more detailed psychopathological criteria. This Kraepelinian concept of MDI was, through the introduction of operational diagnosis in Feighner's criteria[1] (1972)

---

[1] Notably, the Feighner criteria for primary affective disorders (Feighner et al. 1972) include representative symptoms based on the Hamilton Rating Scale for Depression (Hamilton

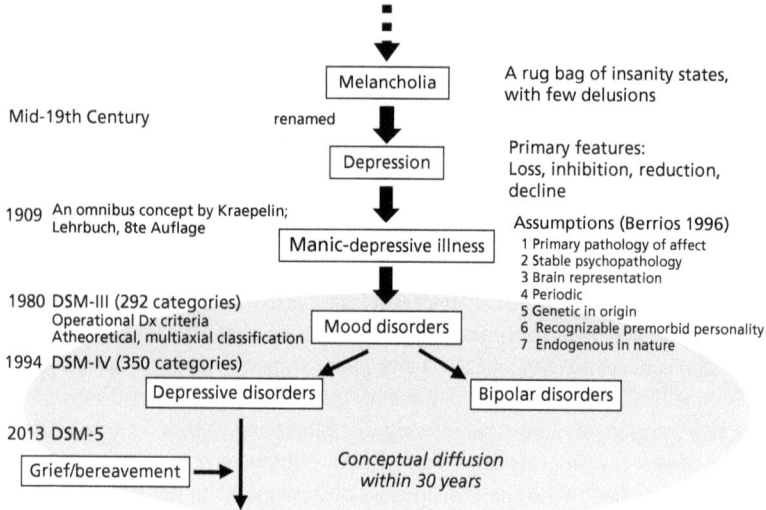

Fig. 35.1 Conceptual history of depression.

and the Research Diagnostic Criteria (1978), translated into mood disorders as classified in the DSM-III (American Psychiatric Association 1980), which were subsequently further divided into depressive disorders and bipolar disorders.[2]

The evolution and significance of operational diagnosis in psychiatry (Sato and Berrios 2001) is discussed separately in this volume (see Parnas and P. Bovet, Chapter 23, this volume), so I will only mention here in relation to depression that: (1) the operational diagnostic criteria in DSM-III and afterwards were intended to improve the reliability of diagnosis across researchers and clinicians; (2) this initiative has had great influence internationally, to the extent that the DSM created by the American Psychiatric Association, rather than ICD, has become the de facto diagnostic lingua franca; and (3) criticism against operationalization has been made from the viewpoint of psychiatry as well as that of the philosophy and history of science (Klerman et al. 1984; Margolis 1994; Saß 1990; Sedler 1994), so far without significant impact on the basic tenets of DSM.

1960), which Hamilton intended "for use only on patients already diagnosed as suffering from affective disorder of depressive type." This rating scale for assessing the effect of treatment thereafter seems to be sometimes mistaken and misused as a diagnostic tool; I have witnessed some psychiatrists in Japan using Hamilton scale scores to validate their diagnoses of depression. This is a telling example of conceptual and diagnostic confusion in clinical practice today.

[2] To simplify this summary of the conceptual history of depression, the relevant concepts of the French school, for example, *forme circulaire de maladie mentale* (Falret), are not included here.

In addition to these general points, it has been claimed that the DSM has gradually enlarged the depression concept by incorporating, under the rubric of major depressive disorder, various forms of depressive syndromes that were previously separately diagnosed, for example, melancholic/endogenous depression, depressive neurosis, depressive reactions (van Praag 1998), with the result that depression today, due to nonspecificity of the major depression concept, poses difficulties in biological research (Mann 2010), is overdiagnosed clinically (Parker 2009), and antidepressants are overprescribed (Healy 1997, 2004). It is beyond the scope of this chapter to argue which of the two nosological conceptualizations is more appropriate: by grouping the depressive syndromes together according to their common features, or differentiating them as previously. It should be noted, however, that this "put them together or put them apart" debate still lingers on, as shown by the recent controversies on the relationship between major depressive disorder and grief.

Based on empirical data (Kendler et al. 2008; Zisook and Kendler 2007), the DSM-5 (2013) has allowed the inclusion (or to be more precise, eliminated the exclusion) of grief and associated bereavement, insofar as they meet the criteria, in major depressive disorder. There have been some objections against this inclusion (Wakefield 2012), but of interest is the fact that criticism also came from outside psychiatry, for example, *The New England Journal of Medicine* (Friedman 2012) and *The Lancet* (2012a, 2012b). In a personal account of his own bereavement following the death of his wife, Kleinman (2012a) regards the inclusion of grief among depressive disorders as a form of medicalization and de facto commercialization, whereby it is deemed legitimate and necessary to treat grief medically, most likely with antidepressants. These criticisms and objections seem to constitute not so much a medical/nosological debate as a sociocultural argument resulting from the discrepancy between a nosological concept within psychiatry, minutely defined in official diagnostic criteria, and a complex notion of a disease in a wider sociocultural context.

35.2.2 Nonmedical Component

The aforementioned *Lancet* editorial (2012a) starts with a question: when should grief be classified as a mental illness?[3] Exactly the same question was addressed

---

[3] From a practical viewpoint, psychiatric help should be (and is being) provided for those afflicted by grief as long as it alleviates their dysfunction and suffering, irrespective of how grief is classified (see Turkheimer's comment in Chapter 36, this volume). The diagnostic controversy surrounding depression seems to be particularly widespread and vehement in the United States, because in the United States, unlike in Europe, Japan, and elsewhere, official listing in the DSM is far beyond a taxonomic issue and is linked closely with wide-ranging social aspects, for example, reimbursement, drug approval, and medicolegal litigation. Perhaps psychiatrists outside the United States tend to practice in less draconian environments, which enable them to act more according to their own clinical judgment.

50 years ago by George L. Engel (1961), who is now best remembered as the academician who proposed the biopsychosocial model, a then new perspective to counterbalance the dominant and narrow biomedical model of disease (Engel 1977). Although the adjective "biopsychosocial" has in the subsequent 50 years become a widely accepted term within medicine, the enormous advances and developments in each specialty have made it extremely difficult for an interdisciplinary biopsychosocial model to work in the hitherto seen enumerative fashion, and a common conceptual framework to integrate all the relevant factors is yet to be found. My approach as summarized in the title of this chapter, therefore, may sound somewhat anachronistic, but for the benefit of clarification let me classify the nonmedical (i.e., outside clinical psychiatry/psychiatric nosology) factors relevant to the depression concept as biological, psychosocial/cultural, and economic/financial. I will focus on the biological and economic/financial factors, as the crucial psychosocial/cultural factors and their analyses (Kitanaka 2012; Lorant et al. 2007; Marmot and Wilkinson 2006; Metzl 2003; Rai et al. 2013; Siegrist 2013; Sakai et al. 2005) are beyond the scope of this chapter.

35.2.2.1 Biological Factors

To highlight the ever widening gap between the clinical practice and a more biological/reductionist view of psychiatry as a clinically applied offshoot of basic neuroscience (Insel and Quiron 2005), biological factors are discussed here within the nonmedical component. Steven Rose (2005, 2006, 2012), himself an excellent biological researcher of memory, has been a consistent critic of neurogenetic determinism. This view purports a clear, simple, and linear causal relationship between genes, the brain, and human behavior, irrespective of its complexity, and promises clear-cut treatment, mostly in the form of pharmacotherapy. It should also be noted that intellectual compartmentalization can take place within the neurosciences per se due to rapid and extensive advance and developments within the ever-expanding field, making it hard to maintain updated knowledge even of the closely related biological domains, let alone clinical realities. This may partly explain why the huge investments made during the "decade of the brain" in the United States have brought so little success, with the result that big pharma, investors, and the market are now withdrawing from central nervous system drug development and hunting instead for a more profitable and promising therapeutic area (Greenslit and Kaptchuk 2012). Very recently, President Obama's "most ambitious scientific research plan to date—the BRAIN (Brain Research through Advancing Innovative Neurotechnologies) Initiative" has started to accelerate the development of new tools to map the activities of the human brain (Editorial 2013). This initiative will boost neuroimaging research, which will undoubtedly involve depression and bring about novel findings that will affect—whether to clarify or complicate—the depression concept further.

35.2.2.2 Economic/Financial Factors

Medicalization nowadays automatically implies commercialization. An obvious example is pharmaceuticalization (Abraham 2010), whereby a targeted new disease concept, coupled with a novel pharmaceutical agent to treat it, is strategically promoted worldwide: direct-to-consumer advertisements encourage patients to ask their doctors to prescribe the new drug, whilst clinical trials showing its efficacy superior to older drugs guide prescribers to choose the drug. It has been claimed that the massive prescription of selective serotonin reuptake inhibitors for depression and social anxiety disorder is a representative example (Healy 2004; Horwitz and Wakefield 2007; Lane 2007).

There are, however, many other evolving fields that are highly profitable—so-called business opportunities—where people rush in. A significant portion of academicians' work these days is, nolens volens, running after and managing research grants: universities are privatized, expected to possess good entrepreneurship, and be concerned about efficient management to fend for themselves (Bok 2003). Hence diverse commodities, from diagnostic criteria (Frances 2013) to neuroimaging facilities, are being commercialized under academic–industry partnerships, encouraged in particular in the United States by the Bayh–Dole Act (Public Law 96-517, Patent and Trademark Act Amendments of 1980) and elsewhere by similar legislation (Mowery and Sampat 2005). An important caveat for commercialization is that the market tends to crowd out nonmarket norms (Sandel 2012). Therefore, the dynamics governing the relationship between the medical/nosological component, a nonmarket norm, and the nonmedical component, in which economic/financial factors including market trends play an increasingly powerful role, seem to be critically important in understanding the depression concept today. However, Abraham (2010) argues that it has not been due to biomedical innovation but to marketing, consumerism, and regulatory policy that massive pharmaceuticalization has taken place. This shows how powerful market trends have become in influencing medicine, so that the nonmedical component tends to outweigh the medical component in conceptualizing depression today.

35.3 Consequences of the Issues Related to the Depression Concept

35.3.1 Multifaceted Sequelae of the Issues Concerning Depression

Let me further summarize this in a historical flowchart (see Figure 35.2).

Conceptual and nosological issues have arguably always been a besetting challenge in psychiatry; it is only natural that such issues lead to diagnostic difficulties, which can subsequently mislead treatment in clinical practice. It was precisely for this reason that operational diagnostic criteria were introduced, with the hope that they would improve at least diagnostic reliability by providing a common language. However, the introduction of rigorous inclusion/exclusion criteria based on the operational diagnostic criteria in clinical trials evaluating the efficacy of antidepressants has been shown to widen the discrepancy between the trial subjects and the broad range of depressive patients actually seen in clinical practice and to whom the antidepressants are prescribed (Zimmerman et al. 2002); in

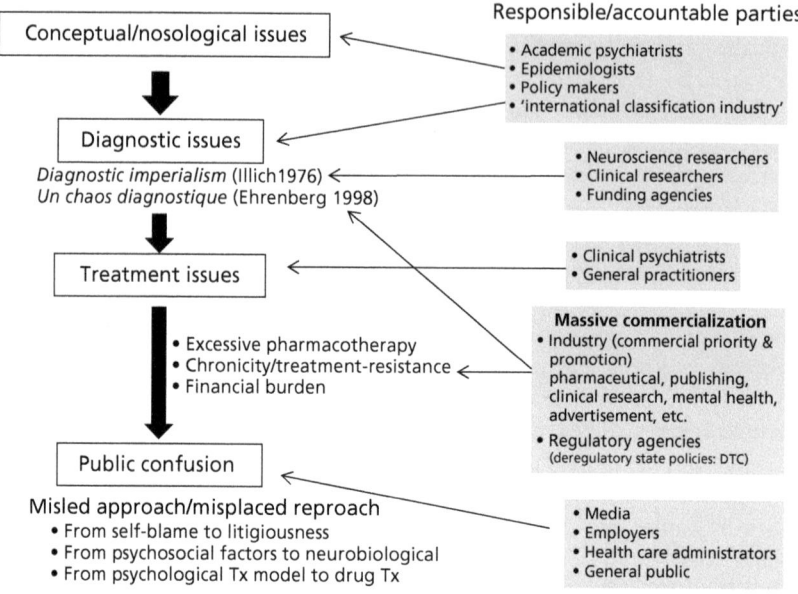

Fig. 35.2 Depression: conceptual issues and its sequelae.

other words, contrary to the original intention, enhanced diagnostic reliability has not necessarily led to actual improvements in diagnosis and treatment in the real world. This is an example in psychiatry of the recent alarming tendency in medicine at large toward a widening disparity between refined clinical research methodologies and the research questions most relevant to clinicians and patients; this disparity leads to what Chalmers and Glasziou call "research waste" (2009). The recent advent of Research Domain Criteria as a neuroscience-based classification, which is an attempt to overcome the problems associated with DSM and ICD (Insel et al. 2010), may in the future cause further confusion among clinicians who are not au fait with the nosological controversies and taxonomic intricacies as to which diagnostic criteria they should follow and which treatment guidelines they should base their practice on.

Confusion in medical practice inevitably affects the general public in turn and thereby leads to further confusion regarding how the public views depression, its treatment, and sufferers. This complex vicious circle involves many people in different professions who, knowingly or unknowingly, play some part in it, and makes it easy for them to attribute the problem to somebody else; academia, industry, government, mass media, and the general public are all part of this mutually critical process. There seems to be a peculiar lack of due awareness on the part of psychiatrists at large of their share of the responsibility for this everlasting confusion, perhaps because blaming others, for example, policymakers, marketers, and media, is always an easy and effective responsibility avoidance. Is it then a mere coincidence that guilt (*Schuldgefühl*) is rarely taken up in depth these days as a core feature of endogenous/melancholic depression (Berrios et al. 1992; Kimura 1965, 1966)? As far as the confusion is concerned, almost everybody seems to be to blame to a greater or lesser degree, with the possible exception only of those with depression themselves. And it is a sad irony that patients with endogenous depression are the very people who tend to blame themselves. A further irony is that melancholic depression is classified merely as a subtype of the major depressive disorder in the DSM, and not as an independent category with distinctly specific psychopathological features, as some claim it to be (Parker et al. 2010).

This summary forces us to confront the fact that, despite conscientious and sound efforts made in each psychiatrist's own area of endeavor, psychiatrists have also played a significant role in this multifaceted confusion resulting from the depression concept today. As an example I recall a most productive professor of psychiatry at the Maudsley Hospital, London, some 20 years ago who told the junior doctors and researchers that he never believed in the DSM, and that he only used it because he would not otherwise be able to get his articles published in first-class journals. At that time I was naïvely impressed by his statement, taking it as the embodiment of the intellectual independence of British psychiatry, but it now seems to me that the de facto acceptance of, and accordance with, DSM under the publish-or-perish zeitgeist, as exemplified by this anecdote, have helped the DSM to achieve its exceptionally dominant position today, where it seems to be beyond criticism.

35.3.2 Conceptual Changes and "market needs"

The conceptual changes illustrated thus far seem, in a strange and unexpected way, to neatly meet the market needs of the globalized economy in the twenty-first century. To recapitulate, first, operational criteria were introduced to standardize diagnosis objectively. This approach invariably led to the minimization or elimination of "subjective" interpretation and individual clinical judgment by trained experts, thereby making it unnecessary to enhance expertise and trust, both of which can only be attained after long experience (Daston and Galison, 2007; Kasahara 2009; Kasahara and Kimura 1975) (Figure 35.3). This implies that we may no longer need experts; in the hierarchy of evidence-based medicine, it is well known that so-called expert opinion is given the lowest status. This undermines, perhaps irretrievably, the autonomy and value of the profession itself.

These regrettable developments in psychiatry correspond well with various managerial practices that are welcomed and encouraged in business administration. If an operation is sufficiently well defined and standardized, with procedures set forth in a manual, it can then be efficiently outsourced to cheap nonexperts, who can be trained to do whatever is stipulated in the manual. The manuals, or standard operating procedures, are defined, revised, and controlled centrally. In this way, expensive experts are no longer required, and all judgments and resulting actions are carried out in accordance with the manual to maximize efficiency and minimize legal liability, that is, errors arising from individually biased judgments made by expensive and independently minded experts are eliminated. The

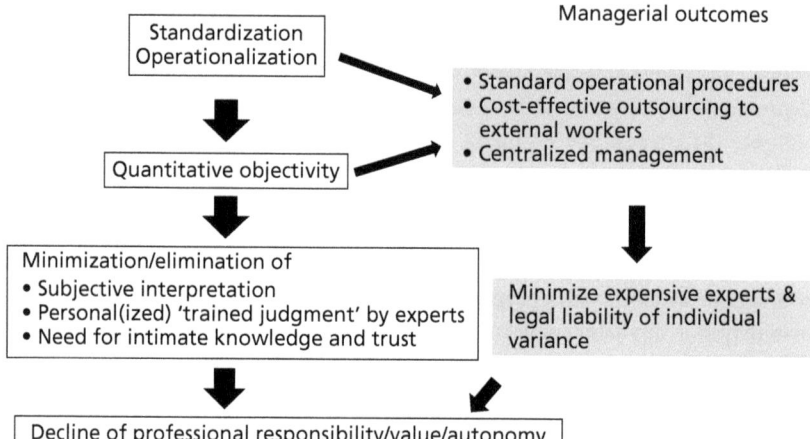

Fig. 35.3 Conceptual changes meet market requirements. Data from Porter (1995), Daston and Galison (2007), and Gaukroger (2012).

recent practice of rating scales and structured diagnostic interviews carried out by nonexperts after somewhat cursory training illustrates this trend in psychiatry and goes against Hamilton's caveat of 50 years ago that the value of his scale depends entirely on the skill of the interviewer (Hamilton 1960).

Incidentally, the past 20 years have seen a constant decline in many countries in the number of medical graduates choosing psychiatry as their profession (Lyons 2013). It may be only natural that aspiring and intellectual junior doctors are not too impressed by a specialty they see as offering less professional autonomy, more centralized regulation, less appreciation of accumulated diverse clinical experience, and more emphasis on quantitative objectification and determinism than others.

The most likely reason why these epistemological changes have taken place within the last 20 odd years, then, is that the business-school parlance and mindset of the globalized economy has so rapidly and deeply affected academicians that culture-sensitive pluralism (see Longino's discussion of pluralism as tolerance of a multiple framework, Chapter 2, this volume) in psychiatry has been replaced by an omnivorous oligarchy of globalized consumerism (Mount 2012).

I have almost finished my task of summarizing the biopsychosocioeconomic factors relevant to the conceptual status of depression today. If these historical changes were historical inevitability, to use the sardonic words of the political philosopher Isaiah Berlin (1954/1997), I might very well stop here and say *quod erat demonstrandum*. However, further discussion seems necessary yet, because the confusion seems to linger on as if nothing had happened, although it has already been well delineated and criticized by erudite scholars, for example, Shorter (2009) and Healy (1997, 2004). There must be something we can still do to improve the situation.

35.4 Paths Forward

35.4.1 The Gauguin Question—D'où venons-nous? Que sommes-nous? Où allons-nous?

It seems that at least two further questions need to be addressed before closing this chapter. First, why have these critiques had so little effect in improving the conceptual confusion of depression, and second, what can be done from here on to deal with the confusion?

First of all, it is worth wondering whether we have been barking up the wrong tree, that is, posing irrelevant questions and/or arriving at incorrect answers. This is not likely. Rather, I believe that we were wrong to believe that barking up the right tree alone would help chop it down. We academicians are often guilty of the vice of wishful thinking: criticism stated coherently and beautifully to the point will automatically awaken an omnipotent *deus ex machina*, who will then descend from heaven and sort out the mess for us at a stroke. This never happens. In other words, we may very well have arrived at the correct etiology and diagnosis of the confusion. If so, we now need to proceed to discussion of suitable treatment for said confusion.

35.4.2 The Singapore Statement for Clinical Research

In planning treatment for our confusion, the Singapore statement (Kleinert 2010), which was made in response to ongoing difficulties and problems in multinational, multisite clinical trial implementation, may be of help (Box 35.1). These principles seem as deceptively simple as some ancient Chinese philosophical aphorisms, but the implication here is that the opposite of these principles has too often been the case, for example, hiding untoward study results, massaging the figures, blaming others, and ducking responsibility if things go wrong, and harsh competition amongst researchers (Elliott 2010). It is worth remembering that elimination of the notion of individual responsibility was a common feature of the various beliefs associated with historical inevitability (Berlin 1954/1997).

Let me apply these principles to our situation.

Box 35.1 Singapore Statement: a global agreement on responsible research conduct (Kleinert 2010)

Principles:
- *Honesty* in all aspects of research.
- *Accountability* in the conduct of research.
- *Professional courtesy and fairness* in working with others.
- *Good stewardship* of research on behalf of others.

35.4.3 Treatment Plan for Conceptual Confusion

Table 35.1 shows the principles, their corresponding target symptoms, and the actual corrective actions to be taken.

Now, a second and final question remains: can we do this on our own? I do not suppose we can, because things do not seem to have significantly improved so far, in spite of all the sensible peer criticisms and suggestions that have been put forward. Therefore, an attempt was made to pick up some of the views of the people outside academic psychiatry on depression at large.

35.4.4 Nonspecialists' Views

Many of us psychiatrists may have allergic reactions to nonprofessional (or nonmedical) writings on mental illnesses, regarding many of them as ill-informed and ill-informing, naïve, and even soppy. This reaction is excusable, because we know that idly romanticizing mental disorders is a luxury we cannot afford in the face of severely ill patients whose lives are at stake. But many serious and admirable works have in fact been published, and it is a moot question as to whether medicalizing, pathologizing, and then commercializing depression is any better than humanizing it, if not romanticizing it. I have examined a haphazard selection of several monographs on depression by nonpsychiatrists (de Botton 2009; Ehrenberg 1998; Földeny 2004; Guardini 2008; Sartorius 2011; Zehentbauer 2011) and have found them illuminating, especially in regard to their sensible objections to, and discomfort with, pathologizing and medicalizing melancholy,

Table 35.1 Suggested treatment plan

Principles from the Singapore statement	Corresponding actions to be taken	Targeted symptoms and signs in psychiatry
Honesty	◆ Transparent publications ◆ Negative results welcomed	◆ Promethean promises (Rose 2012) ◆ Immodest claims of causality (Kleinman 2012b)
Accountability	◆ Acknowledgment of boundaries, culpabilities, and limitations	◆ Responsibility ducking ◆ Manichean vindictive reproach as self-defense
Professional courtesy & fairness	◆ Mutual respect and support ◆ Empathic understanding	◆ Divorce between science and clinical practice (Shorter 2009) ◆ Self-righteousness ◆ Medical hubris (Illich 1976)
Good stewardship	◆ International coordination of multidisciplinary endeavors ◆ Restriction of profit-motivated initiatives	◆ Intellectual crisis and academic oligarchies (Fava 2006) ◆ Excessive short-term commercialization

and thereby belittling its diverse manifestations and personal significance to those who suffer from it.

Many may have found it somewhat hilarious that the British National Health Service has recently suggested that general practitioners should prescribe good self-help books rather than antidepressants to some patients with depression (Brown 2013). This seems like yet another cost-cutting political maneuver, but again it is a moot question as to whether medicalizing or medicating depression is always justified and invariably better than demedicalizing it.

The aforementioned books by nonspecialists as well as the initiative to prescribe books instead of antidepressants may suggest that the general public, general practitioners, and nonpsychiatrists are all beginning to realize that something is deeply wrong with psychiatry today in its handling of depression, because: (1) increasing numbers of people are diagnosed and medicated, yet (2) pharmacotherapy is not as effective as espoused and advertised. In short, we need to take seriously these manifestations of public discomfort, or worse, distrust and exasperation, with what psychiatry provides in medical practice, which in many ways is just the result of confusion within the field.

35.4.5 Der Wanderer über dem Nebelmeer

In closing my attempt to address the confusion of the depression concept, I am reminded of a picture by Casper David Friedrich, *Der Wanderer über dem Nebelmeer* (Wanderer above the Sea of Fog), 1817 (Figure 35.4). This masterpiece depicts where we are now: mist and fog can still be seen beneath our eyes, along with steep cliffs and challenging hills ahead and no easy paths to traverse them; at the same time, however, the sky is high, and the atmosphere clear and inspiring. Zehentbauer uses this exact imagery in *Melancholie—Die traurige Leichtigkeit des Seins*:

> In melancholia, we experience ourselves as limited beings and perceive these limits as a thickly woven wall of fog (*Nebelwand*), which we often believe we can see through. But what exactly lies behind this spiritual wall of fog?—Divinity? The cosmic self? The sacred? Or nothing but a reflection of ourselves? (Zehentbauer 2011, p. 30, translated by the quoting author)

Indeed this conceptual confusion intertwined with so many diverse issues is depressing enough. But we do need to go through this *Nebelwand* in order to rescue our patients from the mist of confusion, at least part of which is our own creation. It is our professional and moral duty now to decrease, not increase, the confusing *Nebelwand* before us. If the conceptualization of an important and grave illness is so confused as to negatively affect clinical practice surrounding it, this is indeed a crisis.

In *Sein und Zeit*, Heidegger (1927/1984) remarked that: "The level which a science has reached is determined by how far it is *capable* of a crisis in its basic concepts" (p. 29).

At stake now, therefore, is whether we psychiatrists are capable of overcoming this *Nebelwand*, namely a crisis in depression research and practice (Fava 2006).

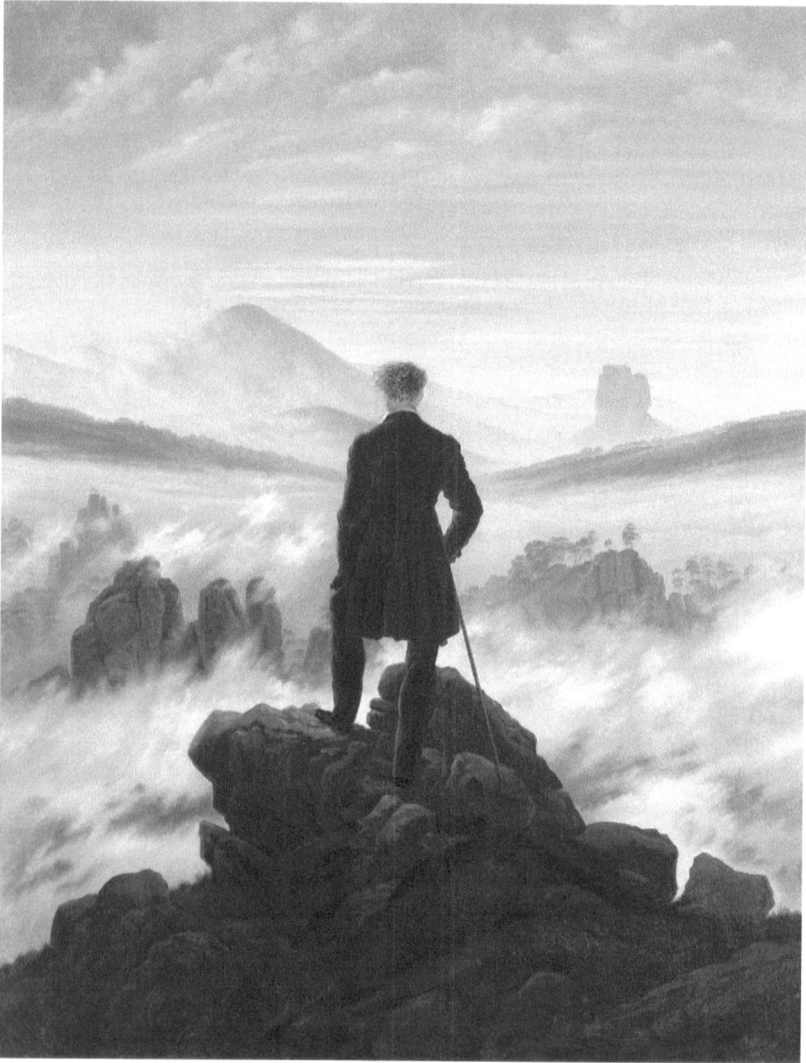

Fig. 35.4 *Der Wanderer über dem Nebelmeer* (Wanderer above the Sea of Fog), 1817, by Casper David Friedrich.

My hotchpotch attempt pales before the incisive scholarship and mesmerizing erudition exhibited by my colleagues in this volume, and yet the grave issues that I have had to take up are extremely unpalatable. I only hope that I have gone a little way toward clarifying some of the issues that are of concern to all of us.

Acknowledgment

The author is immensely grateful to Professor Timothy Minton, Keio University School of Medicine, for his valuable editorial help in finalizing this chapter.

References

Abraham, J. (2010). Pharmaceuticalization of society in context: theoretical, empirical and health dimensions. *Sociology*, 44, 603–622.

American Psychiatric Association (1980). *Diagnostic and Statistical Manual of Mental Disorders* (3rd ed.). Washington, DC: American Psychiatric Publishing.

American Psychiatric Association (2013). *Diagnostic and Statistical Manual of Mental Disorders* (5th ed.). Arlington, VA: American Psychiatric Publishing.

Auden, W.H. (1948). *The Age of Anxiety: A Baroque Eclogue*. London: Faber & Faber.

Berlin, I. (1968). The role of the intelligentsia. *Listener*, 79, 563–565. (Reprinted in Hardy H. (ed.) (2000). *The Power of Ideas*, pp. 125–133. London: Chatto & Windus.)

Berlin, I. (1997). Historical inevitability. In H. Hardy and R. Hausheer (eds.) *The Proper Study of Mankind—An Anthology of Essays*, pp. 91–118. London: Chatto & Windus. (Work originally published in 1954.)

Berrios, G.E., Bulbena, A., Bakshi, N., et al. (1992). Feelings of guilt in major depression. Conceptual and psychometric aspects. *British Journal of Psychiatry*, 160, 781–787.

Berrios, G.E. (1996). *The History of Mental Symptoms*. Cambridge: Cambridge University Press.

Bok, D. (2003). *Universities in the Marketplace: The Commercialization of Higher Education*. Princeton, NJ: Princeton University Press.

Brown, M. (2013). GPs to prescribe self-help books for mental health problems. *The Guardian*, January 31.

Chalmers, I. and Glasziou, P. (2009). Avoidable waste in the production and reporting of research evidence. *Lancet*, 374, 86–89.

Daston, L. and Galison, P. (2007). *Objectivity*. New York: Zone Books.

De Botton, A. (2009). *The Pleasures and Sorrows of Work*. London: Hamish Hamilton.

Editorial (2012a). Living with grief. *Lancet*, 379, 589.

Editorial (2012b). Psychiatry's identity crisis. *Lancet*, 379, 1274.

Editorial (2013). Mapping the mind—smart thinking for brain health? *Lancet*, 381, 1247.

Ehrenberg, A. (1998). *La Fatigue d'être Soi: Depression et Société*. Paris: O. Jacob.

Elliott, C. (2010). *White Coat, Black Hat: Adventures on the Dark Side of Medicine*. London: Beacon Press.

Engel, G.L. (1961). Is grief a disease?—a challenge for medical research. *Psychosomatic Medicine*, 23, 18–22.

Engel, G.L. (1977). The need for a new medical model: a challenge for biomedicine. *Science* 196, 129–136.

Fava, G.A. (2006). The intellectual crisis of psychiatric research. *Psychotherapy and Psychosomatics*, 75, 202–208.

Fava, G.A. (2009). The decline of pharmaceutical psychiatry and the increasing role of psychological medicine. *Psychotherapy and Psychosomatics*, 78, 220–227.

Feighner, J.P., Robins, E., Guze, A.B., et al. (1972). Diagnostic criteria for use in psychiatric research. *Archives of General Psychiatry*, 26, 57–63.

Földeny, L.F. (2004). *Melancholie* (Erw. Neuausgabe.) Berlin: Matthes & Seitz.

Frances, A. (2013). *Saving Normal—An Insider's Revolt Against Out-of-Control Psychiatric Diagnosis, DSM-5, Big Pharma, and the Medicalization of Ordinary Life*. New York: William Morrow.

Friedman, R.A. (2012). Grief, depression, and the DSM-5. *New England Journal of Medicine*, 366, 1855–1857.

Gaukroger, S. (2012). *Objectivity: A Very Short Introduction*. Oxford: Oxford University Press.

Greenslit, N.P. and Kaptchuk, T.J. (2012). Antidepressants and advertising: psychopharmaceuticals in crisis. *Yale Journal of Biological Medicine*, 85, 153–158.

Guardini, R. (2008). *Vom Sinn der Schwermut*. Berlin: Topos Plus.

Hamilton, M. (1960). A rating scale for depression. *Journal of Neurology, Neurosurgery and Psychiatry*, 23, 56–62.

Healy, D. (1997).*The Antidepressant Era*. Cambridge, MA: Harvard University Press.

Healy, D. (2004). *Let Them Eat Prozac: The Unhealthy Relationship between the Pharmaceutical Industry and Depression*. New York: New York University Press.

Heidegger, M. (1984). *Sein und Zeit* (15th ed.). Tubingen: Max Niemeyer Verlag. (Macquarrie, J. and Robinson, E. (trans.) (1962). *Being and Time*. Oxford: Basil Blackwell.) (Work originally published in 1927.)

Hollender, M.H. (1972). Conversion hysteria—a post-Freudian reinterpretation of 19th century psychosocial data. *Archives of General Psychiatry*, 26, 311–314.

Horwitz, A.V. and Wakefield, J.C. (2007). *The Loss of Sadness: How Psychiatry Transformed Normal Sorrow Into Depressive Disorder*. New York: Oxford University Press.

Illich, I. (1976). *Limits to Medicine: Medical Nemesis: The Expropriation of Health*. London: Marion Boyars.

Insel, T., Cuthbert, B., Garvey, M., et al. (2010). Research domain criteria (RDoC): toward a new classification framework for research on mental disorders. *American Journal of Psychiatry*, 167, 748–751.

Insel, T.R. and Quiron, R. (2005). Psychiatry as a clinical neuroscience discipline. *Journal of American Medical Association*, 294, 2221–2224.

Kasahara, Y. and Kimura, B. (1975). Zur Klassifizierung der depressiven Zustände. *Psychiatria et Neurologia Japonia*, 77, 715–735 [in Japanese].

Kasahara, Y. (2009). *Essential Clinical Practice for Depression*. Tokyo: Misuzu Shobo [in Japanese].

Kendler, K.S. and Parnas, J. (eds.) (2012). *Philosophical Issues in Psychiatry II: Nosology*. Oxford: Oxford University Press.

Kendler, K.S., Myers, J., and Zisook, S. (2008). Does bereavement-related major depression differ from major depression associated with other stressful life events? *American Journal of Psychiatry*, 65, 1449–1455.

Kimura, B. (1965). Vergleichende Untersuchungen über depressive Erkrankungen in Japan und in Deutschland. *Fortschritte der Neurologie und Psychiatrie*, 33, 202–215.

Kimura, B. (1966). Schulderlebnis und Klima. *Nervenarzt*, 37(9), 394–400.

Kitanaka, J. (2012). *Depression in Japan: Psychiatric Cures for a Society in Distress*. Princeton, NJ: Princeton University Press.

Kleinert, S. (2010). Singapore Statement: a global agreement on responsible research conduct. *Lancet*, 376, 1125–1127

Kleinman, A. (2012a). Culture, bereavement, and psychiatry. *Lancet*, 379, 608–609.

Kleinman, A. (2012b). Rebalancing academic psychiatry: why it needs to happen—and soon. *British Journal of Psychiatry*, 201, 421–422.

Klerman, K.L., Vaillant, G.E., Spitzer, R.L., and Michels, R. (1984). A debate on DSM-III. *American Journal of Psychiatry*, 141, 539–553.

Lane, C. (2007). *Shyness: How Normal Behavior Became a Sickness*. New Haven CT: Yale University Press.

Lorant, V., Croux, C., Weich, S., et al. (2007). Depression and socio-economic risk factors: 7-year longitudinal population study. *British Journal of Psychiatry*, 190, 293–298.

Lyons, Z. (2013). Attitudes of medical students toward psychiatry and psychiatry as a career: a systematic review. *Academic Psychiatry*, 37, 150–157.

Maj, M. (2012). When does depression become a mental disorder? In K.S. Kendler and J. Parnas (eds.) *Philosophical Issues in Psychiatry II: Nosology*, pp. 221–228. Oxford: Oxford University Press.

Mann, J. (2010). Clinical pleomorphism of major depression as a challenge to the study of its pathophysiology. *World Psychiatry*, 9, 167–168.

Margolis, J. (1994). Taxonomic puzzles. In J.Z. Sadler, O.P. Wiggins, and M.A. Schwartz (eds.) *Philosophical Perspectives on Psychiatric Diagnostic Classification*, pp. 101–128. Baltimore, MD: Johns Hopkins University Press.

Marmot, M. and Wilkinson, R.G. (2006). *Social Determinants of Health* (2nd ed.). Oxford: Oxford University Press.

Metzl, J.M. (2003). *Prozac on the Couch: Prescribing Gender in the Era of Wonder Drugs*. Durham, NC: Duke University Press.

Mount, F. (2012). *The New Few or A Very British Oligarchy: Power and Inequality in Britain Now*. New York: Simon & Schuster.

Mowery, D.C. and Sampat, B.N. (2005). The Bayh–Dole Act of 1980 and university–industry technology transfer: a model for other OECD governments? *Journal of Technology Transfer*, 30, 15–127.

Parker, G., Fink, M., Shorter, E., et al. (2010). Issues for DSM-5: whither melancholia? The case for its classification as a distinct mood disorder. *American Journal of Psychiatry*, 167, 745–747.

Parker, G. (2009). Diagnosis of depressive disorders. In H. Herrman, M. Maj, and N. Sartoirus (eds.) *Depressive Disorders* (3rd ed.), pp. 1–26. Chichester: Wiley.

Porter, T.M. (1995). *Trust in Numbers: The Pursuit of Objectivity in Science and Pubic Life*. Princeton, NJ: Princeton University Press.

Rai, D., Zitko, P., Jones, K., Lynch, J., and Araya, R. (2013). Country- and individual-level socioeconomic determinants of depression: multilevel cross-national comparison. *British Journal of Psychiatry*, 202, 195–203.

Rose, H. and Rose, S. (2012). *Genes, Cells and Brains: The Promethean Promises of the New Biology*. London: Verso.

Rose, S. (2005). *The Future of the Brain: The Promise and Perils of Tomorrow's Neuroscience*. New York: Oxford University Press.

Rose, S. (2006). *The 21st Century Brain: Explaining, Mending and Manipulating the Mind*. London: Vintage Books.

Sakai, Y., Akiyama, T., Miyake, Y., et al. (2005). Temperament and job stress in Japanese company employees. *Journal of Affective Disorders*, 85, 101–112.

Sandel, M. (2012). *What Money Can't Buy: The Moral Limits of Markets*. New York: Allen Lane.

Sartorius, M. (2011). *Die hohe Kunst der Melancholie*. Gütersloh: Gütersloher Verlagshaus.

Saß, H. (1990). Operationalisierte Diagnostik in der Psychiatrie. *Nervenarzt*, 61, 255–258.

Sato, Y. and Berrios, G.E. (2001). Operationalism in psychiatry: a conceptual history of operational diagnostic criteria. *Seishin Igaku (Clinical Psychiatry)*, 43, 704–713 [in Japanese].

Scull, A. (2009). *Hysteria: The Biography*. Oxford: Oxford University Press.

Sedler, M.J. (1994). Foundations of the new nosology. *Journal of Medicine and Philosophy*, 19, 219–238.

Shorter, E. (2009). *Before Prozac: The Troubled History of Mood Disorders in Psychiatry*. New York: Oxford University Press.

Siegrist, J. (2013). Berufliche Gratifikationskrisen und depressive Störungen: Aktuelle Forschungsevidenz. *Nervenarzt*, 84, 33–37.

Van Praag, H.M. (1998). The diagnosis of depression in disorder. *Australia and New Zealand Journal of Psychiatry*, 32, 767–772.

Wakefield, J.C. (2012). Should prolonged grief be reclassified as a mental disorder in DSM-5?: reconsidering the empirical and conceptual arguments for complicated grief disorder. *Journal of Nervous and Mental Disorders*, 200, 499–511.

Zehentbauer, J. (2011). *Melancholie: Die traurige Leichtigkeit des Seins*. Berlin: Peter Lehmann.

Zimmerman, M., Mattia, J.I., and Posernak, M.A. (2002). Are subjects in pharmacological treatment trials of depression representative of patients in routine clinical practice? *American Journal of Psychiatry*, 159, 469–473.

Zisook, S. and Kendler, K. (2007). Is bereavement-related depression different than non-bereavement-related depression? *Psychological Medicine*, 37, 779–794.

Chapter 36

What do we want from a depression diagnosis?

Eric Turkheimer

On National Public Radio on January 21, 2014, the singer Jennifer Holliday was interviewed by Robin Young about her career, including her experience with depression. She has also struggled with her weight, and the following exchange ensued (<http://hereandnow.wbur.org/2014/01/21/jennifer-holliday-returns>):

> Young: Did that issues [sic] around the weight compound the depression or did the depression compound the issues around the weight or ...
> Holliday: I think that the weight came upon as the depression and then added to it. Now, I had clinical depression, so that's actually a medical condition. I now live with and suffer with multiple sclerosis.
> Young: Oh, no. Yeah.
> Holliday: The side effect of that is also depression. So a lot of things have various factors involved with depression.

Ms. Holliday perceives that there is something important about the designation of her depression as "clinical", and in this brief response to Professor Sato's erudite review of the historical, cultural, and scientific contributions to the evolution of the construct of depression (Chapter 35, this volume) I will explore that perception. Why do we care so much about the official, DSM-encoded, clinical definition of depression? There are, of course, many good reasons to care, as Sato's chapter reminds us. But there are also important domains in which it doesn't matter very much, and life might be easier for everyone concerned if theoretical and empirical questions about the nature of psychiatric disorder were isolated from the quotidian concerns of clinical practice.

As Sato documents, the long historical discussion about depression as a disorder has recently reached an apotheosis in a narrow but heated disagreement about the so-called grieving exception. The latest version of the DSM allows that under some circumstances the typical, normal, one might say necessary responses to the death of a loved one may qualify as a disorder. In theory, it makes sense. If it means anything to say that grieving is a *function* of human cognition, then it ought to be possible for that function to fail. Presumably psychotic delusions would not represent the normal function of grief, however understandable they might be in the recently bereaved. Yet at the same time, it would be difficult not to worry about the medicalization of ordinary human grief that is enabled by the exemption's expiration. History has taught us all too well how these matters proceed, as what begins with exceptional treatment of frank disorder ends with ubiquitous methylphenidate in the morning and zolpidem at bedtime. My goal is to sort out these competing theoretical demands. The answer, I think, is a limited psychiatric libertarianism.

I begin with another example of reaction to depression from the sufferer's point of view, this one close to home. When my late mother was dying from the lung cancer that had invaded her bones, she was in great physical pain, but she was also anxious (not a sufficient word for what she was feeling), depressed, and unable to sleep. She was, one might say, mourning her own death, and the most reliable comfort she could find was from Xanax® (alprazolam). She took it regularly. I don't know where it came from; presumably her primary care physician prescribed it. Was she suffering from "clinical" depression or anxiety, from something that had not been exempted from the current version of the DSM? Who cares? My mother certainly didn't and neither did I. She was suffering, Xanax® relieved it, and that was that.

It seems safe to say that fear of impending death is a normal function of the human mind, and the universality of this fear is the very reason empathy exists. "Some things may never happen:" said Philip Larkin, "this one will" (<http://www.poetryfoundation.org/poem/178058>). But by the argument about grieving, if fear of death is a function it can also fail to function properly, and one can imagine reasoned discussion and empirical investigation of the circumstances in which fear of death might be considered a disorder. Are you going to have a heart attack today? Most of the time, however, whether one's fears about death are functional or dysfunctional doesn't matter. Dying people suffer, and we grant them the right to choose how they relieve their suffering. They might take Xanax®, they might pray, they might see a grief counselor, or read a book about accepting death, and any or all of these things may or may not work for them. How well they work on average and what their risks might be is a topic for empirical research, and as professionals we might advise patients about their relative costs and benefits, but to even think about diagnosing normal and abnormal behavior under sentence of death is, in any imaginable situation, just too much.

Less of this little analysis than one might think depends on mortality as a cause of human distress. Jennifer Holliday had experienced great success following her role in *Dreamgirls*, but afterwards her weight shot up to almost 400 pounds. Her record company released her and she couldn't get a job performing. She was diagnosed with multiple sclerosis. She was—never mind DSM—depressed, and who could blame her? But did she "meet criteria" for "clinical" depression? There are many reasons not to care. Like my mother she was suffering, and like my mother she had a variety of options. She could take medication, see an analyst or a cognitive behavior therapist, read a book, visit a website, whatever. Such options may be more or less effective for people in general, and more or less effective given Ms. Holliday's individual constitution and needs, but when all is said and done it was up to her. It would be rare for a diagnosis or the absence of one to carry enough information to be of serious assistance in helping Ms. Hudson decide what to do. We in the clinical professions don't like to say it, but treatment with selective serotonin reuptake inhibitors (SSRIs), as opposed to cognitive behavior therapy or reading a book, doesn't work better in depression cases that happen to meet DSM criteria. SSRIs affect depression in the same sense that Xanax® affects fear and loathing, albeit probably less successfully in the short run. Drugs have effects, under some circumstances those effects are desirable, and all drugs come with attendant risks. It is no different for psychoanalysis, substituting relationships for drugs.

Libertarian thinking of this kind can untie a lot of difficult knots in psychiatry. I'll work one more example: alcohol. It is almost universally accepted by now that alcohol abuse and dependence are disorders, and in the terms I have suggested here, of course they are. If alcohol consumption can be normal, it can also be abnormal. But the question of *who* has this disorder, and what the implications of having it ought to be, is perpetually fraught at both the general level and for individual cases. I enjoy a glass of wine in the evening, but I often do without one and hopefully don't qualify as disordered. My parents, in the fashion of the *Madmen* generation of which they were a part, favored a couple of stiff cocktails every single night, and they did not tolerate abstention cheerfully. Did they meet criteria, given their overall high level of functioning and the boozy standards of the time? You know my answer: who cares? People drink. Some people drink more than others. People who do drink derive some benefits and suffer some consequences. People who, in their own opinion or the opinion of others, drink too much and want to drink less can find a variety of methods to help them, as usual ranging from the pharmaceutical to the psychotherapeutic to the cultural to the religious. For most clinical purposes, exceptions to follow, the question of who has a disorder and who doesn't can be safely ignored.

There are, needless to say, good reasons why questions of disorder matter. The first, which I won't dwell on with this audience, is that the nature of psychiatric disorder is just an interesting and difficult theoretical problem, practical irrelevance notwithstanding. Beyond that, the most obvious reason to care about diagnosis is money. I don't know how my mother's Xanax® was paid for, but if Medicaid was involved, questions of whether the prescription was justified by a clinical diagnosis would have played an important role. A second class of reasons is legal, involving compulsion to treatment or exculpation from criminal behavior. If a person becomes suicidal at the end of life or a family wants to compel a member into alcohol treatment, clinical diagnosis provides at least an officially prescribed route through the nearly impossible tangle of ethical conundrums that are involved. Practical considerations such as these are undeniably important, especially to clinicians who earn a living providing treatment or patients who need to pay for it, but it is ironic that so many of the reasons we care about diagnosis are ultimately mercenary, and so removed from the core mission of comprehending, empathizing with, and alleviating human suffering.

But that is too easy, because there is one other good reason to care about diagnosis, and it is relevant to both our deepest theoretical questions and the real concerns of doctors and patients. It is, in fact, what Jennifer Holliday was referring to. Her response to Young's question about the role of weight in her depression was actually an objection. After acknowledging that her weight and her depression may have been mutually causal, she changed course, reminding Young that she had *clinical* depression, which is "actually a medical condition." What did she mean by this? She meant, I think, that as a medical condition her depression has the same status as her multiple sclerosis, a neurological condition that descended on her, which as such was not entangled in the web of intentional causes and effects that made up her psychological life and her experience of the many personal difficulties she was having at the time. She was almost certainly encouraged to think this way by her clinician, probably in the customary lay language of chemical imbalances in her brain.

What we all—clinicians and patients alike—want from diagnosis is relief from the Sisyphean burden of understanding the relationship between our bodies and our intentions. Why we suffer in the aftermath of great success, why it is so hard to lose weight, why our drinking habits are so hard to change, are questions of such enormous philosophical, clinical, and personal difficulty that they eventually exhaust us, once again doctors and patients together. Melancholia, obesity, and alcohol use are not—sorry—simply genetic or neurological conditions inflicted on us like multiple sclerosis, awaiting medical treatment if anyone could only figure out how. Neither, of course, are they simply lifestyles, matters of immediate and straightforward will. Perhaps nothing is. What, exactly, such conditions are, how in Holliday's words, "the weight came upon to the depression and then added to it," is a question that has not been answered: not philosophically, not medically, not psychologically, not personally. If it sometimes offers us relief from our collective clinical and personal uncertainty to act as though human struggles are just diseases, and our efforts to overcome them just treatments, so be it. I wouldn't want to deny anyone the professional security or personal comfort that comes from believing that it is so, but at the same time we must bear in mind that it is also an oversimplification.

Honesty about our clinical and personal oversimplifications compels an explanatory humility that will be well served by a default libertarian philosophy of how we regulate our clinical interactions. Empirical investigation can certainly contribute to our understanding of how people grieve, how we might alleviate the unbearable pain grief can bring, and even to the diagnosis and classification of grieving gone awry. The controversy caused by the expiration of the grieving exception, I would suggest, is not rooted in antiempiricism, but instead in skepticism about the clinical professions' willingness to abstain from clinical overreach once a disorder has been legitimized. The empirical scientific foundations of our notions of disorder remain incomplete, and even as they are completed, their application to individual cases remains extraordinarily difficult. Until there exists hard scientific knowledge to support or undermine the notion that some form of grieving in a particular person at a specific time is pathological, it is best to leave the question out of our discussions with patients, and instead guide them in seeking relief from their problems according to the unique configuration of their own desires.

Section 13
The shaping of autism

Chapter 37

Introduction to "On the ratio of science to activism in the shaping of autism"

Josef Parnas

Autism or Asperger's syndrome, as it was called from the 1940s, was once a very rare developmental disorder. Today, it has become a not infrequent and lifelong condition, renamed in the DSM-5 as autistic spectrum disorder. Some people even talk about an "epidemic of autism." This syndrome represents a good subject for a discussion trying to clarify the roles of scientific and extrascientific factors in the "shaping" of the concept of autism.

Ian Hacking's chapter on this issue deserves to be read together with the subsequent commentary from Kenneth Kendler (Chapter 39). These two texts form an interesting exchange, not only on the substantial issues but also in styles and perspectives. Ian Hacking, a celebrity among philosophers of science, paints his picture with broad strokes of his philosophical and sociological brush and is mildly skeptical of the empirical arguments proposed by the psychiatric community. Kenneth Kendler, himself with widely respected scientific credentials, gives a careful comment written by a meticulous scientist, personally involved in the construction of the DSM-5.

Chapter 38

On the ratio of science to activism in the shaping of autism

Ian Hacking

38.1 "Shaping"

Autism has notoriously evolved from the 1940s, when it was a very rare developmental disorder of children, to the present day, when it is a not uncommon, but lifelong, condition. How autistic people think of themselves has changed. How families relate to members with autistic traits today is very different from a previous generation. Schools, social services, surroundings: everything is new, and much is still in flux. We now speak of autism spectrum disorders, or (to conceal our ignorance) acronymically as ASDs. The "spectrum" itself has evolved in the living memory of many people.

It is by no means clear that autism is one thing, or even some small and specific number of things. The very group (or groups) of people involved has been shaped over the course of some 70 years. This chapter argues that autism activists have done most of the shaping, and not scientific inquiry—except that for a critical period in the shaping of autism, many of the scientists were also activists.

You might suppose that the central part of the shaping of autism is the framing of formal definitions, epitomized by the successive *Diagnostic and Statistical Manuals of Mental Disorders* (DSM). In the case of autism spectrum disorders, I see the DSM as a bureaucratic record. It makes a big difference to who gets what kind of help for autism, whether or not they satisfy a DSM definition, but the shaping has already happened by the time a DSM is negotiated.

38.2 **The Ratio**

I will state the innuendo of my title in an overly sensational way:

> The ratio of science to activism in the shaping of autism has been 1:99.
> 1% science, 99% activism.

There are several reasons for making such an outrageous statement.

First, the "internal" and the "external" factors that have shaped autism overlap. The most influential and effective experts—what after Feinstein (2010) I shall call the pioneers—were often involved in autism in their personal lives. I am filing science practiced by activists on the side of the activists, not science. That is of course to load things in favour of my thesis, but it is an exaggeration intended to emphasize an anomaly in the history of medicine.

In the case of most diagnoses, it is easy enough to distinguish the people-known-about as opposed to the knowers. The patients ("passive") as opposed to the doctors ("active"). Or more generally those who are ill, and the experts and authorities who try to help them get better or at least carry on. It is not quite like that with autism, because so many of the pioneering figures in autism research have been personally involved, with an autistic child of their own.

I apologize for introducing an abbreviation to express this. I shall speak of a person being p-c-a if they are *p*ersonally *c*onnected to an *a*utistic person, by a family bond or other intimate relationship. I do not want to pry into private lives. The abbreviation serves to distance what is often a deeply emotional relationship:

> p-c-a = personally connected to an autistic person, (usually by familial bonds)

Being at heart a logician, I count self-identity as a connection, and hence I count people who are themselves autistic as p-c-a. Well-known figures such as Temple Grandin, Donna Williams, and Jim Sinclair are "limit cases" (as we logicians say) of people who are p-c-a.
Before I proceed to some generalizations, please remember the adage:

> If you've met one autistic person,
> You've met one autistic person.

A *first* reason, then, why autism is unusual is that so many of the pioneering scientists who sculpted the diagnosis have been p-c-a.

A *second* reason has to do with activists and advocacy groups. It is to be expected that activists are p-c-a. What is unusual is the extent to which they have been effective in shaping the perception and the experience of autism.

A *third* unusual feature of autism is that there are very great cleavages among advocacy groups, pursuing very different agendas, and having very different ideas about what autism "is".

38.3 Ignorance of Causation

A *fourth* feature of autism is that we know virtually nothing about what causes autism, to the point that some knowledgeable people doubt we are talking about one thing. Our remit for this conference spoke of "our knowledge of the nature and causes of psychiatric illness." I recall a panel at the 1998 convention of the American Psychiatric Association (APA) in Toronto; it included Robert Spitzer, chief editor of the DSM-III. He was defending the fact that DSM continued to classify by symptoms, not causes. His most telling example was autism, and he asserted that we know nothing about the causes of autism but still need it in the DSM. One could make exactly the same observation today, defending DSM-5 against the criticism that it is too noncausal.

We do know that the ratio of males to females among those diagnosed with ASDs is four to one. That has been a constant ever since the 1950s. But we have no explanation, although Simon Baron-Cohen (2002, 2003) conjectures that autism is an extreme in a range of traits far more common among males than females, and he has gestured at testosterone levels at certain stages of fetal development. He gets a certain amount of flak for what is claimed to be arrant sexism, but at least he addresses one of the very few stable generalizations about autism. Collaborators in Baron-Cohen's research group do take seriously the thought that ASDs in girls may be seriously underdiagnosed; see, for example, Lai et al (2012). Gender differences were a major topic at the International Meeting for Autism Research, May 2–4, 2013, which included brain imaging results reported by Meng-Chuan Lai.

We know that to some extent autism runs in families, and research for autism genetics has become extremely well funded. We can only suppose that autism is a neurological disorder, and so we search for abnormalities in the brain. Speculations such as these fuel research, and in the opinion of most experts are almost certainly true, but we still don't know much.

We don't know the nature or causes of autism, to the point that although it is filed as a disorder in DSM-IV and the new DSM-5, there is a powerful 'neurodiversity movement" that contends it is just a difference, not a disorder, let alone an illness. The slogan is, "Autism: it's a Difference, Not a Disease."

I shall return to neurodiversity, which is connected with "Autism Pride," evidently descended from other pride movements, beginning with Black Pride and Gay Pride. The central doctrine is that there are two kinds of people: neurotypicals—that's most of us—and autistic. The defect in this movement is that it tends to downplay the varying degrees in which autistic people differ from neurotypicals. Many, perhaps most of those now diagnosed as on the autistic spectrum can, with a little help, fend for themselves in a neurotypical world, even if it is none too easy. But the most severely affected really have great difficulty carrying on in *any* world.

38.4 **Summary of Oddities**

To sum up, autism is unusual because, among many other things:
1. Many leading scientific experts on autism have been p-c-a.
2. Activists (mostly p-c-a) have been amazingly effective in shaping autism.
3. Different advocacy groups have very different agendas.
4. We still know next to nothing about what causes autism.

In confirmation of these observations, I may cite two fairly recent books. Adam Feinstein's *A History of Autism: Conversations with the Pioneers* (2010) includes countless helpful vignettes of pioneers; these confirm how many of the second wave of pioneers were p-c-a. By the first "wave" I mean only Leo Kanner, Hans Asperger, and a few other contemporaries who were not p-c-a. Yet even in the case of Kanner, he relied to a quite unusual extent on written reports and diary entries by the parents of the few children he used as the basis for his initial study. He outsourced his research to p-c-a family members.

A more recent book is Chloe Silverman's *Understanding Autism: Parents, Doctors and the History of a Disorder* (2012). "Parents, doctors"—could the history of any other disorder be written around that pair? Feinstein and Silverman are complementary in a number of ways. First, because Feinstein really did converse with pioneers around the world, but his perspective is British. Silverman's focus is American. A great many of Feinstein's pioneers are manifestly p-c-a. Silverman's "parents and doctors" forewarns us that the history of the disorder is a dual story of experts (doctors) and the p-c-a folk, the parents. Moreover, the usually disjoint categories, parents and doctors, remarkably overlap in that many of the original doctors were parents of autistic children. In her chapter 4, "Brains, pedigrees, and promises," Silverman (2012) reports on research on the neurobiological and genetic nature of autism, and shows pretty clearly that there is a lot of hype, prompting a great deal of hope, but very little knowledge.

Moreover, Feinstein himself instantiates the phenomenon I am presenting, namely the ubiquity of being p-c-a in work on autism. He is the father of a 20-year-old autistic son. His research was sponsored by Steve Shirley (Dame Stephanie Shirley) who was a brilliant IT entrepreneur and also had an autistic son who died at the age of 35 (see Shirley 2012.) Steve made a veritable fortune with her self-founded company, which she is now ploughing back into autism research and education.

38.5 An Aside: My Own Interest in Autism

I am just a kibitzer. But I hope I am of a low-level and relatively harmless kind. Autism invites a great deal of highbrow speculation about the nature of the human mind. Autistic people often feel they are just specimens available for endless tests.

So I had better backtrack, and explain my own interest. I have long been fascinated by the ways in which classifications influence people, and the ways in which classifications change as the people classified change. I call this my "Making up People Project," and I will not elaborate on it. I say only that autism is an amazing story of the making and molding of a new classification hand-in-hand with the making and molding of the people who fall under the classification. There is an extraordinary back-and-forth looping effect between the category of autism and autistic people. Any of you slightly familiar with my project will recognize phrases such as "making and molding" and above all "looping." Moreover, autism is not yet some one definite thing scientists are trying to find out about, it is a "moving target" (Hacking 2007).

The project, and especially the phrase "looping effect" seems to have caught on and spawned many studies by other hands, and even workshops and conferences. My way of talking—"making up"—might seem to imply that we would all be better off if autism had never come into being as a way of being a person. On the contrary!

The social movement to diagnose, recognize, rethink, and extend the boundaries of autism has enormously benefitted a very great many individuals. I recently saw a photo of a child padlocked to a tree in a Somali village because it was the only way the family could control her outbreaks of tantrums and her inability to socialize or even talk coherently. That was a child born into extreme third-world poverty, but she is a powerful *metaphor* for the state of many children in the past, who would now be diagnosed as autistic. Autism activism has unchained a great many children and now adults.

And for those who know my book about multiple personality (*Rewriting the Soul*) or the one about fugue (*Mad Travelers*), I do *not* think autism is a transient mental illness. What might possibly turn out to be transient is our present grouping of criteria with the implication that they are all interconnected, in short, that autism is just one kind of thing. That conception may disappear. Perhaps it will be remembered as a magnificent "political" strategy for creating a common front among individuals with very different but unusual needs.

38.6 An Exclusion: Talk of an Epidemic

I shall ignore the most popular general interest question about autism: why does the incidence of diagnosis keep on going up and up? Is there an epidemic? Not in any literal sense. For all the debates, this is briefly and precisely established by Gernsbacher et al., "Three reasons not to believe in an autism epidemic" (2005). (By the way, Gernsbacher is p-c-a.)

It may be useful to mention dissonances that muddy the waters. The MIND Institute affiliated with the University of California, Davis is one of the best funded autism research organizations. It was formerly called the M.I.N.D. Institute, short for Medical Investigation of Neurodevelopmental Disorders. In its publicity newsletter a few years ago we read that "UC Davis M.I.N.D. Institute study shows California's autism increase not due to better counting, diagnosis." It refers to us to a study in *Epidemiology* (Hertz-Picciotto and Delwiche 2009), and writes that:

> "It's time to start looking for the environmental culprits responsible for the remarkable increase in the rate of autism in California," said UC Davis M.I.N.D. Institute researcher Irva Hertz-Picciotto, a professor of environmental and occupational health and epidemiology and an internationally respected autism researcher. (<http://www.ucdmc.ucdavis.edu/welcome/features/20090218_autism_environment/>)

Yet when we turn to Hertz-Picciotto and Delwiche (2009), said to be the basis of this assertion, in this published (and refereed) paper, there is not a word about the causes of "California's autism increase"—be they counting, diagnosis, or noxious chemicals—only an argument that there is an increase. I am not disparaging work seeking environmental influences; these researchers have studied many conjectures, even the dangers of a fetus with a mother living near a freeway. I say only that the relation between publicized assertions and data is often slender.

In a more figurative sense, yes of course there is an "epidemic" of autism diagnoses, but this does not mean that a greater proportion of children are affected with autism spectrum disorders today than 20 years ago—or, so far as we know, in the seventeenth century.

38.7 Some External Factors

Eyal et al. (2010) does bring out all sorts of rather "external" aspects of the story, such as the symbiotic relationship between autism and the disability movement, the de-institutionalization of the mentally ill, the ways in which "retarded" got captured by "autistic," and in general the symbiosis between "special needs" support in the classroom and autism. Eyal (2013) and further work not yet published also re-emphasizes the role of parents learning how to take care of their children, becoming responsible for therapy, for instance, learning how to practice Ivor Lovaas' "Advanced Behavioral Analysis" (ABA).

"Special needs" was fostered by an "external" coincidence: J.F. Kennedy's sister Rosemary was, in the lingo of the day, "retarded." This led Eunice Kennedy Shriver to be a powerful advocate for the 1962 establishment of the US National Institute of Child Health and Human Development. She egged on the presidential address of February 5, 1963, "Mental retardation ranks with mental health as a major health, social, and economic problem in this country. It strikes our most precious asset, our children." Diagnosing with hindsight, a number of experts have suggested that the Kennedys were p-c-a (viz. Rosemary was autistic.)

Rather than the question, "Is this an epidemic?" (answer, "No"), my interest is in how a new kind of person came into being, how a new way of human life emerged. Of course there have been people, whom we would now diagnose as autistic, for a very, very long time. But only in the past few decades has that become a way to conceive of oneself, of one's children, of one's friends.

38.8 The Internet

The most important single "external" item that has to do with the recent shaping of autism is the Internet. Autism lives on the Internet. Everyone has heard the self-propagating canards: "geeks are autistic," "computer nerds are autistic." Yes, many of them do have autistic traits. But there is much more to it than that. Autistic people have all sorts of difficulties communicating with others, and many positively avoid face-to-face contact, especially eye contact. But many autistic people, including some who are severely handicapped, open up on a keyboard (Hacking 2010).

A few years ago, one of the most familiar sights at some gatherings of autistic people was that half of them were happily chattering away on keyboards. Times have moved on: lots of texting, iPads, etc. Nowadays at conferences that include autistic people, they are encouraged to tweet to ask questions and otherwise participate, rather than speaking out, which may, for many seriously autistic people, be difficult or impossible. (This might be a good idea for all conferences, at least it would put a 140-character limit on stupid questions!)

Thus something external, the Internet, has been integral to the shaping of autism. Or *is* it external? Suppose one was to argue that the Internet and its auxiliaries were the outcome of autistic traits shared by a largish group of youngish people?

To return to my main interest, there is now a new way to be a person, and to think of yourself and those you care about—various words involving autism and "Asperger." If you want a new kind of person, type "Aspie" into a search engine. DSM-5 has deleted Asperger's disorder as a diagnosis, but I expect that the culture of Aspies is too entrenched to be deleted by the stoke of a pen.

Only in the past decade have events like this become possible:

AUTISM NETWORK INTERNATIONAL
presents Autreat 2013
Living Life the Autly Way
August 5–9, 2013
4 p.m. Monday to 1 p.m. Friday
California, Pennsylvania

The organizers go out of their way to say that all autistic people are welcome, no matter how severely limited they may be in this or that aspect. It is part of "autism pride" to insist that autistic people are just different. But a note of reality creeps in if you read the full announcement. Some autistic children, one might say, are more different than others. When it comes to practical matters:

> The daily charge for children and teens includes room and board & a daytime activity program for children under 18. Staff:child ratio is approximately 1:6. If your child needs more support than this, please bring an aide for your child, or contact ANI about hiring extra staff for an additional fee.

38.9 Organization

There are many more curious features of autism than it is possible even to mention in a short chapter. I shall now proceed as follows.

1. Brief observation on the beginning of autism as a diagnosis. No p-c-a involved.
2. Scientific leaders who are p-c-a get into the act.
3. Divergent activisms.
4. Autism still in flux.
5. A speculation about the unparalleled efficacy of autism advocates.

38.9.1 The Beginning of Autism as a Diagnosis. No p-c-a Involved

There is not the slightest reason to think that either Asperger or Kanner had an autistic family member. But as already mentioned, Kanner's vignettes of autistic children relied heavily on lengthy reports sent to him by parents of the children he was thinking about. Hence right from the start there was intense p-c-a involvement.

38.9.2 Scientific Leaders who are p-c-a get into the Act

Kanner noticed that the parents of the children he diagnosed tended to be rather uptight competitive professionals (just the sort of folk who bring their kids to pediatric clinics). He conjectured that the children grew up in a cold emotional climate, which contributed to their problem. This was the heyday of Freudian psychology in America. He coined the phrase "refrigerator mother" which undoubtedly caused untold harm. In fact Kanner's observations jibe well with Simon Baron-Cohen's observations that the parents of autistic children tend to excel in engineering, mathematics, male-oriented, emotion-free activities. They also tend to be *driven* with well-defined goals. (This will be emphasized in my later section 38.9.5.)

Kanner may not have been so far off. Alas, Bruno Bettelheim picked up the wrong end of Kanner's stick, and convinced a generation of Americans that autism was the result of bad mother–child bonding.

Revenge of the p-c-a! The first voice to speak out loud and clear was that of the San Diego psychiatrist, Bernard Rimland. He founded what became the Autism Society of America in 1965, the first American autism advocacy group. He also published the first book about autism, insisting that it was a neurological condition even in its title: *Infantile Autism: The Syndrome and Its Implication for a Neural Theory of Behavior* (Rimland 1964). Yes, he had an autistic son.

The first British autism advocacy group was founded a few years earlier, in 1962, first regionally for North London, and then became the (UK) National Autistic Society. One of the founding members was Lorna Wing, who became a NHS "consultant" = specialist in pediatric psychiatry. Yes, she had a troubled daughter. But unlike most of Kanner's children, her daughter did not have much of a problem with language. Wing read Hans Asperger's 1944 paper, and decided her daughter was like his children. And so a new diagnosis was born.

The name "Asperger's syndrome" was actually settled at tea involving Lorna Wing, Elizabeth Newsome, and another woman whose name I regret I do not know. Wing proposed that the subdisorder be named after Asperger. Her two companions, I was told, favored "able autism" as the name, partly on the ground that English parents would not want an ailment for their children with a nasty German name. Happily, Wing won the day.

Wing, mother of a daughter with many autistic traits, wonderfully exemplifies my claim (2). Not only did she give Anglos Asperger's ideas, but she had a strong hand in the thought that Autism is a "spectrum disorder," now made official in DSM-5. Rather than defending "her" syndrome—Asperger's—she decided in the end it was not a good idea. It prompted fruitless debates as to how "high-functioning autism" differs, or not, from Asperger's. She also fostered the valuable idea of a "triad" of difficulties as characterizing the difficulties of autistic people.

A person is "on the spectrum" if and only if the following behavioral criteria are present:

A qualitative impairment in social interaction.
A qualitative impairment in communication.
A markedly restricted repertoire of activities and interests.

This does not give the whole picture. Remember that many autistic people are subject to seizures—are hypersensitive to loud sounds, bright lights, itchy surfaces, and so on—find arm flapping helpful—engage in "stimming"—have tantrums in reaction to unexpected change—repeat what's just been said: echolalia. Nevertheless, the triad is so much more meaningful than the 1994 DSM-IV menu for autism! Happily that is somewhat simplified in the 2013 DSM-5.

The triad tells the story so much more clearly than the manuals. DSM-IV is the hardest to take in. ICD is easiest to understand because it is less of a menu. But one feels that the triad has something to do with people, whereas the DSMs have been written by accountants. (Which, in a sense, is true in North America. To get your treatment for any mental "disorder" paid for by your insurance company or by your public health insurance in Canada, you have to be coded by DSM.) Note that I am not claiming that the panels who wrote the final definitions of autism, Asperger's, and ASDs are likely to be p-c-a. I am claiming only that only for those who shaped the disorders.

I have mentioned only two of the early movers and shakers who are p-c-a because I don't want to get personal. But these two, Rimland in the United States and Wing in the United Kingdom, serve to set the stage. Note that in both the United States and the United Kingdom, autism got in on the ground floor of the emerging field of child psychiatry, what with Kanner having the first American clinic of pediatric psychiatry. Michael Rutter, another leading pioneer, was the first British professor of the subject.

38.9.3 Divergent Activisms

The closest thing to an umbrella organization for autism advocacy is *Autism Speaks*. It was founded in 2005 by Suzanne and Bob Wright. It has grouped together *The National Alliance for Autism Research* and *Cure Autism Now*. It has become the engine of charities for autism research in the United States, and is now assuming that role in the United Kingdom. Wright is CEO of NBC Universal, and a powerhouse in the corporate world. "The May 2004 merger of NBC and Vivendi Universal was the highlight of Wright's business career, which included one of the longest, most productive tenures of any [US] media company chief executive." Why did the couple found *Autism Speaks*? He is often quoted: "I want my grandson back!" He's using the not-uncommon metaphor that his once normal happy little boy was abducted—by aliens—and has become an alien (Hacking 2009). Many autistic people deeply resent this way of thinking.

On August 9, 2007 *Nature* ran an article on a recent extravaganza mounted by *Autism Speaks*: Lincoln Center featuring stars of stage and screen, for which the cheapest seats cost $1500. This one benefit event yielded $1.5 million. *Nature* went on to say that autism was stripping the larder bare, every year getting a larger and larger slice both of the charity pie and the National Institutes of Health pie for research on children's illnesses. The success story continues.

CAN: Cure Autism Now was founded in 1995 by Portia Iverson and her husband, who have an autistic son. Portia Iverson's *Strange Son: Two Mothers, Two Sons, and the Quest to Unlock the Hidden World of Autism* (2006) is a book about her own son and Tito Mukhopadhyay, whom she brought to America with his mother. Mukhopadhyay has been acclaimed as a poet; he hardly speaks but writes eagerly on a keyboard. He wrote a review of Iverson's book on Amazon (USA): "The book *Strange Son* felt like a 'slap' on my face." He hates statements by Iversen such as, "When I left their apartment that day I felt as if I'd glimpsed into the mind of an alien being" (p. 129). "My actions" writes Mukhopadhyay, "have been mentioned as 'beastly', 'alien being', 'possessed by a demon.'"

Before merging in 2007 into *Autism Speaks, CAN* had provided $50 million for research, much of it genetic. It established *AGRE*: a DNA depository and registry of phenotypic and genotypic information, and of brain tissue, available for research. The neurodiversity movement hates *CAN* and the very word "cure." It likes the slogan, "Cure Ignorance, not Autism!"

The *Autism Research Institute*, founded by Bernard Rimland, established *DAN: Defeat Autism Now*, with a quite different message. It strongly advocated diet as a road to improving autism. It embraced Andrew Wakefield, the British doctor who started the vaccine scare, who in the end was stricken from the UK medical register, and who migrated to Texas. A *DAN* conference was always surrounded by companies selling various kinds of dietary supplements. *ARI* has, however, stopped holding *DAN* conferences, but the various dietary wings of the autism movements are still flourishing.

I have mentioned the notice of an Autreat later this year, "live life the autly way." It is organized by *Autism Network International*, which is descended from *GRASP: The Global and Regional Asperger Syndrome Partnership*, itself found by an aspie, Jim Sinclair, famed for a much reprinted talk "Don't mourn for us" given at a conference in Toronto in 1995. Then there is *Aspies for Freedom*, founded 2004, whose membership by 2007 had grown to 20,000. It is against the very idea of a cure, and a whole gamut of "abuses' such as crazy diets, electroshock, chelation, and opposed to the rote training of Lovaas' ABA, a form of behavioral modification.

Enough. One of the causes of the divisiveness is that many parents feel they have a normal happy child whom they have grown to love more and more, and then something goes awry. They are desperate for help, and will embrace all sorts of nostrums. For every nostrum there is a success story, and also failures aplenty. One of the attractions of the neurodiversity movement is that it encourages acceptance and support whenever needed, without raising false hopes. I have wanted to weep when I have been at meetings of parents reminiscent of a 12-step program. A parent gets up to tell his tale: "Hi, I'm Jimmy, proud parent of Ben, my son who's recovering from autism." One knows that sooner or later, Jimmy (and Ben) is going to have to make their peace. Ben is not recovering. Despite a few counterexamples, autism is for life.

One of the roots of the divisive tendencies among autism families is that autistic people are so different from one another, and what is good for one is not necessarily a good thing for another. This is felt most strongly by parents of really severely impaired children. Alison Singer, a former vice president of *Autism Speaks*, wrote in a blog about her daughter Jodie and a friend Haley:

> Many days it is hard to believe that the challenges Haley faces with regard to her Asperger Syndrome and those Jodie struggles with are related under the same DSM-IV diagnosis. At one end of the autism spectrum we often find lower functioning persons like my daughter who cannot speak, have violent tantrums and can be self-injurious, while at the other end we have persons who struggle with very significant, but very different, predominantly social issues.

(Singer resigned from *Autism Speaks* because it would not cease funding research into vaccines as causal agents.)

38.9.4 Autism still in Flux

Autism has been on the move for decades and it has not settled down yet. It is merely symptomatic that the biggest media furor surrounding the DSM-5 (released in May 2013) has been about autism. Most psychiatric diagnoses are pretty firmly in the control of the experts. This is simply not true for autism.

The most notable feature is that DSM-5 deleted Asperger's as a distinct disorder. The outcry over the new criteria has two causes. One is practical. In many jurisdictions, parents of children with autistic traits have benefited enormously from being diagnosed as autistic, and getting all sorts of special help in school and daily life. In California, parents get significant time off by having their child babysat by a specially trained babysitter. So there is fear that different criteria are going to delete some parents/children from the rolls. In general, the APA maintains that studies show that pretty much everyone captured by DSM-IV will be captured by DSM-5, but other studies show the opposite. Although there is a vast battery of "validated" diagnostic and screening procedures, the fact that there is such disagreement reminds us how fluid the whole diagnosis is.

There is a quite different concern about deleting Asperger's. Many young people define themselves as Aspies. That in itself has become a whole way of life. It helps to say "who you are/what you are." I have already stated my expectation that "Aspie" will continue as a way to be a person, no matter what the APA says.

There is also a nagging doubt, voiced in various tones of voice, as to whether "autism" is rightly a psychiatric diagnosis at all. The manifestations are so different, that one wonders if we have not simply got a very mixed up syndrome, behind which lie many unrelated causes.

There is a vast amount of genetic sequencing of autistic persons going on right now. Most spectacular is BGI's promise to do a complete sequence for 10,000 autistic people by the end of the decade and probably much sooner. BGI, formerly Beijing Genomics, located in Shenzhen, China, is by far the best funded (and best staffed) sequencing outfit in the world. The directors of BGI know that *if* they can produce a sort of genetic map of autism, it will be heralded around the world. (BGI is at least as competitive as a California start-up.)

These efforts will doubtless show innumerable genetic oddities associated with subclasses of autistic people. My own hunch is that by themselves they will have very little direct influence on our understanding of autism.

What we *may* see is a return of a nineteenth-century research program, which had the disparaging name of "degeneracy." The thought was that a family of "deviancies" was heritable, with different ones showing up in successive generations. Jean-Martin Charcot is often reviled for being anti-Semitic (which he was), paying particular attention to deviancies in Jewish families. That was not stupid, as at the time, say the 1870s, Jews in or arriving in Paris formed a relatively closed gene pool. The picture was that in a family line one might see dipsomania in one generation, folie circulaire (bipolar) in the next, melancholia in another branch, kleptomania in the next generation, etc.

We have had a resurgence of this picture (with no mention of the old idea) first in a Scottish family over four generations which seems to have exhibited just about every psychiatric disorder, and whose members have a unique genetic variation at one locus. Most recently we have had "Identification of risk loci with shared effects on five major psychiatric disorders: a genome wide analysis" (Cross-Disorder Group of the Psychiatric Genomics Consortium 2013): "We aimed to identify specific variants underlying generic effects shared between [...] ASD, ADHD, bipolar disorder, major depressive disorder, and schizophrenia" (p. 1371).

As for other current research projects, we may note the "Autism Phenome Project" run by the previously mentioned MIND Institute. MIND was founded by p-c-a families, especially a TV anchor and her very successful building contractor husband. Extremely well funded, it self-describes as the leading research institute of its kind in the world. The head researcher of the Phenome Project, David Amoral, thinks that "The tremendous variation in autism leads us to believe that it is a group of disorders rather than a single one." Hence the Project, which will study a largish sample, 900 children aged 2–4 who are diagnosed as autistic, 450 children with other developmental difficulties, and 450 neurotypicals. Each child will have an in-depth analysis including genetics, neurology, immunology, metabolism, and behavior analyzed along as many vectors as are manageable. The hope is that the children will fall into a number of distinctive clumps.

You might say that a positive result would be welcomed by the neurodiversity movement—more diversity! On the contrary, the movement vigorously resists any attempt by neurotypicals to split and divide autistic people.

Autism, as I have said, is in flux.

38.9.5 A Speculation about the Unparalleled Efficacy of Autism Advocates

A fundamental chapter in the history of autism will be about advocacy groups. Is there anything unusual about autism advocacy? I shall make a suggestion that will not be universally welcomed. It combines two observations: (1) impressionistic and (2) controversial.

The impressionist observation begins with the fact that many of the leading early makers and shapers of autism diagnosis and treatment were p-c-a. Add to this the remarkable qualities of influential advocates. I first mentioned Steve Shirley (2012), who must be unique in the United Kingdom: a *woman* who starts an *information technology* company from nothing, and when she sells it can write a £50 million pound check for autistic causes. Moreover she does her best to employ only women in the company, having to fight sex-discrimination laws. Just imaginable in California, but in *Britain*?

Next take the founders of *Autism Speaks*, one of whom, as I reported earlier, is described as the outstandingly successful, long-running executive in a cut-throat industry. With an autistic grandson.

The largest single autism philanthropist is James Simons, whom the *Financial Times* characterizes as the world's smartest billionaire. He is a gifted creative mathematician who went on to found a hedge fund which cleared him $10 billion (and his math undoubtedly contributed to the near-failure of capitalism). He is putting up more than $100 million for autism research, with the MIND Institute as a major recipient. He is very discreet about his private life, which I respect. I note only what is regularly reported on the Internet, including Wikipedia, without denial. One son died early from drowning in Bali, and another riding a bicycle that was hit by a car—and Simons has provided family DNA for autism research.

My controversial observation (2) is the Baron-Cohen conjecture that autism is an extreme case of systematizing brains, most of which are male. Systematizing brains are given to the construction of impersonal structures, great attention to detail, and absolute single-mindedness. This type of brain is heritable; it runs in families, mostly showing up in the male line. Even those who accuse Baron-Cohen of gross male chauvinism when he distinguishes types of brains have to admit he is the rare researcher who attends to a simple fact: most autistic children are male.

Baron-Cohen collects statistics on the family trees of autistic people and confirms, on a grand scale, the first impressions of Kanner and Asperger about the parents of autistic children. They have family trees overloaded with single minded, goal-directed systematizers.

My speculation is that the success of autism advocacy movements is owing in part to the autistic traits of the leaders. This should not be heard as a negative remark but as a positive one. People in the Neurodiversity Movement urge that "We have talents that you neurotypicals lack." I am suggesting a generalization on that theme, that relatives of autistic people may be possessed of quasi-autistic talents, which helps account for their success in moving autism from the rare to the common.

So suppose autistic *traits* are heritable, without necessarily being disabling. Such traits in p-c-a activists could help explain the curious efficacy of autism advocates. They are *driven* to one and only one end.

References

American Psychiatric Association. (2013). *Diagnostic and Statistical Manual of Mental Disorders* (5th ed.). Arlington, VA: American Psychiatric Publishing.

Baron-Cohen, S. (2002). The extreme male brain theory of autism. *Trends in Cognitive Sciences*, 6, 248–254.

Baron-Cohen, S. (2003). *The Essential Difference: Men, Women and the Extreme Male Brain*. London: Allen Lane.

Cross-Disorder Group of the Psychiatric Genomics Consortium; Genetic Risk Outcome of Psychosis (GROUP) Consortium. (2013). Identification of risk loci with shared effects on five major psychiatric disorders: a genome-wide analysis. *The Lancet*, 381(9875), 1371–1379.

Eyal, G., Hart, B., Onculer, E., Oren, N., and Rossie, N. (2010). *The Autism Matrix: The Social Origins of the Autism Epidemic*. Cambridge: Polity Press.

Eyal, G. (2013). For a sociology of expertise: the social origins of the autism epidemic. *American Journal of Sociology*, 118(4), 863–907.

Feinstein, A. (2010). *A History of Autism: Conversations with the Pioneers.* Oxford: Wiley-Blackwell.

Gernsbacher, M.A., Dawson, M., and Goldsmith, H.H. (2005). Three reasons not to believe in an autism epidemic. *Current Directions in Psychological Science*, 14, 55–58.

Hacking, I. (2007). Kinds of people: moving targets. *Proceedings of the British Academy B*, 151, 285–318.

Hacking, I. (2009). Humans, aliens and autism. *Daedalus*, 138, 44–59.

Hacking, I. (2010). Autism fiction: a mirror of an Internet decade? *University of Toronto Quarterly*, 79, 632–655.

Hertz-Picciotto, I. and Delwiche, L. (2009). The rise in autism and the role of age in diagnosis. *Epidemiology*, 20, 84–90.

Iverson, P. (2006). *Strange Son: Two Mothers, Two Sons, and the Quest to Unlock the Hidden World of Autism.* New York: Riverhead Books.

Lai, M.-C., Lombardo, M.V., Ruigrok, A.N., Chakrabarti, B., Wheelwright, S.J., Auyeung, B., et al. (2012). Cognition in males and females with autism: similarities and differences. *PLoS One*, 7(10), e47198.

Rimland, B. (1964). *Infantile Autism: The Syndrome and Its Implication for a Neural Theory of Behavior.* Englewood Cliffs, NJ: Prentice Hall.

Shirley, S. (2012). *Let It Go!* Luton: Andrews.

Silverman, C. (2012). *Understanding Autism: Parents, Doctors and the History of a Disorder.* Princeton, NJ: Princeton University Press.

Chapter 39

The shaping of autism and other psychiatric disorders: an alternative perspective

Kenneth S. Kendler

In a creative and evocative style, Hacking explores the social context of the diagnostic conceptualization of autism in Chapter 38. The self-declared focus of this conference was to clarify how, from an historical perspective, the field of psychiatry responds to internal (aka scientific/empirical) versus external (aka social-cultural) influences. Hacking boldly declares that for autism the ratio has been 1:99.

39.1 Progress in Autism Research

Hacking raises many issues in his chapter and in the limited available space, I must, in my response, prioritize them. In the interest of disclosure, I should note that I have spent my life in the field of psychiatric research with a special focus on genetics. In my view, Hacking substantially underestimates the progress made in our understanding of the etiology of autism. His proposed ratio of 1:99 is not an accurate reflection of the emerging current understanding of autism. As Hacking notes, one important observation in the so-called epidemic of autism is how rising rates of autism are often mirrored by falling rates of mental retardation (MR) in the same population. Perhaps the most important molecular genetic advance in autism research has been the identification of large genomic deletions or insertions (called "copy number variants" or CNVs) that are significantly associated with autism spectrum disorders across several large studies (Devlin and Scherer 2012). However, recent analyses has shown that most of these CNVs are not specific to autism but have been associated with a range of developmental disabilities including more typical MR and, in some cases, adult schizophrenia. So both epidemiological and genetic research are pointing toward close links between autism and broader disabilities including what would have traditionally been called MR. Science is contributing much more than 1% to shaping psychiatry's current ideas about autism.

39.2 Shaping a Psychiatric Disorder

But let me turn to two broader questions around which I will structure this response. First, what does it mean to "shape" a psychiatric disorder? Hacking claims that that nature of autism was largely shaped by individuals who are PCA (persons connected to autism). I want to challenge that view and then show that the shaping of psychiatric disorders by affected individuals or persons connected (PC) to them has occurred before in modern psychiatry. Second, I want to review the concept that autism spectrum conditions represent a difference and not a disorder, and try to put these issues in a broader psychiatric context. Then, I will close with some reflections about how Hacking's essay relates to the overall themes of this volume.

Let me begin with a small bit of field work. On receiving a preliminary version of Hacking's chapter, I was surprised at his claim that PCA individuals were largely responsible for the shaping of our concept of autism. This was not consistent with the history of psychiatry (e.g., the role played by Kanner and Bleuler) or my personal experience with leading autism researchers. I wrote to Dr. Susan Swedo, who chaired the DSM-5 work group on pervasive developmental disorders. This was the group who, after an extensive review of the empirical literature and many consultations with various constituencies, made the controversial proposal to eliminate the prior separate diagnoses of autistic and Asperger's disorders that were present in the DSM-IV (American Psychiatric Association 1994) and meld them into an autism spectrum disorder in the DSM-5. If this wasn't "shaping" autism, I was hard put to think what was. I asked Susan what proportion of her workgroup was PCA—giving her Hacking's definition. Her response was 1/15 or 6.6%. I asked how much the concept of the autism spectrum came from the advocacy groups, which Hacking is surely right are strongly influenced by and often led by individuals who are PCA. She said that the advocacy groups were not pushing the spectrum concept and that indeed, as Hacking notes, the Asperger's groups strongly opposed the concept.

From the perspective of both academic and clinical psychiatry, in the United States, the DSM is the ultimate "shaper" of psychiatric disorders. It is the DSM criteria that are taught to all American medical students and psychiatric residents. It is these criteria that are used for clinical evaluations, research papers, and grant applications. So how does this jive with Hacking's claim that nearly all of the shaping of autism came from PCA individuals? Surely, we are using the term "shaping" in distinct ways, likely informed by our different perspectives. I attend DSM and psychiatric research meetings. Hacking attends autism conventions and Asperger's ("Aspies") support groups. He is using a broader concept of "shaping"—in a cultural context, setting an agenda for change. Needless to say, I don't think Hacking's view that for autism spectrum disorders, the DSM is best seen as a "bureaucratic record," accurately reflects how the DSM works in the psychiatric world.

That said, let me turn to something more interesting. Given that PCA individuals played a role in shaping the concept of autism, how unique is this in the history of psychiatry? Are there other examples of disorders where affected individuals, or their relatives, shaped a disorder and got it officially recognized? The clearest example of which I am aware is post-traumatic stress disorder (PTSD). The process, that lead to the creation of this disorder and its acceptance into DSM-III, was well told in a 1990 paper by Wilbur Scott (Scott 1990). While a bit overdramatic, the following quote from early in his paper gives you a flavor of Scott's approach to the story:

> Like the disappearance of the disorder of homosexuality from DSM-II, the story of how PTSD appeared in DSM-III is one that belies the cool clinical language in which the manual's diagnoses and syndromes are described [...] the struggle for recognition of PTSD by its champions was profoundly political, and displays the full range of negotiation, coalition formation, strategizing, solidarity affirmation, and struggle both inside various professions and "in the streets." (p. 295)

The main facts are not in dispute. While adverse psychological reactions to war go back far into human history, the current concept of PTSD emerged in a very particular time, place, and context—in the late 1970s in the United States, still divided over the history of the Vietnam War and the treatment of its veterans. The entry of this diagnosis into the DSM was critically influenced by an organized lobbying effort of veterans' groups, including many affected by PTSD, who argued that without official recognition by the DSM, affected individuals would receive insufficient care and be ineligible for the disability payments that they deserved. This effort was aided by a group of largely liberal psychiatrists, who Scott suggests acted out of a complex set of scientific, personal, and social-political motivations to support the inclusion of PTSD into DSM-III (Scott 1990). So in the shaping of PTSD as a "real" disorder, due to combat exposure (rather than pre-existing disorders) deserving of care and, if necessary, service-connected disability, much of the action was carried out by individuals who were either "PC-PTSD" or just plain folks with PTSD.

Of course, there is another oft-described example of diagnostic shaping going "the other way." The movement to remove homosexuality from the DSM-II—of "re-shaping" homosexuality from a disorder into a difference—was predominantly driven by gay individuals and their supporters, inside and outside of the psychiatric profession (PC-Gay, I guess) (Drescher and Merlino 2007; Zachar and Kendler 2012).

Lest we get carried away, I am unaware of any recent efforts of sufferers from major depression, generalized anxiety disorder, schizophrenia, or antisocial personality disorder, or their friends and family, to "shape" the disorders either at a broader cultural or more specific psychiatric level. So, such processes have impacted on what is probably only a small proportion of all psychiatric disorders. But, I can bring this short section to a close with a perhaps rather obvious conclusion—consistent with the point that I think Hacking was trying to make. These three stories—autism, PTSD, and homosexuality—would together totally undermine any strong positivist view of psychiatric nosology in practice. Such a view would be something like "The nature of psychiatric disorders and changes introduced thereto by the official manuals (aka DSM and ICD) are decided solely by science and empirical findings, with no appreciable influences arising from social and cultural factors." While this might be a desirable proscriptive statement, as a description of the world in which we live, it is surely inaccurate.

39.3 Defining being Disorders and some Field Work

This makes for a smooth transition to the final topic on which I want to comment. We have no tight, concise, and operational definition of a psychiatric disorder. By operational, I mean a gold standard definition against which you could test proposed conditions and come away with a clear, unambiguous answer that it either is, or is not, a disorder. I helped to "lightly" revise the DSM-IV criteria for a psychiatric disorder and readers may want to consult the resulting definition (Stein et al. 2010). It does do some work but you will see that it is too woolly to function in a practical way in most cases.

If it were not so serious, we might chuckle at the situation before us. We have some conditions where the sufferers were not classified in the DSM but wanted to be, such as PTSD. (Also, note in Chapter 41 in this book that a number of critics to the acceptance of premenstrual dysphoric disorder into the DSM-IV believed that more women self-diagnosed themselves with this condition than actually had it—so they might count here, as well.) But then we also have disorders that are in the DSM, such as homosexuality and Asperger's syndrome, but individuals with those conditions want to get out and see their condition as a difference, not a disorder.

I again did some field work on this question—on the Internet. First, I went to the website of the North American Man/Boy Love Association (NAMBLA). Here is how this organization is described in Wikipedia:

> The North American Man/Boy Love Association (NAMBLA) is a pedophile and pederasty advocacy organization in the United States that works to abolish age of consent laws criminalizing adult sexual involvement with minors, and for the release of all men who have been jailed for sexual contacts with minors that did not involve coercion. (<http://en.wikipedia.org/wiki/Nambla>)

This description accurately recounts the content on their website, which argues that consensual homosexual contact with minors is normative and cites historical precedents (e.g., ancient Greece). They are in the DSM and want out (but are also in criminal codes and want out from those, but I will not address that issue) but this is very unlikely to happen.

Next, I went to <http://www.intervoiceonline.org/> a website for what is commonly called the "Hearing Voices Movement." Here is a small selection of the texts available there:

> Working across the world to spread positive and hopeful messages about the experience of hearing voices. If you hear voices, know someone who does or want to find out more about this experience—then this site is for you [...] Because hearing voices is a much stigmatised experience we wanted to create a safe place where you can find out more about hearing voices and to create an interactive online community where you can let us know about your point of view or experience. Here, you will find a very different way of thinking about the meaning of hearing voices. We understand "voices" to be real and meaningful, something that is experienced by a significant minority of people, including many who have no problems living with their voices [...]. Our

research shows that to hear voices is not the consequence of a diseased brain, but more akin to a variation in human behaviour, like being left-handed.

This is about as clear a description of a "different but not disordered" viewpoint as one might hope to find. Here, however, there is a long history of a debate within psychiatry (well documented in a magisterial volume by another contributor to this volume [Berrios 1996]) about whether normal people can have hallucinations. The majority opinion (now supported by a range of general population studies [van Os et al. 2009]) is that they can. The features of the hallucinations seen in disordered and nondisordered people differ widely, and I would wonder what a careful psychiatrist would say after a careful evaluation of a group of members of the Hearing Voices Movement. At least some substantial proportion of individuals in this movement would belong in (DSM) and, like the "Aspies," want out.

Then, I tried to find a web site for obsessive–compulsive disorder (OCD) that took the "different but not disordered" approach. I failed after a moderately thorough search. The website that kept coming up (<http://www.ocfoundation.org/>) clearly accepted the "disordered" model.

What characteristics might be shared by individuals who want a disorder that they have removed from the DSM? I would posit four factors. First, the symptoms are ego-syntonic. That is, they feel comfortable, part of who they are, and are not "imposed" on the person. Second, the "experiences" under debate are not, when they actively occur, unpleasant. They don't feel bad. Third, the individuals involved see no benefits from being able to assume the "sick role." Fourth, (and this criteria—often the point the rubber hits the road, needs qualification—see below), the experiences are not inherently associated with impairment in doing things that most normal people want to do. I used the term "inherently" here to mean that the symptoms themselves are impairing, rather than the impairment arising as a result of how society responds to individuals with those symptoms.

Let's apply these four criteria to some of the conditions we have considered. Homosexuality clearly meets the first three criteria and most of the debate focused on the fourth criteria, where the data supported the view that homosexuality was not inherently associated with disordered functioning in the world. Clearly, pedophiles would claim the first three (although some affected individuals are indeed tortured by their impulses that they actively try to resist). They would also argue the fourth, but most mental health professionals disagree, arguing that having sex with minors, even without overt coercion, is inherently abusive, harmful to the minor, and, hence, worthy of condemnation and punishment in the perpetrator. OCD wouldn't get past first base because affected individuals perceive the compulsions as being imposed on them and they are unpleasant, causing intense anxiety if resisted. It is hard to argue that spending hours washing ones hands or checking dozens of times for locked doors or gas burner switches is not impairing. They want to be treated and get better. I would bet, but have no data on this, that the hallucinators, who join the hearing voices movement, would argue that they meet all four criteria. Subjects with PTSD, by contrast, fail all the criteria. Symptoms are intrusive, aversive, and impairing, and they wanted treatment and some felt they deserved benefits of the sick role.

Now what about autism? No one answer will work. For the severely affected individuals I saw during my training (nonverbal, head banging, flapping, etc.), they so obviously fail the third and fourth criteria (they are impaired and need treatment) that the issue is moot. For someone with mild Asperger's, they would clearly make the first two criteria, and could see themselves as different, but not disordered. It would then come down to how "impaired" they are in the real world. If it means being awkward in social situations and having trouble talking to strangers, but being really good at computer programming and comfortable with texting and email, maybe they would make that criteria too.

The most difficult problem here is best illustrated by another condition we have not yet considered: deafness. Although I risk being politically incorrect, I consider it obvious that the third and fourth criteria are not met. Not being able to hear is maladaptive. If you are deaf, getting some special training to cope in the world and learning sign language will increase your ability to adapt. Note, I claimed nothing about whether sign language can be as expressive as spoken speech, or that deaf culture cannot be as full or vibrant as hearing culture. So seen from one perspective, deafness is clearly disordered. But from the other, you could reasonably want them to praise the difference and cherish it.

The biggest problem with such patient movements to get out of the DSM is that general human and, particularly, psychiatric experience teaches us that individuals are often very poor judges of their level of impairment. People can be disordered without feeling like they are. We call this "lack of insight." It is common in psychiatric illness. Anders Breivik felt he was doing a noble deed, saving Norway by killing scores of innocent teenagers and expressed no regret for his actions. I have seen manic patients who run naked in the street, screaming that they were God's anointed, after spending their family into ruin on unneeded furniture and cars, who felt everything was fine. I suggest that any readers who are in doubt of the veracity of my claim should volunteer at the nearest emergency room with a busy psychiatric service. A few nights in such an environment will convince you of the painful truth that individuals can be seriously disordered with no insight into the nature or severity of their condition.

39.4 Conclusions

Where does this leave us? The large majority of human differences, thankfully, are not disorders. But psychiatric disorders exist. Individuals who are considered disordered have the right to voice an opinion that they are not. Nor should we assume that official psychiatry always gets the boundary between illness and "benign difference" exactly right. We should worry about labeling people who are merely different as disordered because of moral or cultural factors. It is a very hard problem. But contrary to some conspiratorial theories, most psychiatrists want to spend time treating people who they can really help. There are already too few of us to treat well those with the bad disorders. And, even if a person is disordered, being proud of, or trying to benefit from, the unique perspectives that their disorder can bring to them and to their world is a good thing.

In closing, let me outline two issues of relevance in this discussion to the themes of this book. First, this exchange illustrates in a general manner how nonscientific issues can impact on the important question of what kinds of disorders or differences belong in, or out, of our manuals. I have not here touched on the large effort made to bring science to bear on what changes should be made in the DSM-5 (Kendler 2013) and how such efforts relate to the questions we have here posed. That discussion is for another day. We will see these general themes taken up in the chapter by Zachar and Kendler on PMDD in the DSM-IV and DSM-5 (Chapter 41, this volume). Second, this discussion illuminates a potentially finer point relating to Hacking's broader agenda of his "Making up People Project" and his looping concept. Classifying people into psychiatric disorders is not like putting animals into species. People may seek out classifications and own them, or they may reject them as either not applicable to them or as a mischaracterization of their behavior and experience. These actions can then impact on future classifications as was seen so clearly in the PTSD story. This is a process rarely discussed in psychiatric nosology and deserving of more attention.

Acknowledgment

Dr. Peter Zachar provided helpful comments on an earlier draft.

References

American Psychiatric Association (1994). *Diagnostic and Statistical Manual of Mental Disorders* (4th ed.). Washington, DC: American Psychiatric Association.

Berrios, G.E. (1996). *The History of Mental Symptoms: Descriptive Psychopathology Since the Nineteenth Century*. Cambridge: Cambridge University Press.

Devlin, B. and Scherer, S.W. (2012). Genetic architecture in autism spectrum disorder. *Current Opinion in Genetics and Development*, 22(3), 229–237.

Drescher, J. and Merlino, J.P. (2007). *American Psychiatry and Homosexuality: An Oral History*. New York: Routledge.

Kendler, K.S. (2013). A history of the DSM-5 Scientific Review Committee. *Psychological Medicine*, 43(9), 1793–1800.

Scott, W.J. (1990). PTSD in DSM-III—a case in the politics of diagnosis and disease. *Social Problems*, 37(3), 294–310.

Stein, D.J., Phillips, K.A., Bolton, D., Fulford, K.W., Sadler, J.Z., and Kendler, K.S. (2010). What is a mental/psychiatric disorder? From DSM-IV to DSM-V. *Psychological Medicine*, 40(11), 1759–1765.

Van Os, J., Linscott, R.J., Myin-Germeys, I., Delespaul, P., and Krabbendam, L. (2009). A systematic review and meta-analysis of the psychosis continuum: evidence for a psychosis proneness-persistence-impairment model of psychotic disorder. *Psychological Medicine*, 39(2), 179–195.

Zachar, P. and Kendler, K.S. (2012). The removal of Pluto from the class of planets and homosexuality from the class of psychiatric disorders: a comparison. *Philosophy, Ethics, and Humanities in Medicine*, 7(1), 4.

Section 14

The decision to include or exclude a diagnosis in psychiatric nosology: the case of premenstrual dysphoric disorder

Chapter 40

Introduction to "A DSM insiders' history of premenstrual dysphoric disorder"

Josef Parnas

Chapter 41 presents a kind of in vivo case study of the interactions between science and extra-scientific processes involved in the construction of nosological categories of psychiatry.

The very first medical report on a cluster of symptoms, regularly affecting some women over their menstrual cycle, the so-called syndrome of premenstrual tension, appeared in 1931. The name changed with time to premenstrual syndrome, subsequently renamed as late luteal phase dysphoric disorder (LLPDD) and currently known as the premenstrual dysphoric disorder (PMDD). It was listed as a psychiatric disorder in the DSM-III, but in the DSM-IIIR and the DSM-IV it was moved to the section on the condition deserving further study (aka the "appendix"). In the DSM-5, PMDD returned to the main section of the manual devoted to depressive disorders as a diagnosis approved for routine clinical use.

PMDD is an ideal-type condition to stimulate a controversy about its justification as a psychiatric disorder. By its nature it affects only females (here, feminist issues may arise); it is clearly linked to physiological rhythm (is it not a somatic issue?); does it exist as a distinct behavioral abnormality or is it just a variant of female experience?: does it need to be treated pharmacologically? (the issues of medicalization and "big pharma").

Zachar and Kendler provide a detailed narrative on the vicissitudes of this psychiatric nosological category. Their account is not only based on a careful study by interested outsiders but is crucially enriched by the insights of one of the participants of the very process of DSM construction.

Chapter 41

A DSM insiders' history of premenstrual dysphoric disorder

Peter Zachar and Kenneth S. Kendler

41.1 Premenstrual Syndrome, Premenstrual Dysphoric Disorder, and the DSM

Premenstrual dysphoric disorder was first described by Robert Frank (1931) as *premenstrual tension* and later renamed premenstrual syndrome (PMS) by Raymond Greene and Katherine Dalton (1953). Its psychiatric symptoms are irritability, affective lability, depression, and anxiety. These symptoms begin during the last week of the luteal phase of the menstrual cycle and remit after onset of menses. Interest in the condition increased in the 1980s after Dalton helped acquit a woman of murder by testifying that she suffered from severe PMS.

According to Figert (1996) the original impetus for including distress and impairment related to menstruation in the DSM-III-R came from Robert Spitzer, the architect of the DSM-III revolution. Spitzer reported to her that he had been invited to several conferences on premenstrual syndrome, a condition about which he had limited information. What interested Spitzer was that PMS had caught the attention of mental health professionals.

As the chair of the Work Group to revise DSM-III, Spitzer saw it as his responsibility to make sure that they considered all the conditions that were of concern to mental health professionals, leading him to convene a premenstrual syndrome advisory committee. The story of what happened next has been told many times (Caplan 1995; Figert 1996; Spitzer et al. 1989).

Classifying a menstruation-related mental disorder was not acceptable to some of the psychiatrists at the meeting because of their fear that it would stigmatize a normal part of a woman's monthly cycle, but the advisory committee nevertheless recommended that the newly name *premenstrual dysphoric disorder* (PDD) be included in the manual. Soon thereafter those psychiatrists, Jean Hamilton and Teresa Bernardez, began an intense letter writing and media campaign warning of the dangers of PDD. The opposition quickly grew in intensity, aided in part by participation of psychologists such as Lenore Walker and Paula Caplan who were also concerned about other newly proposed disorders, specifically masochistic personality disorder and paraphilic rapism. Over the next year, there were closed-door debates, public debates, additional oversight committees, and protests.

When the DSM-III-R was published in 1987, PDD was not included as an official disorder; rather, it was renamed late luteal phase dysphoric disorder (LLPDD) and placed in a new section called appendix A—as a proposed disorder in need of further study. In fact, the DSM appendix was created largely to contain this syndrome. This was the outcome that Spitzer wanted whereas the opposition wanted the disorder completely eliminated from the DSM.

41.2 Overview of DSM-IV and DSM-5

Work on the DSM-IV began soon after the DSM-III-R was published. According to Michael First (personal communication, February 8, 2012), the leaders of the DSM-IV Task Force knew that LLPDD was going to be a hot button issue, and by the time the process was concluded it had the greatest amount of press coverage and had created the most angst in the organizers (Kendler 2012).

The LLPDD Work Group was formed to make recommendations for the diagnosis in DSM-IV. They had different opinions on whether to move the disorder to the main section of manual, keep it in the appendix, or eliminate it (Endicott 2000; Frank and Severino 1995). When two senior psychiatrists were asked by the DSM-IV leadership to review the documentation prepared by the Work Group, they recommended retaining it in the appendix. After a vigorous debate, the majority of the DSM-IV Task Force agreed with them.

In 1988, psychologist Paula Caplan was asked to be an advisor to the LLPDD Work Group, but later discontinued her involvement when she concluded that her scientific input was not wanted (Caplan 1995). After she heard about the decision to retain the disorder in the appendix, she organized a petition campaign, sent notices to electronic discussion groups, alerted the media, and began speaking against classifying menstruation-related distress as a mental illness. The goal of the protest was to have the disorder eliminated entirely from the manual. It was not successful. LLPDD was renamed premenstrual dysphoric disorder (PMDD) and kept in the appendix.

When the DSM-5 was published in 2013, PMDD was moved to the main section of the manual as a diagnosis approved for routine clinical use. Interestingly, in the age of the Internet, the public and professional controversies about the DSM-5 revision greatly outnumbered those of previous revisions, but the status of PMDD was not among them.

Why was there such a dramatic change in the reactions to the status of PMDD in the DSM-5? Given that PMDD has been a contested construct, one should expect that there has been progress in the research base justifying the classification of PMDD as an official disorder. However, considering the depth of the controversy, the many social and cultural issues that are enmeshed with the scientific issues, and the nature of psychiatric disorder constructs themselves, we do not believe that this change can be reducible to a straightforward narrative of scientific progress.

Our reasoning is historically based. In the history of science—including both the Newtonian and the Darwinian revolutions—when new findings are mired in controversy, nonempirical considerations often play an important role in influencing what truth claims a community accepts. Nonempirical considerations cannot make psychiatry's claims about PMDD true, but they can support or oppose people's willingness to accept those claims.

We begin this chapter by giving these assumptions some philosophical heft. Next we will turn to an examination of the factors that influenced the decision makers during the DSM-IV revision.

41.3 Decision Vectors

In her book *Social Empiricism*, Miriam Solomon (2001) proposed a normative model for understanding how consensus and dissent should be distributed to support scientific progress. In doing so she integrated insights into the nature of cumulative scientific progress articulated by Philip Kitcher (1993) with broader considerations such as how a scientific community is best structured to be objective as described by Longino (1990) and with the factors influencing a community's willingness to accept new truth claims as argued by sociologists of scientific knowledge such as Bruno Latour (1987) and Harry Collins (1992).

Solomon's normative model utilizes the idea of a decision vector. A decision vector is any factor that influences the outcome of a scientific decision such as accepting or rejecting a theory. Solomon also distinguished between empirical and nonempirical decision vectors.

An empirical decision vector is any factor that leads scientists to prefer theories with empirical success. This includes predictive success, explanatory success, and descriptive success. For example, if one were to assume that a valid disorder construct should predict response to treatment, and a diagnosis of PMDD accurately does predict response to particular treatments, this would be an empirical reason for favoring this diagnostic construct.

Nonempirical decision vectors are any other factors leading a community to prefer one theory (or diagnostic construct) over another. These include economic, social-political, and ethical considerations, as well as psychological traits like conservativeness and peer pressure. For example, if placing PMDD in the manual makes it is more likely that research studying the condition will be funded, those who conduct such research might be more inclined to support inclusion. If a PMDD diagnosis encourages women to blame their bodies rather than their social situations for their distress, those who are concerned about the empowerment of women may prefer the construct not be included.

Previous generations of philosophers might have referred to empirical decision vectors as rational considerations and nonempirical decision vectors as biasing factors, but Solomon argued that they can both contribute to successful science and are inevitably part of any scientific change. During scientific controversies, competing perspectives (e.g., PMDD is a unique disorder versus PMDD is misinterpreted depression versus PMDD reflects only normal premenstrual mood fluctuations) may each have some empirical success, and therefore dissent can be useful. According to Solomon (2008), nonempirical considerations should not be used to support theories with no empirical validity, but if competing claims have some empirical success, then nonempirical decision vectors should be equally distributed among those claims (i.e., ideally empirical success should tip the balance).

41.4 The DSM-IV Task Force and the LLPDD Work Group

The DSM-IV revision process was divided into the Task Force and the Work Groups. The Task Force—or leadership team—had 30 members and was chaired by Allen Frances. Reporting to the Task Force were 13 different Work Groups. Work Groups had 5 to 16 members and were responsible for specific sections of the manual, such as Mood Disorders or Personality Disorders. The LLPDD issue was considered to be so important that it was assigned a Work Group of its own.

In addition to reviewing the published literature on the controversies that occurred after the initial PMDD proposal was made, we asked many of the participants in the DSM-IV revision to both reflect on that process and offer their perspectives about what had changed by the time of the DSM-5 proposal. Those who were interviewed are listed in Table 41.1. The interviews were conducted by phone by Kenneth Kendler and occurred between October 19, 2011 and February 8, 2012. After the first draft of the chapter was written, a copy was sent to the participants, offering them the opportunity to suggest corrections, which were then incorporated into the final draft of this chapter and a previously published article (Zachar and Kendler 2014).

On the LLPDD Work Group, Barbara Parry, Jean Endicott, and Ellen Frank all supported moving the disorder to the main section of the manual. Michael First agreed with them. Judith Gold and Sally Severino believed that it should stay in the appendix, as did Allen Frances and Harold Pincus. Nada Stotland favored eliminating the disorder from the manual altogether.

Table 41.1 List of people interviewed

Name	Role
Jean Endicott, PhD	Member of the DSM-III-R and DSM-IV LLPDD Work Groups
Michael First, MD	Editor of text and criteria for the DSM-IV
Allen Frances, MD	Chairperson of the DSM-IV Task Force
Ellen Frank, PhD	Member of DSM-IV Task Force and Mood Disorders WG consultant to LLPDD Work Group
Judith Gold, MD	Chair of the LLPDD Work Group and DSM-IV Task Force Member
Barbara Parry, MD	Member of the DSM-III-R DSM-IV LLPDD Work Groups
Harold Pincus, MD	Vice-Chairperson of the DSM-IV Task Force
Sally Severino, MD	Member of the DSM-III-R DSM-IV LLPDD Work Groups
Nada Stotland, MD	Former chair of the APA Committee on Women and member of LLPDD Work Group
Kimberly Yonkers, MD	Member of DSM-5 Mood Disorders and PMDD Work Groups

Our listing of the vectors, presented in Table 41.2, is based largely on the interviews. We make no pretension to having identified a complete list of vectors; rather, our goal was to develop a list that is comprehensive enough to represent the primary issues of dispute during the controversy. We have sorted these decision vectors into three categories, reflecting the options that were available to the Work Group.

When studying controversies that have been closed, it is easier to distinguish between empirical and nonempirical decision vectors. When a controversy is ongoing, however, one of the issues being debated is what implications "the evidence" has for diagnostic constructs, or what it is *evidence for* (Kendler 1990; Zachar and Kendler 2010). For instance, does the fact that the onset and remission of symptoms occurs as described in the diagnostic construct confirm that PMDD is a distinct disorder? Perhaps it means instead that a woman's reaction to ongoing difficulties is being exacerbated by the menstrual cycle. If a controversy is intense, then what counts as fact and what counts as artifact may also be subject to debate. For these reasons and in order to not prejudge the issues, we identify decision vectors without sorting them into the empirical and nonempirical boxes.

41.5 Vectors for Moving PMDD to the Main Body of the DSM-IV

41.5.1 Agreement on Symptoms and Time Course

Many of the DSM-IV work groups conducted literature reviews of the research that had occurred on their assigned disorders following the publication of the DSM-III. The results of these literature reviews were published in the *DSM-IV Sourcebooks* (Widiger et al. 1996). With respect to their literature review, the members of the LLPDD Work Group recalled that there was general agreement about the factual material (Frank and Severino 1995; Gold et al. 1996).

For example, according to the literature review, 3–6% of the population report symptoms consistent with PMDD. This suggested to the committee that it was neither a trivial diagnosis, nor a normal part of most women's menstrual cycles. They also agreed that there are women who meet criteria for the disorder with respect to

Table 41.2 DSM-IV decision vectors

Move to main DSM-IV section	Retain in the appendix	Delete from the DSM-IV
Agreement on symptoms	Philosophical ideas about disorder	The problem of false positives
Benefits of treatment	Higher standard of evidence	Questionable diagnostic validity
The biomedical model	The politics of DSM	Feminism and negative social consequences
	Peer pressure consensus	
	Reaction to public opposition	Criticisms of pharmaceutical industry

symptoms and time course, and that do not have another co-occurring disorder, which are standard validators in psychiatry according the criteria proposed by Robins and Guze (1970). The symptoms of PMDD are also associated with clinically significant distress and impairment—which is part of the DSM definition of mental disorder. The Work Group added one symptom to the criteria used in DSM-III-R—involving feeling overwhelmed—and reorganized the criteria so that depression and anxiety were listed first.

The evidence also indicated that if hormonal levels are altered, the symptoms still occur during the time of the month that normally would be the late luteal phase. Not being the manifestation of a late luteal phase hormonal profile, the Work Group recommended changing the name to premenstrual dysphoric disorder.

41.5.2 Benefits of Treatment

The research reviewed by the Work Group indicated that anxiolytics and antidepressants were more effective than a placebo for treating many premenstrual symptoms. Suppression of ovulation by chemical means was a promising approach. Although not an acceptable treatment approach, when ovulation is surgically eliminated symptoms are also eliminated.

The consensus view of those who wanted to move the diagnosis to the main section of the manual was that there are clearly women who are impaired by PMDD and placement of the disorder in the main section would facilitate proper diagnosis and treatment. It would also encourage further research. Parry in particular reported being surprised that anyone would oppose putting this in the manual given the magnitude of the scientific evidence, and its potential benefits to women. She believed that the criteria were quite narrow, identified the small group of women who were actually ill, and would reduce stigmatization as a whole. According to Frank, the more certain benefits of being able to educate women about the nature of their symptoms outweighed the vague concerns about potential harms (Frank and Severino 1995).

In psychiatry both clinical and personal experience can be decision vectors. For example, Barbara Parry said that as a resident she encountered a case of severe PMDD in a high-functioning health services provider. The symptoms included a florid psychosis that remitted after the onset of menses. This case was what got her interested in studying menstruation and recurrent psychiatric disorders.

Several members of the Work Group mentioned what they saw as a campaign of intimidation used by some opponents of the diagnosis. With respect to these opponents, Endicott stated that she was not intimidated because both she and her mother had PMS-related symptoms. According to her, these kinds of problems were a valid part of her experience and congruent with her reading of the empirical data. She also emphasized that many women at this time believed that such problems should be looked into and that the feminist opposition did not speak for all women.

41.5.3 The Biomedical Model of Psychiatric Disorders

A concept like PMDD was a good fit for an era in which the biological perspective in psychiatry was gaining dominance (Andreasen 1984; Guze 1992). Tied as it was to cyclical changes in a woman's monthly cycle, PMDD was readily seen as a biologically based mood disorder. For instance, in addition to a predictable monthly onset and remission of symptoms, PMDD symptoms also disappear during pregnancy and after menopause. There was also evidence that higher levels of premenstrual tension ran in families, and resemblance was higher among monozygotic than dizygotic twins (Gold et al. 1996).

The Work Group specifically noted that the condition was an important exemplar of a biologically based psychiatric condition (Gold et al. 1996). It may even, they said, help call attention to the endocrinological aspects of other psychiatric disorders. Keeping it in the manual, it was believed, would be an important boost to current and emerging biomedical research programs.

41.6 Vectors for Deleting PMDD from the DSM-IV

41.6.1 The Problem of False Positives

The Work Group's report in the *DSM-IV Sourcebook* noted that there was a tendency among some women to seek treatment for normal premenstrual distress (PMS) and even to label it premenstrual syndrome, but not actually meet the more stringent criteria for a diagnosis of PMDD (Gold et al. 1996). Furthermore, they noted that symptoms identified with PMDD might better be accounted for by the exacerbation of a preexisting disorder, such as depression and dysthymia, an anxiety disorder, a somatoform disorder, a substance use disorder, bulimia, or a personality disorder. Finally, there was a concern that women may prefer the more socially desirable PMDD diagnosis even if they would be more accurately diagnosed with another psychiatric disorder. In epidemiological terms, there was a high risk of false positive PMDD diagnoses.

Nada Stotland reported that her primary concern was that PMDD would be a diagnosis that many women would seek even if they did not actually have PMDD. Although the criteria were written tightly to eliminate these kinds of false positives, she believed that because the diagnosis could be made provisionally (before daily ratings to confirm the symptom pattern were completed), it would be.

(Another important concern of Stotland's was that the evidence for the maladaptive effects of male hormones on violence and aggression was much stronger than the assumptions about female hormones and depression, but there was no corresponding disorder for men being considered.)

With respect to the issue of false positives, clinical experience and the relevance of salient data also played a role. Stotland said that she once saw a high-functioning woman who was seeking a prescription to treat her "PMDD." This woman believed that PMDD was responsible for her strong negativity toward her husband and her son, and was worried about harming her son psychologically. Stotland agreed to write the prescription, but 6 weeks later the woman returned and declared that she was feeling better every day not just during her premenstrual phase. She had decided that she was really depressed and did not have PMDD.

41.6.2 Questionable Diagnostic Validity

Severino noted that most of the research reviewed by the LLPDD Work Group studied PMS, not PMDD (Frank and Severino 1995). According to her, much of what was believed to be known about PMDD was an extrapolation from PMS. Those who were more skeptical of the disorder contended that the symptoms are mostly physical and occur during menstruation; the psychiatric symptoms are not limited to the late luteal phase and might represent normal problems-in-living that are exacerbated by physical discomfort (Caplan 1995, 2008; Severino and Gold 1994).

Although there were suggestive findings of differences between women with and without PMDD in levels of neurotransmitters and hormones, these differences were not tightly correlated with the onset and remission of symptoms as one might expect. Undermining the notion that PMDD was validated as a biological disorder, Parlee (1994) observed that the diagnosis of PMDD is made only on the basis of self-report, not biological markers.

Another concern acknowledged by the LLPDD Work Group was that both PMS and PMDD were deeply embedded in cultural assumptions about gender roles. Of particular concern was the assumption that women are less prone to anger than men, and also more emotionally responsive than men. When adhering to these norms, a woman's anger would have a lower threshold for being considered inappropriate and therefore, pathological. A mental disorder diagnosis could even teach women to experience their anger and irritability as being more severe and troubling than they otherwise would.

41.6.3 Feminist Values and Negative Social Consequences

In *The Female Malady*, Elaine Showalter (1985) described the long and contentious relationship that exists between feminism and psychiatric diagnosis. For example, in the late nineteenth century, women who advocated for professional and sexual freedom were diagnosed as hysterics and degenerates. In the next century, Karl Abraham and later Freud came to believe that a woman's aspiration to enter a traditional male profession represented a manifestation of her castration complex.

We would be remiss to not mention that for many generations, the various symptom clusters classified under hysteria were explained by one or other version of the uterine theory (Micale 1990; Scull 2009). Although the literal belief that hysteria was the result of a wandering womb was abandoned by the seventeenth century, it was replaced by the theory that the symptoms of hysteria were caused by vapors that arose from the female reproductive system. Given this history, a new diagnostic category that traces psychiatric distress to menstruation readily looked like a repackaged and updated version of the uterine theory. What concerned feminists is the persistent tendency of mental health professionals to perceive women as being less capable than men, and to reify that perception by tracing it to biology.

During the development of both the DSM-III and the DSM-III-R, the feminist movement was succeeding in changing attitudes about the roles of women in society, especially attitudes about educational opportunities, employment options, and the fair distribution of childcare responsibilities. As the implementation in the 1890s of the Jim Crow laws (targeting black people) had shown, gains in rights and liberties can readily be undone. For example, the rights to vote and be elected to public office that black people had enjoyed for 30 years after the American Civil War were practically eliminated by these laws. With respect to women's issues and the DSM-IV, in the United States, the defeat of the Equal Rights Amendment in the 1980s by antifeminists such as Phyllis Schlafly was still fresh in people's minds. Also, the Christian fundamentalist organization called "The Moral Majority" had recently become prominent in the Republican Party. Their advocacy of a woman's proper role as wife and mother suggested to others that the progress that had been achieved needed to be assertively defended.

Many of those who favored deletion were concerned about PMDD being a disorder that by its very nature would be limited to women, and could be used against women. For example, those who opposed equal opportunity in the workplace argued that the menstrual cycle makes women more emotionally unstable and dysfunctional every month. If PMDD became an official diagnosis, the opponents could also say that this was not only their *opinion*, nor was it bigotry; rather, it was "science" as demonstrated by the fact that it is in the DSM.

Another worry was that PMDD would serve to mask the actual reason for a woman's anger and distress. With PMDD in the manual, natural and justified reactions to abuse and mistreatment could be labeled a mental disorder. Rather than seeing the problem as being due to a negative external situation, the problem would be seen as located inside the woman's body.

On the Work Group, a variety of attitudes regarding feminism played a role in what members thought should happen in the DSM-IV. The person most obviously associated with women's groups was Nada Stotland—who was the Chair of the American Psychiatric Association (APA) Committee on Women. Although Stotland favored deleting the disorder, several of the members of the Work Group stated that during their deliberations Stotland had a nuanced view of the proposed disorder and did not evaluate it in black and white terms. She saw it as her duty to both represent her constituency and to work within the system.

Sally Severino was newer to feminism. Many members of the Work Group recalled that during this time, Severino's exposure to feminism was a profound consciousness-raising experience for her. Severino herself reported that her training in psychoanalysis did not include a feminist perspective, and she did not have a serious encounter with feminism until she was promoting a book she had written on PMS (Frank and Severino 1995; Severino and Moline 1989). One can see a reflection of this new way of thinking for Severino in a book chapter she wrote as the DSM-IV process was winding down (Severino 1994). In this chapter she discussed the patriarchal myth that women are naturally subordinate to men, and that a woman's proper role was to be a good mother and wife. She argued that the disputes about PMDD, including how to name it, reflect the fact that society is increasingly questioning the patriarchal myth. The perception of several Work Group members was that at this time Severino shifted more toward Stotland's views, although she did not support eliminating the diagnosis from the manual.

Ellen Frank considered herself a feminist of long standing. Frank reported that she was exposed to feminism in college and it was a part of her personal and professional identity (Frank and Severino 1995). She did not believe that being a feminist required her to oppose moving PMDD to the main section of the manual. In her view, narrow-minded people who believed that women are less capable would not change their minds if PMDD was eliminated from the manual.

41.6.4 The Role of the Pharmaceutical Industry

A final issue of contention that existed both inside and outside the committee structure was the belief that the diagnosis of PMDD was being pushed by the pharmaceutical companies because categorizing PMDD as a mood disorder would open a large and new market for antidepressant medication.

Severino in particular was skeptical of the pharmaceutical industry, and of the neutrality of those scientists whose research programs were being funded by the industry. She noted that she too had worked on research projects funded by pharmaceutical companies, but her support was discontinued when she found a high placebo response rate. In contrast, Parry claimed that such concerns were irrelevant. The main concerns she said were deciding what is best for the patients and doing the best science possible.

41.7 Vectors for Retaining PMDD in the DSM-IV Appendix

41.7.1 Philosophical Assumptions about the Nature of Psychiatric Disorders

Some members of the Work Group believe that Severino's exposure to feminism led her to change her opinion about what should occur in the DSM-IV, but Severino claimed that she did not switch her opinion on PMDD during the process, and that she cannot be grouped with either the advocates for the diagnosis or with the opponents. Her concerns, she observed, were more philosophical—relating to the nature of a psychiatric disorder. In her opinion, if PMDD is not an exacerbation of a pre-exiting disorder, then it is also a kind of thing that is distinct from a mood disorder. Many of its key symptoms such as sensations of bloating are not properly "psychiatric." She reports that her opposition to what happened in the DSM-IV was a disagreement about listing PMDD in the mood disorders section as an example of a Mood Disorder Not Otherwise Specified (NOS) and giving it an official Mood Disorder NOS code number in the appendix. This, she claimed, essentially moved PMDD into the main body of the manual.

Another philosophical dispute that served as a decision vector occurred largely between Barbara Parry and Allen Frances. In a philosopher's terms, Frances (2013) is a committed instrumentalist who believes that disorders are constructs that clinicians find useful rather than real entities out there in the world. Parry claimed that this "philosophy" influenced Frances' decision to not move the disorder into the main body of the manual. If disorder constructs are primarily clinical instruments, then nosologists need to consider the practical consequences of making or not making the diagnosis. Frances's primary concern was with potential negative social consequences for women. Parry disagreed with his emphasis—noting that the assumption of the PMDD diagnosis is that it is a tightly demarcated phenomenon with specific physiological basis, and therefore an entity out there in the world that should be classified.

41.7.2 Higher Standard of Evidence

One of the arguments of the advocates for moving the diagnosis into the mood disorders section was that the evidence for the validity of PMDD was better than for many of the disorders already in the DSM. For example, one of the problems with past research on PMDD was the use of retrospective reports of symptoms, which tend to be inflated. Making a DSM-III-R diagnosis required prospective daily ratings of symptoms—a much more rigorous assessment than is required for other DSM disorders. Symptoms must also have been present for at least two consecutive cycles and be greatly reduced following menses.

The counter argument of the opponents was that the comparative superiority of evidence for PMDD does not mean that PMDD should be moved to the main section of the manual; rather, it means that the evidence for a large number of psychiatric disorders is inadequate.

Both Judith Gold and Sally Severino favored keeping PMDD in the appendix because they believed that the risk that the diagnosis would be used against women meant that PMDD *should* have higher standards of evidence for inclusion. Their concern was that there was not yet enough research using these higher standards to separate PMDD from PMS or from an exacerbation of another psychiatric disorder. This meant that Gold and Severino joined Stotland in opposing moving the disorder to the main section of the manual, with their three opinions countering those of Parry, Endicott, and Frank, who argued that psychiatrists can neither predict nor control what corporations, lawyers, and other people will do and that scientific decisions should not be made with them in mind.

41.7.3 The Politics of DSM-IV

Several members of the LLPDD Work Group suggested that they were set up to fail from the very beginning, but this was disputed by Allen Frances and Harold Pincus. Supporting the latter opinion, Figert (1996) reports conversations with Jean Hamilton (who was a leading figure in the DSM-III-R protests) and Robert Spitzer that occurred prior to the emergence of the DSM-IV controversy in which both of them hypothesized that the LLPDD Work Group had been set up in order to get PMDD into the main body of the manual.

After the literature review and the many months of deliberation was complete, Frances spoke with the Work Group to try to reach consensus. When it became clear that there was not going to be agreement on what to do, Frances created a subcommittee composed of John Rush and Nancy Andreasen—two prominent research psychiatrists. Rush and Andreasen reviewed the Work Group's report and recommended to the Task Force that it did not meet the higher standard for being moved to the mood disorders section. During the Task Force's discussion, Ellen Frank, Robert Spitzer, Janet Williams, and Kenneth Kendler opposed this recommendation, but they were in the minority. After the majority of the Task Force agreed that the disorder should remain in the appendix, Frances left it to the Work Group to prepare the PMDD section.

Michael First reported that he was in favor of moving PMDD to the main section. Allen Frances, however, wanted to keep it in the appendix. In this Frances was joined by Mel Sabshin, who was the medical director of the American Psychiatric Association from 1974 to 1979. Pincus noted that opposing both Frances and Sabshin would have no chance of succeeding; hence, he supported its remaining in the appendix.

Frances believed that the scientific support for the disorder was being overestimated by the advocates, but several members of the Work Group believe that Frances was risk aversive and did not want to repeat the DSM-III-R controversies or the DSM-II era controversy about the deletion of homosexuality (Bayer 1981; Zachar and Kendler 2012). We should add that Allen Frances has a long history of being genuinely concerned about how diagnostic categories could be misused, so arguments against moving PMDD because of its potential for harm would readily appeal to him.

The most adamant opponent of the decision to keep PMDD in the appendix remains Parry, who believes that the LLPDD Work Group and the Task Force were too afraid of controversy and simply made the wrong decision. Endicott in contrast believes that the concerns about how the diagnosis would be misused were exaggerated and not shared by all women, but understands why Allen Frances did not support it in order to protect the overall DSM process. The third member of the Work Group who opposed this decision, Ellen Frank, was very distressed at that time by the unwillingness of the Work Group to let science lead the way. She was also upset by the intimidation tactics of the opposition and, in retrospect, agrees with Frances' political decision to not support its inclusion at that moment in history. In her interview Judith Gold was quite surprised to hear that some members believed that the Work Group thought they had failed. From her perspective, they decided to be more scientifically rigorous about PMDD criteria in comparison to other DSM-IV disorders.

41.7.4 Peer Pressure Consensus

The guiding assumption of the entire DSM-IV process was called "the consensus model." Rather than committees deciding an issue by voting, the architects believed that if the data were clearly laid out, reasonable people would agree on its implications for the DSM. Frances's notion of consensus was not limited to scientific consensus. It also included clinical consensus and organizational consensus. Requiring such consensus was a strategy for being cautious about proposed changes.

When Frances and Sabshin put together the Work Group, they wanted a diversity of perspectives and also people who they believed would be fair-minded. Looking back, every member of the work group agreed that if fair-mindedness was the goal, the architects were particularly successful in selecting Judith Gold to chair the Work Group. Under her leadership, the Work Group was very cohesive. For example, Endicott reported that after the final decision to keep PMDD in the appendix had been made, she was having lunch with Nada Stotland. One of her colleagues came upon them and was incredulous that they were interacting. Endicott told her she and Stotland were friends who agreed to disagree.

Some members also suggested that wanting to find points of consensus may have led to disagreements among the Work Group members being minimized at the end. In support of this claim, Paula Caplan (1995) reported that before the final vote, Stotland told her that she did not believe that the diagnosis should be in the manual at all, but that she did not know how to stop it from being retained.

41.7.5 Reaction to Public Opposition

Given that the LLPDD Work Group (reluctantly in some cases) agreed on a consensus final opinion, the people interviewed generally held that much of the opposition came from outside the DSM process and largely from psychology. Paula Caplan (1995), who later wrote a book titled *They Say You're Crazy: How the World's Most Powerful Psychiatrists Decide Who's Normal*, figures prominently here.

Referring to these events as PMSgate, Caplan (1995) noted that she did not believe that the scientific evidence supported the validity of a mental illness related to menstruation. Furthermore, the foreseeable harms to women that would be contingent upon such a diagnosis were alarming to her. Given her reading of the scientific evidence and the values issues, she saw no reason to compromise. As a result, during the time that the LLPDD work group was active, other critics had a more important influence on the Work Group's deliberations.

Caplan began appearing in public debates with Judith Gold whose job it was to speak for the Work Group to the Task Force, to the critics, to concerned professionals, and the press. In her role as the public face of the opposition, Caplan charged those directly involved with the DSM-IV revision with serious distortions of the truth and outright lies. She also suggested that many women were immersed in a belief system which taught them that women are inferior and that their inferiority is closely linked to biology. They failed to understand, she suggested, that according to the evidence, mood problems prior to menstruation are not caused by being premenstrual.

Late in the process Caplan and her colleagues sent a letter to all the members of the APA Legislative Assembly and the APA Board of Trustees warning that psychiatrists would be legally liable for the harm done by giving a psychiatric diagnosis that is not justified by research. The letter also claimed that the consequence of retaining the diagnosis in the appendix would lead to increases in malpractice insurance and to public embarrassment to the profession of psychiatry as a whole. Many observers believed that the combination of personal attacks and dramatic warnings, especially about lawsuits, lost the opposition credibility in the larger psychiatric community.

41.8 The DSM-5: Opposition does not Emerge

When we examine the DSM-5 revision in light of the history just reviewed, two things stand out. One, this revision involved more professional and public controversy about the recommended changes than occurred in either the DSM-III-R or DSM-IV. These controversies included proposals to eliminate the bereavement exclusion for major depressive disorder, eliminating many of the personality disorders, eliminating the diagnostic category of Asperger's syndrome, adding a psychosis risk syndrome, and introducing a new mood dysregulation disorder for children. There was, however, very little said in the public media about the decision of the Mood Disorders Work Group to move PMDD from the appendix into the main section of the manual.

41.8.1 FDA and Sarafem®

Those interviewed suggested that a key factor in reduction in the level of controversy was a ruling by the US Food and Drug Administration (FDA) in the year 1999. According to Endicott et al. (1999), in 1998 a panel of 16 experts were brought together to review and discuss newly available evidence on PMDD and concluded that it was a distinct clinical disorder that differed from other mood and anxiety disorders. Much of the new research focused on the efficacy of blocking serotonin re-uptake for about 50–60% of the women diagnosed with PMDD. Once the experts came to believe that PMDD was worthy of being considered as an indication for specific treatments, and Eli Lilly presented the results of their clinical trial using the PMDD diagnostic criteria, the FDA approved Prozac® (fluoxetine) for the treatment of PMDD. Eli Lilly later repackaged it as Sarafem® (Greenslit 2005).

Allen Frances, who was a major force in the opposition to many proposed DSM-5 changes, specifically noted that he was not aware of what the current research on PMDD indicated, but that he chose to not ring the alarm bell about its being moved to the main section of the manual because the FDA action made the status of PMDD in the DSM largely irrelevant with respect to how the pharmaceutical companies target their drugs. At this point, believed Frances, moving it to the main section of the manual wouldn't do much harm.

41.8.2 Dire Consequences do not Emerge

One point that was very specifically mentioned by several people interviewed was that the predicted negative social consequences did not materialize after Sarafem® was introduced. They took this as evidence that the concerns about negative consequences were exaggerated and some of them simply unfounded.

41.8.3 DSM-5 Politics

Many of the debates that occurred during the DSM-5 revision were related to the intention of the architects to revolutionize psychiatric classification by implementing dimensional models in which psychiatric disorders lie on a continuum with normality (Kupfer et al. 2002). Included in these proposals were categories for classifying milder subthreshold conditions as vulnerability conditions along the lines of hypertension. Rather than concern about the social and political consequences of false positive diagnoses, the goal was to let science lead the way to a better taxonomy. This represented an important internal shift in politics. The politics of DSM-IV (avoid harm) served as a vector for keeping PMDD in the appendix whereas the politics of DSM-5 (make revolutionary changes) supported moving it into the main body of the manual. Furthermore, in adopting a dimensional model, PMDD can be seen as continuous with PMS—and all the research conducted on PMS becomes directly relevant to PMDD.

41.8.4 Next-Generation Feminism

Jean Endicott believes that Sarafem® normalized the treatment of PMDD. She noted that popular women's magazines discuss PMS by giving recommendations for lifestyle changes. If that does not work, the magazines tell women to go see their doctor. They also inform women this is a real entity and they do not need to feel ashamed by it.

Endicott, Ellen Frank, and Kimberly Yonkers (who headed the DSM-5 Gender and Cross-Cultural Issues study group) also suggested that there has been a generational change among feminists. According to them, professional women who were born in the 1970s and 1980s are more secure than those Baby Boomers born in 1945–1960. Less intimidated and less fearful of losing their status, they represent the kind of feminism that Frank felt that she possessed during the DSM-IV revision process.

41.8.5 Additional Research on Validity and Treatment Benefits

The Mood Disorders Work Group for DSM-5 asked a panel of eight experts in women's mental health: (1) to evaluate the DSM-IV criteria for PMDD, (2) to assess whether there is sufficient empirical evidence to support its being moved out of the appendix, and (3) to suggest changes to the diagnosis that are supported by the research conducted since the DSM-IV. The panel recommended that PMDD should be moved to the main section of the manual and suggested changes in criteria (Epperson et al. 2012). The reasons for this recommendation emphasize, in Solomon's terms, what the committee considered new empirical vectors supporting the validity of PMDD. These include:

The consistent prevalence rates of PMDD across countries.
The rapid efficacy of SSRIs when taken only during symptomatic periods.
Clear distinction between PMDD and other mood and anxiety disorder, for example, those diagnosed with PMDD are less likely to have a co-occurring personality disorder.
The negative response to hormonal add-back only for those with a PMS history.

Let us briefly examine the issue of hormonal add-back. As was the case for the research available during the DSM-IV revision, no clear pattern of hormonal differences is associated with PMDD. This was taken as evidence against the validity of PMDD. There later emerged additional evidence that the key factor is not differences in levels of hormones, but different central nervous system responses to fluctuating levels of hormones (Epperson 2013). For example, if normal levels of hormones like progesterone are blocked, when those hormones are "added back in," women with a history of PMDD experience the typical psychiatric symptoms, but those without a history do not.

41.9 Science-in-the-Making or Ready-Made Science?

Ready-made science is a term used by Bruno Latour (1987) to describe what occurs after a scientific controversy on some topic is closed and nature is seen as having spoken. Prior to this development, fact claims that are in the process of being established are open to scrutiny and critically examined. For example, prior to the acceptance of the Copernican theory, Galileo's inferences about moons orbiting other planets could be challenged. Later, they were taken to be observations, not inferences. Occasionally, already agreed upon facts can again become a matter of dispute. For instance, psychologists' "observations" of the intellectual inferiority of women and black people in the early part of the twentieth century are now considered to be "illegitimate inferences" from test scores (Gould 1996).

Hillary Putnam (1990) has argued that the concept of a fact includes the notion of an obligation. To call something a fact is to declare that others have an epistemic obligation to accept it, no matter what their preferences may be. To assert that the facts now support the validity of PMDD is also to say that our epistemic obligations have been better specified.

A plurality of obligations are relevant in psychiatry (epistemic, ethical, political, etc.). Alongside their obligations to science and obligations to patients, many professional women accept that they have an obligation to support feminist values. These obligations likely influence what facts are considered most relevant and how other facts are interpreted.

In general, feminists believe it is important to not blame women for their distress—which psychiatric constructs such as hysteria and borderline personality subtly do. This raises a specific set of obligations and directs attention to a particular set of facts. For instance, if borderline patients are those who it is considered acceptable to dislike, this might increase the extent to which manipulative behavior is considered a defining feature of the disorder (Potter 2009). Viewing the term manipulation as a potentially sexist term of disparagement, however, might lead one to interpret those behaviors differently.

Feminist scholars who specialize in the philosophy of psychiatry believe that it is important to acknowledge that a woman's psychiatric distress and impairment is mediated by historical and cultural factors, but is also genuine (Potter 2006, 2009; Radden 2009). For example, to say that the emotional lability and irritability of PMDD are best understood as reactions to physical symptoms such as headaches could be construed as blaming a woman for lacking coping skills. Not merely dismissing a woman's psychiatric distress as "all in her head" is also a kind of obligation that makes other "facts" relevant.

In that light consider the following quote from a young woman who experiences severe physical and emotional symptoms 7 days out of every month:

> One of the things I find frustrating about modern feminist critique [...] is that I'm expected to be tough no matter what my body deals me, otherwise I'm giving in to patriarchy. What if sometimes, I'm in pain and I can't do it on my own. What has to happen to make that acceptable? (Vargas-Cooper 2012)

Nor is it so simple as just accepting that there has been a generational shift among feminists. In what one of our colleagues has called third-generation feminism, some young women believe that being a feminist means they can choose to stay at home and raise the children, wear lipstick and high heels—and perhaps take a pill for premenstrual distress. It is not clear that these women have accepted any feminist obligations at all.

As we saw earlier, women who might be called next-generation feminists are more confident in their hard-earned social status and do not feel obligated to constantly defend it, but as Stotland noted, to claim that sexism is no longer an issue because women have done so well is analogous to claiming that racism was no longer an issue after Barack Obama became the US President. One could question whether not wanting to call attention to sexism out of fear that one will be seen as a complainer and lose credibility is an advance

To some, the lack of opposition might suggest that the facts have spoken and science has won out, although many advocates for the diagnosis believed the PMDD controversy should have been closed during the DSM-IV process. It may be that empirical considerations should now be seen as having led the way to the PMDD controversy being closed, but that outcome was made easier because the science came to be more supported by a host of nonempirical considerations than it was opposed by them. According to Solomon's model, an unequitable distribution of nonempirical vectors is not an ideal way for controversies to be settled.

According to the interviews, one key nonempirical factor, the approval of Sarafem®, played a key role in the DSM-5 outcome. So did giving PMDD an official code number in the DSM-IV and listing it in the main text as an example of Mood Disorder Not Otherwise Specified. By the time that the DSM-5 development process began, PMDD was no longer a new diagnosis, and *conservativeness* favored keeping it a disorder subject to routine clinical use, hence moving it to the main section of the manual.

Quite likely a shift in the level of passion and commitment was also an important factor. During the DSM-III-R debate, the opposition to PMDD was energized by opposition to masochistic personality disorder and paraphilic rapism. In the DSM-IV it was energized by the heir of masochist personality disorder, specifically, self-defeating personality disorder. Neither of these two constructs was considered for the DSM-5.

The passion of the DSM-5 opposition was largely focused upon the expansion of psychiatry into the fuzzy boundary between normal and abnormal, and largely driven by men who did not emphasize the similarities between the reputed proposals to "make normal grief a mental disorder" and "make a normal part of a woman's monthly cycle a mental disorder." If one scans the many critiques of various DSM categories that have been published in the literature since the DSM-IV, especially those critiques of the expansion of the DSM into conditions that are on the border of the normal and the disordered, PMDD does not get much, if any space (Horwitz 2002; Horwitz and Wakefield 2007; Kutchins and Kirk, 1997). To speculate about why this is the case—clearly it is a delicate issue to summarily dismiss a diagnostic construct that many women are invested in—so it is judicious to not include it in one's list of problematic diagnostic categories (especially if the writer is male).

What happened with the DSM-5 cannot be reduced to a claim that the new evidence silenced the opposition. In an article in *Ms. Magazine*, Caplan (2008) argued that one of the consequences of the Mood Disorder Work Group's appointing a panel of experts was that those experts' ties to the pharmaceutical industry were not subject to the same scrutiny as were those of the Work Group proper. Furthermore, given that research has still not found consistent hormonal differences between women with and without PMDD, Caplan continued to assert that the diagnosis of PMDD with its false assumption of a hormonal etiology leads women to ignore the real causes of their distress. It is, she is quoted by Vargas-Cooper (2012) to say, "an invented mental illness."

One could even claim that the new facts/evidence can be used to call the validity of PMDD into question. For example, women tend to rate the physical symptoms as more severe than the psychiatric symptoms. Furthermore, the more important psychiatric symptoms are affective lability and irritability/anger, not dysphoria (Epperson et al. 2012). Why then, is the disorder considered a premenstrual *dysphoria*?

One always has to worry about the extent to which a controversy is closed because the advocates for one side have successfully recruited enough allies to foreclose the debate. For example, the people at Elli Lilly brought Nada Stotland in with the hope of convincing her to end her opposition to Sarafem®, but they were was not successful. When ally-building is successful, the debate ends because the remaining dissenters come to see little gain in continuing to expound effort on their critical activities, especially if they have been boxed up as fringe figures. Perhaps this is one reason that Stotland suggested in her interview that feminism is dead.

Or perhaps the issue is that the opposition was never very large. More often than we realize, influential public opposition and protests tend to be fueled by a relatively small group of committed people who are less prone to compromise. The opposition to keeping the disorder in the DSM-IV was largely driven by Paula Caplan and most of the opponents from the DSM-III-R battle did not participate. For instance, Jean Hamilton reported feeling emotionally battered by the DSM-III-R controversy and played no role in the DSM-IV protests (Figert 1996).

Initially Caplan resumed her protest and criticized the plan to move PMDD into the main section of the DSM-5, but got little notice. Even this most outspoken opponent of the construct was weary. Just prior to the official publication of the DSM-5, Caplan (2013) reported that her recent silence was partly related to an existential nausea about her long battle with the powerful people who develop the DSM. With respect to other potential opponents, according to Stotland, the problems with the construct are much the same—they are just tired of fighting.

The status of PMDD in the DSM-5 did not become controversial for a plurality of reasons, only some of which we have addressed. The story we have told here has included more information than did a briefer journal article previously published, but this chapter too is a partial representation of events and is largely dependent on the memories and perspectives of those interviewed, all of whom were insiders to the DSM process. One of the advantages of interviewing insiders is that it offers insight into the ongoing tension between discovery and interpretation in formulating mental disorder constructs. We are cognizant that the formulation of disorder constructs always occurs in multifaceted historical and cultural frameworks, and that these frameworks are subject to alternative interpretations. It is our hope than when additional interpretations that enhance and deepen this history are offered, the various perspectives of those who made the history will still be considered informative.

Acknowledgments

A shorter version of this chapter was published as Zachar, P. and Kendler, K.S. (2014). A Diagnostic and Statistical Manual of Mental Disorders history of premenstrual dysphoric disorder. *Journal of Nervous and Mental Disease*, 202(4), 346–352. Sections from that that article are reprinted with permission here.

Nancy Potter, Ginger Hoffman, Andrea Solomon, and Jennifer Hanson offered helpful suggestions on an earlier version of this chapter.

References

Andreasen, N.C. (1984). *The Broken Brain: The Biological Revolution in Psychiatry.* New York: Harper & Row.

Bayer, R. (1981). *Homosexuality and American Psychiatry: The Politics of Diagnosis.* New York: Basic Books, Inc.

Caplan, P.J. (1995). *They Say You're Crazy: How the World's Most Powerful Psychiatrists Decide Who's Normal.* Reading, MA: Addison-Wesley.

Caplan, P.J. (2008). Pathologizing your period. *Ms. Magazine*, Summer, 63–64.

Caplan, P.J. (2013). My recent silence and a voice that matters. *Psychology Today*, May 21. [Online]. Available at: <http://www.psychologytoday.com/blog/science-isnt-golden/201305/my-recent-silence-and-voice-matters>.

Collins, H. (1992). *Changing Order: Replication and Induction in Scientific Practice.* Chicago, IL: University of Chicago Press.

Endicott, J. (2000). History, evolution, and diagnosis of premenstrual dysphoric disorder. *Journal of Clinical Psychiatry*, 61, 5–8.

Endicott, J., Amsterdam, J., Eriksson, E., et al. (1999). Is premenstrual dysphoric disorder a distinct clinical entity? *Journal of Women's Health & Gender-Based Medicine*, 8, 663.

Epperson, C.N. (2013). Premenstrual dysphoric disorder and the brain. *American Journal of Psychiatry*, 170, 248–252.

Epperson, C.N., Steiner, M., Hartlage, S.A., et al. (2012). Premenstrual dysphoric disorder: evidence for a new category for DSM-5. *American Journal of Psychiatry*, 169, 465–475.

Figert, A.E. (1996). *Women and the Ownership of PMS*. New York: Aldine de Gruyter.

Frances, A. (2013). *Saving Normal*. New York: William Morrow.

Frank, E. and Severino, S.K. (1995). Premenstrual dysphoric disorder: facts and meanings. *Journal of Practical Psychiatry and Behavioral Health*, 1, 20–28.

Frank, R.T. (1931). The hormonal basis of premenstrual tension. *Archives of Neurology and Psychiatry*, 26.

Gold, J.H., Endicott, J., Parry, B.L., et al. (1996). Late luteal phase dysphoric disorder. In T.A. Widiger, A. Frances, H.A. Pincus, et al. (eds.) *DSM-IV sourcebook volume 2*, pp. 317–394. Washington, DC: American Psychiatric Association.

Gould, S.J. (1996). *The Mismeasure of Man*. New York: W.W. Norton & Company.

Greene, R. and Dalton, K. (1953). The premenstrual syndrome. *British Medical Journal*, 1, 1007–1014.

Greenslit, N. (2005). Dep*ession and consum*tion: Psychopharmaceuticals, branding, and new identity practices. *Culture, Medicine, and Psychiatry*, 29, 477–502.

Guze, S.B. (1992). *Why Psychiatry is a Branch of Medicine*. New York: Oxford University Press.

Horwitz, A.V. (2002). *Creating Mental Illness*. Chicago, IL: University of Chicago Press.

Horwitz, A.V. and Wakefield, J.C. (2007). *The Loss of Sadness: How Psychiatry Transformed Normal Sorrow into Depressive Disorder*. New York, Oxford University Press.

Kendler, K.S. (1990). Toward a scientific psychiatric nosology. *Archives of General Psychiatry*, 47, 969–973.

Kitcher, P. (1993). *The Advancement of Science*. New York: Oxford University Press.

Kupfer, D.J., First, M.B., and Regier, D.A. (2002). *A Research Agenda for DSM—V*. Washington, DC: American Psychiatric Association.

Kutchins, H. and Kirk, S.A. (1997). *Making Us Crazy: DSM: The Psychiatric Bible and the Creation of Mental Disorders*. New York: Free Press.

Latour, B. (1987). *Science in Action*. Cambridge, MA: Harvard University Press.

Micale, M.S. (1990). Hysteria and its historiography: the future perspective. *History of Psychiatry*, 1, 33–124.

Parlee, M.B. (1994). Commentary on the literature review. In J.H. Gold and S. K. Severino (eds.) *Premenstrual Dysphorias: Myths and Realities*, pp. 149–167. Washington, DC: American Psychiatric Press.

Potter, N.N. (2006). What is manipulative behavior, anyway? *Journal of Personality Disorders*, 20, 139–156.

Potter, N.N. (2009). *Mapping the Edges and the In-Between*. Oxford: Oxford University Press.

Putnam, H. (1990). *Realism with a Human Face*. Cambridge, MA: Harvard University Press.

Radden, J. (2009). *Moody Minds Distempered: Essays on Melancholia and Depression.* Oxford: Oxford University Press.

Robins, E. and Guze, S.B. (1970). Establishment of diagnostic validity in psychiatric illness: its application to schizophrenia. *American Journal of Psychiatry*, 126, 983–986.

Scull, A. (2009). *Hysteria: The Disturbing History.* Oxford: Oxford University Press.

Severino, S.K. (1994). Commentary: late luteal phase dysphoric disorder-disease or dis-ease. In J.H. Gold and S.K. Severino (eds.) *Premenstrual Dysphorias: Myths and Realities*, pp. 213–228. Washington, DC: American Psychiatric Press.

Severino, S.K. and Gold, J.H. (1994). Summation. In J.H. Gold and S.K. Severino (eds.) *Premenstrual Dysphorias: Myths and Realities*, pp. 530–538. Washington, DC: American Psychiatric Press.

Severino, S.K. and Moline, M.L. (1989). *Premenstrual Syndrome: A Clinician's Guide.* New York: Guilford Press.

Showalter, E. (1985). *The Famale Malady.* New York: Pantheon Books.

Solomon, M. (2001). *Social Empiricism.* Cambridge, MA: MIT Press.

Solomon, M. (2008). Norms of dissent. *Technical Report 09/08 CPNSS, LSE*. [Online] Available at: <http://www.lse.ac.uk/CPNSS/research/concludedResearchProjects/ContingencyDissentInScience/DP/SolomonNormsOfDissent0908Online.pdf>.

Spitzer, R.L., Severino, S.K., Williams, J.B., and Parry, B.L. (1989). Late luteal phase dysphoric disorder and DSM-III-R. *American Journal of Psychiatry*, 146, 892–897.

Vargas-Cooper, N. (2012). The billion dollar battle over premenstrual disorder. *Salon*, February 26. [Online]. Available at: <http://www.salon.com/2012/02/26/the_billion_dollar_battle_over_premenstrual_disorder/singleton/>.

Widiger, T.A., Frances, A., Pincus, H.A., Ross, R., First, M. B., and Davis, W. (eds.) (1996). *DSM-IV Sourcebook: Volume 2.* Washington, DC: American Psychiatric Association.

Zachar, P. and Kendler, K.S. (2010). Philosophical issues in the classification of psychopathology. In T. Millon, R.F. Krueger, and E. Simonsen (eds.) *Contemporary Directions in Psychopathology*, pp. 126–148. New York: The Guilford Press.

Zachar, P. and Kendler, K.S. (2012). The removal of Pluto from the class of planets and homosexuality from the class of psychiatric disorders: a comparison. *Philosophy, Ethics, and Humanities in Medicine*, 7. [Online] Available at: <http://www.peh-med.com/content/7/1/4.

Zachar, P. and Kendler, K.S. (2014). A Diagnostic and Statistical Manual of Mental Disorders history of premenstrual dysphoric disorder. *Journal of Nervous and Mental Disease*, 202(4), 346–352.

Chapter 42
The construction of a diagnosis is not a scientific issue

Robert Michels

A famous throwaway line, usually misattributed to Bismarck, is that laws are like sausages—they should never be seen in the making. In Chapter 41, Zachar and Kendler make clear that the same is true of diagnoses, or at least DSM diagnoses. They trace the rich, complex, tangled, conflicted skein of social, cultural, professional, political, and other determinants that shape and reshape the process of constructing a DSM category.

However, there is one important difference between laws and sausages on the one hand and diagnoses on the other. No one has ever suggested that laws or sausages have anything to do with science!

Diagnoses are different. It is not that they have much to do with science; it is that many people believe that they do. To their credit, this was not a problem for the creators of the DSMs. They were explicit that "Our highest priority has been to provide a helpful guide to clinical practice" (DSM-IV; American Psychiatric Association 1994, p. xv).

Different goals lead to different methods. Scientists, and scientific research, want diagnostic categories that are clear, distinct, and have sharp boundaries. Educators want diagnoses that relate to interesting theories and conceptual models. Clinicians are much more pragmatic. They would like to have clear, crisp categories, but their diagnoses must encompass everyone who seeks help and whom they treat, and they know that many seeking help will not fit neatly into precisely defined categories. They would like diagnostic categories that relate to interesting theories—if nothing else they are easier to remember, but that is not as important as having useful guidelines for selecting the optimal treatment. The diagnoses that are most useful for the clinician may not be best for educators or scientists, but faced with this dilemma the creators of the DSM made a choice and communicated it to us quite clearly. Therefore it isn't quite fair to discuss their process as that of making a scientific decision.

Zachar and Kendler tell an important and interesting story, and they tell it well. My only addendum is to emphasize that it is a story about the history of a diagnosis, and that it has little to do with science. It is true that science is not totally irrelevant. It has high status and therefore great rhetorical value in debates that are not inherently scientific. One can imagine scientific research that leads to knowledge that makes a powerful argument for or against a specific diagnosis. However, today this is seldom the case in psychiatry—perhaps a few rare genetic syndromes or conditions secondary to toxic or organic causes. Not premenstrual dysphoric disorder (PMDD).

The nonscientific nature of the issue is clear from the beginning of the story. Interest in PMDD begins when the diagnosis influences a murder trial. Mental health professionals then become interested, and that is enough for the DSM work group. Proponents, opponents, campaigners, and so on emerge soon after. This is the stuff of social discourse and conflict, but not of science.

Zachar and Kendler distract us by their extended discussion of Miriam Solomon's concept of decision vectors that influence "the outcome of scientific decisions" without alerting us that here this is only a metaphor. We are not discussing a scientific decision. The vectors they discuss make this clear: "benefits of treatment," "politics of DSM," "peer presser consensus," "reaction to public opposition," "feminism," and "criticism of pharmaceutical industry." These are not notions at home in scientific discourse.

The most we might hope for is that the formulation of diagnostic categories has space to consider science which might be relevant along with the many other appropriately relevant issues.

Reference

American Psychiatric Association. (1994). *Diagnostic and Statistical Manual of Mental Disorders* (4th ed.). Washington, DC: American Psychiatric Association.

Index

fn indicates footnotes

A
acedia 30
acroagonines 128
activism 326-7, 328, 334-6
adrenocorticotropic hormone 129
advocacy groups 78, 327, 328, 333, 337-8
aggression research 8, 10, 13, 16, 17, 22
agnotology 69
AIDS, *see* HIV/AIDS
alcohol abuse/dependence 321
alienism 34, 107-8
anachronism 39
analytical statements 9
anatomoclinical model 41, 108, 109
Andreasen, N.C. 133, 166, 200-1
anomalies 13
antidepressants 305, 307, 321
antipsychiatry movement 88, 97, 195
antipsychotics 130, 131, 132, 284, 287-8
antiscientific realists 14
anxiety disorders 31
"anything goes" science 6
apperception 156, 158
applied research, disagreement in 63-4, 73-4
archetypes 264-5
Ash, M.G. 153
Asperger's syndrome 333, 336, 343
assumptions 14, 15, 16
atavism 265
atheoretical descriptivism 34
attachment 266
aural hematoma 30
authority, distrust of 12; *see also* expert authority
autism, shaping of 325, 326-38, 341
  activism 326-7, 328, 334-6
  advocacy groups 327, 328, 333, 337-8
  autism pride 328, 332
  causation 327-8
  epidemic of 330
  gender differences 327-8, 338
  genetic research 336-7, 340
  on the Internet 331-2
  leaders 332-4, 337-8
  maternal factors 332-3
  neurodiversity (difference not disease) movement 328, 335, 337, 338, 343-5
  Phenome Project 337
  "special needs" and 330-1
  spectrum disorder 333
  systematizing brain theory 338
  triad of difficulties 333
autonomic regulation 126, 127

B
Bacon, F. 73
Bard, P. 126
Baron-Cohen, S. 327-8, 338
basic emotions 251
basics symptom model 28-9
behavior
  evolution and 261-2
  genetic versus cultural determinism 265-7
  plasticity 262
behaviorism 11
Bentall, R. 97-8
best evidence 62
big pharma xvii, 290
biological coherence 240-1
biological determinism 234
biopsychosocial model 306
Bleuler, M. 197
Blondel, C. 28
bon sens 16
borderline personality 177-8
brain
  in autism 338
  plasticity 275
  in schizophrenia 133, 231-2, 285-6
  symptom formation 41, 52
BRAIN Initiative 306
breast screening debate 64-6, 67, 68, 69, 74-7
Breivik, A. 200 *fn*, 205*fn*, 345
Brenner, B.A. 69
Bridgman, P.W. 191-2, 213, 214-16
Bumke, O. 154
business opportunities 307

C
Cambridge change 33
Cambridge model 28, 41-3, 110, 112
Cannon, W. 126
Caplan, P.J. 351, 362, 367, 368
case social constructionists 83, 88-9
case studies 128
catatonia 31
categories of being 33
category social constructionists 83, 88-9
causal construction 88

causality
  behavioral genetics 249–51
  in medicine 111–12
Cerletti, U. 128–9
change
  Cambridge change 33
  classification 40
  defining 27, 32–4
  events 32–4
  as exchange 35, 40
  ideal type 33
  mental symptoms 30–1, 40–1
  phenomenic 35
  psychopathology 34–5, 39–40
  qualitative 40
  quantitative 40
  structural 40
  transcendental 40, 53
  see also scientific change
chlorpromazine 130, 131, 132
classification
  of change 40
  influence of 329
  purpose-dependent 22
clinical guidelines 67
clinical history-taking 43
clinical interlocutor 42, 43
clinical judgment 197
clinical neuroscience, psychiatry as 124, 134–5, 166, 227
clinical research
  operational diagnostic criterion in 307–8
  research waste 308
  Singapore Statement 311
coherence criterion 240–1
commercialization, depression 306–7
concepts
  as experimental practices 248–9
  prototype-based 206
  semantically inspired 249
configurators, symptoms 41–2, 43
confirmation 9
consciousness 203–4
  hard problem of 28, 202, 218
consensus 60, 63, 64, 361–2
constitutive construction 88
contextualism 6, 14–18, 21–3
continuants 33
convergence 39–40, 121, 127–8, 129–32, 141–2
Copenhagen interpretation 246, 248–51
crisis of identity 151–2
Crow, T.J. 233
cultural assumptions 357
cultural determinism 265–7
cultural neuroscience 112
cultural transmission 268

D

Darwinian theory 31, 36
data
  hypotheses and 15
  salience 61
Davis, K.L. 285
deafness 345
death, fear of 320
decision vectors 57–8, 61–2
  dopamine hypothesis of schizophrenia 287–90, 295–7
  premenstrual dysphoric disorder 352–3, 354–63
  screening mammography 65–6
degeneration 35, 36, 247
Delay, J. 127, 130
delusions 200
depression 302–14
  antidepressant prescribing 305, 307, 321
  biological factors 306
  biopsychosocial model 306
  caring about the diagnosis 319–22
  clinical trials on 307–8
  conceptual history 303–4
  economic factors 306–7
  enlargement of concept 305
  grief and 305–6, 319
  market needs 309–10
  medical/nosological component 303–5
  multifaceted sequelae to concept 307–9
  nonmedical component 305–7
  nonspecialist views 312–13
  operationalization 301, 304, 307–8, 309–10
  overdiagnosis 305
  self-help books 313
Der Wanderer über dem Nebelmeer (Friedrich) 313, 314
determinism
  biological 234
  genetic versus cultural 265–7
  Laplace's 246, 247–8
developmental psychiatry 178
developmental systems theory 267–8
diagnosis/diagnostic criteria
  accuracy of 155, 157
  index or constitute the disorder 189
  operationalism and 195–6, 198–200
  polythetic 206–7
  science and 371–2
  structured interviews 207
  symptom counting 199, 207
  typification 205
Diagnostic and Statistical Manual of Mental Disorders, see DSM headings
dialogue, symptom formation 43
diencephalon 121, 123–35, 274
  animal experiments 126
  autonomic regulation 126, 127
  electroshock therapy 127, 128, 129
  emotion regulation 126, 127
  endocrine system 129
  as an epistemic object 124
  experimental studies on 125–6

posterity of 132–4
psychiatry's interest in 125–7
psychosomatic disorders 126, 128
territory of convergence 127–8, 129–32, 141–2
difference versus disease (neurodiversity) movement 328, 335, 337, 338, 343–5
discontinuants 33–4
divorce, heritability 233, 236
dopamine hypothesis of schizophrenia 91, 92, 281–2, 283–93
  conservative hypothesis 297
  decision vectors 287–90, 295–7
  degenerative research program 293
  final common pathway 286–7, 295
  historical background 283–4
  historical contextualization 291–2
  lack of genetic correlation 286
  lack of viable competing hypotheses 296
  modified versions of 285, 286–7, 289, 295
  pharmaceutical industry and 290
  poorly specified theory 285, 289
  popularity of 282
  scientific developments 284
  simple hypothesis 297
drugs
  antidepressants 305, 307, 321
  antipsychotics 130, 131, 132, 284, 287–8
  HAART 92, 95
  Sarafem® 363
DSM
  purpose of 70
  shaping of psychiatric disorders 341
DSM-III 194–7
DSM-III+ 190, 199, 200–1, 202
DSM-IV, premenstrual dysphoric disorder 351, 353–63
DSM-5 189
  Asperger's syndrome deletion 336
  grief in 305–6
  premenstrual dysphoric disorder 70, 351, 363–5
Duesberg, P. 94, 95–6
Duhem, P. 14–15, 95

E

economic factors, depression 306–7
Einstein, A. 214–16
electroshock therapy 127, 128, 129
emotions
  basic emotion theories 251
  diencephalon and 126, 127
  evolutionary approach 262–3
empirical decision vectors 57, 58, 61, 62
  dopamine hypothesis of schizophrenia 287–9
  premenstrual dysphoric disorder 352
  screening mammography 65–6
empiricism
  logical 5, 8–11

  social 60, 61, 62, 66, 73, 77–8, 297, 352
encephalitis lethargica 126
Endicott, J. 353, 355, 360, 361, 362, 363, 364
endocrine system 129
environment
  environmentalists in psychopathology 232
  etiology and 224–5
  genetic versus psychosocial meaning 13
environment of evolutionary adaptation 262, 264
epigenesis 246, 268, 275
epistemic objects 124
epoché 206
essentialism, basic emotions 251
etiology
  characterization of disorders 91–2
  environment and 224–5
  specific genetic 237
events
  change 32–4
  symptoms as 36–9
evidence 61, 62
evidence reports 68
evolution 259–70
  atavism and 265
  cultural transmission 268
  Darwinian 31, 36
  developmental systems theory 267–8
  emotions and 262–3
  of evolutionary psychiatry 275–6
  human behavior 261–2
  human mind 260–1
  meanings 35–6
  niche construction 267
  of science 121
evolutionary psychiatry 257
  evolutionary psychology and 263–5
  evolution of 275–6
  neuroscience and 274
  psychopathology in 257–8
  scientific legitimacy of psychiatry 273
evolutionary psychology 259, 263–5
Examination of Anomalous Self-Experience (EASE) 100–1
exaptation 262
exclusionary social constructionism 83, 87, 93–8
experimental psychology 153–4, 155–7, 158–9
expert authority 61, 63–6, 67, 68, 69, 74–7, 78
expertise, operational criteria and 309–10
explanatory gap 28, 182, 202, 218
Ey, H. 274
Eyal, G. 330–1

F

factor analysis 239
facts, obligations and 365
Faraone, S.V. 233
Feighner criteria 196

Feinstein, A. 328, 329
feminism 357-9, 364, 365-6
Feyerabend, P. 6, 11, 13
financial factors, depression 306-7
First, M. 353, 361
first-rank symptoms 28
Fodor, J. 258
Foerster, O. 126
Frances, A. 353, 360, 361-2, 363
Frank, E. 353, 355, 359, 360, 361, 364
Freud, S. 173, 175-6
Friedrich, C.D. 313, 314

G
Gadamer, H. 42
Gagel, O. 126
Galton, F. 228-9
genetics 227-42, 245-52
  autism 336-7, 340
  causality 249-51
  Copenhagen interpretation 246, 248-51
  cultural determinism and 265-7
  empirical concept of a gene 248-9
  gene for X research program 250
  genome and 263
  heritability 223, 232-4, 246-7, 249
  personality 239-40
  risk factors 223-4, 225
  schizophrenia 231, 237, 286
  twin method 229-31
  variation and mechanism 224, 225, 236-9
  weak and strong role 225
genome 263
genome-wide association studies 286
German psychiatry 149-60
Gestalt 204-6
Gold, J. 353, 360, 361, 362
Goodman, S.N. 69
good sense 16
gray areas 68
grief 305-6, 319
Griesinger, W. 152
Grinker, R.R. 126-7
group selection 263
guideline synthesis 67

H
HAART 92, 95
Hacking, I. 88, 89, 99
hallucinations 38, 53, 343-4
Hamilton Rating Scale for Depression 303-4 *fn*
Hanson, N.R. 11
hard problem of consciousness 28, 202, 218
Hayward, R.A. 68
health, normative concept 260
Hearing Voices Movement 343-4
Helicobacter pylori theory of ulcers 291-2
Hempel, C.G. 193-4, 213-14, 216

heritability 223, 232-4, 246-7, 249
  coefficient 231
HIV/AIDS 87, 90-1, 92, 101-2, 292
  dissenters 93-6
holism 5, 11-14, 20-1
  pragmatic 218-19
Holliday, J. 319, 320, 321-2
homosexuality 260-1, 342, 343, 344
Howes, O.D. 286
Hughlings Jackson, J. 36
human nature 241-2
  as a process 268-70
Huntington's disease 235-6
Hyman, S.E. 89, 201
hypnotism 154
hypotheses, observation and 9, 14-15
hypothetico-deductivist reasoning 9-10

I
ICD-10 190190, 197-8, 199
ideal type 33
improper linear model 62
inclusionary social constructionism 83, 84, 86, 96-7, 99, 102
incommensurability
  of measurements 17
  of theories 12, 13, 14, 20-1
incompatible theories 12, 14, 20-1
individual differences 223-4
insight 345
instrumentalism 14
Internet, autism on 331-2
INUS conditions 91, 112
Iverson, P. 334

J
James, W. 268
Jammer, M. 215-16

K
Kapur, S. 286
Keedwell, P. 264
Kendler, K.S. 91, 240-1, 250, 361
Kennedy family 331
Koch's postulates 94
Kraepelin, E. 146, 155-8
Kuhn, T. 5, 11, 12, 13, 216

L
lack of insight 345
Lange, F.A. 153
Laplace determinism 246, 247-8
latent class analysis 98
lethargic encephalitis 126
levodopa 284
Lewis, A. 213-14
Lewontin, R.C. 234
limbic system 130
lobbyists, *see* advocacy groups
localization theories 159

logical empiricism 5, 8–11
looping effects 99, 329
Lotze, H. 35

M
McHugh, P.R. 103
Mackie, J. 91 *fn*
Maggiore, C. 93
mammography screening debate 64–6, 67, 68, 69, 74–7
manuals, standardized procedures 309–10
market needs 309–10
medicine
  as applied science 60
  causality in 111–12
  consensus conferences 64
  disagreement in 63–6, 67, 68, 69, 74–7, 78
  progress in 86, 90, 101–2
mental acts, symptoms as 32, 39, 52
mental symptoms
  atoms of madness 34–5
  basic symptom model 28–9
  Cambridge model 28, 41–3, 110, 112
  change of 30–1, 40–1
  concept 109–10
  configurators 41–2, 43
  counting 199, 207
  dialogue 43
  as events 36–9
  mental acts 32, 39, 52
  natural kinds 36
  neurobiological model 40–1, 43, 51–2, 53
  passive nature 32, 39
  pragmatic characteristics 43
  prototypical Gestalt 204
  received view of 40–1
  secular changes 30, 31–2
  as signs 38
  social factors 112
  as things 27–8, 36–9
  time-related changes 30
  treatment-related changes 30
mere observation 194
metamorphosis 27, 32, 40
metaphysics, exclusion of 151–2
methodological hierarchies 68
microbial theory of disease 291
monism 11, 13, 16

N
naive materialism 155
natural kinds 31, 32, 36
natural science 242
natural selection 259
nature
  change in 31
  debate 235–41
  human nature 241–2, 268–70
  meaning of 241–2
  nature–nurture debate 223–4, 228–9, 235

neo-Kraepelinians 146, 195–6
Nesse, R.M. 262–3
neurobiology of symptom formation 40–1, 43, 51–2, 53
neurodiversity (difference not disease) movement 328, 335, 337, 338, 343–5
neuroleptics 130, 131, 132, 284, 287–8
neuropsychoanalysis 176, 177
neuroscience 306
  cultural 112
  evolutionary psychiatry and 274
  psychiatry as 124, 134–5, 166, 227
neurotransmitters 129, 131–2, 284
neurotypicals 328
new psychology 153–4
Newtonionism 34
next-generation feminism 364, 366
niche construction 267
nonempirical decision vectors 57–8, 61–2
  dopamine hypothesis of schizophrenia 289–90, 296–7
  premenstrual dysphoric disorder 352–3
  screening mammography 66
nonessentialism, basic emotions 251
normal science 13
normative concepts 260–1
North American Man/Boy Love Association (NAMBLA) 343
nosology
  depression 303–5
  Kraepelin on 155, 156–7
  pluralism 22

O
object of psychiatry 31, 203–4
obligations 365
observation
  holism 11
  hypothesis and 9, 14–15
  as an operation 194, 214*fn*
  statements 9
  units of 9
obsessive–compulsive disorder 344
operationalism 187–8, 190–208, 213–14
  aggression 8, 10, 22
  concept of operational definition 167–8, 193–4
  depression 301, 304, 307–8, 309–10
  diagnosis 195–6, 198–200
  DSM-III 194–7
  DSM-III+ 199, 200–1, 202
  epistemiological considerations 202–7
  ICD-10 197–8, 199
  influences 188
  introduction of operational definitions 194
  observation and 194, 214*fn*
  ordinary linguistic meaning 200
  origins 191–3
  psychiatric terminology 199, 216–17

operationalism (*Cont.*)
  significance 190
  symptom counting 199, 207
  virtues 188
Overholser, W. 132

P
paradigms 11, 13
Parkinson's disease 284
Parry, B. 353, 355, 359, 360, 361
pedophilia 343, 344
peptic ulcer disease 291-2
perception
  conceptually informed 205
  as events 37
personality 239-40
personality disorders 146-7, 177-8
Perspectives model 103
pharmaceutical industry
  depression 306-7
  dopamine hypothesis of
    schizophrenia 290
  premenstrual dysphoric disorder 359
phenomenal-experiential realm 99-101
phenomenological reductionism 206
phenomenology 180-1, 197, 206
phenotypic null hypothesis 240
phobias 266
physiological psychology 158-9
Pincus, H. 353, 360, 361
pluralism 11, 13, 16-17, 20, 21-3
policy issues 63
political issues 360-1, 364
polythetic diagnosis 206-7
positivism 10
positron emission tomography,
  schizophrenia 285-6
post-traumatic stress disorder 341-2, 344
pragmatic holism (emergence) 218-19
preformationism 246
premenstrual dysphoric disorder 58-9,
  69-70, 349, 350-68, 371-2
  biomedical model 356
  cultural assumptions 357
  decision vectors 352-3, 354-63
  diagnostic validity 357
  DSM-IV 351, 353-63
  DSM-5 70, 351, 363-5
  in DSM appendix 70, 251, 359-63, 364
  false positive diagnoses 356-7
  FDA and 363
  feminist view 357-9, 364, 365-6
  hormonal add-back 364
  name changes 350
  peer pressure consensus 361-2
  pharmaceutical industry 359
  philosophical assumptions 359-60
  political issues 360-1, 364
  public opinion 362-3
  ready-made science 365-8

Sarafem® for 363
standard of evidence 360
symptoms 354-5
timecourse 355
treatment benefits 355, 364-5
presentism 39, 121-2
Pressman, J. 132-3
Price, J. 264
process
  human nature as 268-70
  perceptions as 37
professionalization 64
professional self-interest 291
progress
  in medicine 86, 90, 101-2
  in psychiatry 85-6, 113-14
  in science 86, 89, 90
proleptic rhetoric 140-1
proscription 13
prototype 204-6, 207
psychiatry
  as clinical neuroscience 124, 134-5, 166, 227
  disagreement in 58-9, 63-4, 69-70
  endocrinology and 129
  historical construction in 107-8
  interdisciplinary nature 150-60, 165-8,
    182, 208
  object of 31, 203-4
  progress in 85-6, 113-14
  scientific legitimacy 272-4
  secular change in psychiatric
    knowledge 31-2
  social construction in 87-90
  social factors in history of 110-12
  terminology, operational nature 199, 216-17
psychoanalysis 171-2, 173-9, 180-3
  in academia 175
  neuropsychoanalysis 176, 177
  and psychiatric research 177-8
  research in 176-7, 182
psychology
  evolutionary 259, 263-5
  experimental 153-4, 155-7, 158-9
  "new" 153-4
psychopathology
  change in 34-5, 39-40
  environmentalists in 232
  evolutionary psychiatry 257-8
  normativity in 260-1
  social construction 261
psychophysical parallelism 154, 158-9
psychophysics 153-4, 155
psychosocial model 195
psychosomatic disorders 126, 128
public policy 63
purist view 5

Q
qualitative change 40
Quanstrum, K.H. 68

quantitative change 40
quantum physics 247-8

R
rank 266-7
rationalists 78
rational reconstruction 10
rational science 12
rational treatment 92-3
ready-made science 365-8
reduction, theory change 10
reductionism 202, 206, 217-18, 234, 238, 245
reframing 67-8
reification 201
relativity theory 10
replacement 10, 32
Research Diagnostic Criteria 145, 196
Research Domain Criteria (RDoC) 89, 147, 201-2, 218, 308
research waste 308
revisionist historians 149, 150
Rheinberger, H.-J. 124
Rimland, B. 333, 335
Ripke, S. 286
Rose, S. 306

S
Sacks, O. 53
St Louis criteria 196
Santa Barbara School 263-4
Sarafem® 363
Sawyer, E. 96-7
schizophrenia
 amphetamine effects 285
 brain imaging 285-6
 brain pathology 133, 231-2
 change and 31
 as a construct 88-9
 dissenters 97-8
 dopamine in, *see* dopamine hypothesis of schizophrenia
 etiology 91-2
 genetic factors 231, 237, 286
 looping effects 99
 reification 201 *fn*
 self and 100-1
 social constructionist approach 88-9, 91, 92, 97-8, 102
 subjective experience of 99-101
 surveillance definition 91
Schnädelbach, H. 151
Schwarz, S.C. 231
science
 "anything goes" 6
 diagnosis and 371-2
 evolution of 121
 normal 13
 as practice 16
 progress in 86, 89, 90
 rational 12

ready-made 365-8
values in 12, 13, 17, 22-3
scientific change
 contextualism 6, 14-18, 21-3
 holism 5, 11-14, 20-1
 internal versus external forces 5, 7, 11, 13, 17
 logical empiricism 5, 8-11
 as theory change 10
scientific disagreement 58, 60-71
 agnotology and 69
 applied research 63-4, 73-4
 benefits of 60
 causes 61-2
 decision vectors framework 57-8, 61-2
 guideline synthesis 67
 managing 67-9
 meaning 62-3
 methodological hierarchies 68
 norms of 62
 premenstrual dysphoric disorder 58-9, 69-70
 reframing 67-8
 screening mammography debate 64-6, 67, 68, 69, 74-7
 social structure 63
 trust 68-9
scientific imperialism 257, 259, 266
scientific knowledge
 dynamic conception 16
 logical empiricist view 10
scientific legitimacy 272-4
scientific models 21-2, 23
Scott, W.J. 341-2
screening mammography debate 64-6, 67, 68, 69, 74-7
selective serotonin reuptake inhibitors 307, 321
self-experience, schizophrenia 100-1
Selye, H. 129
serotonin 131-2
Severino, S. 353, 357, 358-9, 360
sham rage 126
shaping disorders, *see* autism, shaping of
Shirley, S. 329, 337
shock therapy 127, 128, 129
Showalter, E. 357
significance, empiricist criterion 9
signs 38
 prototypical Gestalt 204
 see also mental symptoms
Silverman, C. 328-9
Simon, H. 218
Simons, J. 338
Singapore Statement 311
Singer, A. 335-6
Slavney, P.R. 103
social constructionism 85-103
 case approach 83, 88-9
 category approach 83, 88-9
 causal construction 88

social constructionism (*cont.*)
  of a concept 84
  constitutive construction 88
  of an entity 84
  exclusionary 83, 87, 93–8
  HIV/AIDS 87, 90–1, 92, 93–6, 101–2
  inclusionary 83, 84, 86, 96–7, 99, 102
  medical progress 101–2
  in psychiatry 87–90
  psychopathology 261
  schizophrenia 88–9, 91, 92, 97–8, 102
  scientific change 12, 13
  scientific progress 89
social empiricism 60, 61, 62, 66, 73, 77–8, 297, 352
social factors 84, 86, 110–12; *see also* social constructionism
"special needs" 330–1
Spitzer, R. 196, 350, 361
standard operating procedures 309–10
statements, analytical/synthetic 9
statistical indices 249
status 266–7
Stevens, A. 264
Stotland, N. 353, 356–7, 358, 360, 362, 366, 367
stress exposure 134
structural change 40
structured diagnostic interview 207
subjectivity
  ontological status of 202–3
  in schizophrenia 99–101
supra-biological features 110, 111
surveillance definitions 90–1
Swain, G. 135
symptoms, *see* mental symptoms
synthetic statements 9
systematizing brain 338
Szasz, T. 97

T
technology 267–8
tensed/tenseless time 33
terminology, operational nature 199, 216–17

territory of convergence 39–40, 121, 127–8, 129–32, 141–2
thalamus 130, 133, 181
theory change 10
theory-ladenness of meaning 5, 11–12, 14
third-generation feminism 366
thought experiment (Fodor) 258
time, tensed/tenseless 33
token 33, 38, 83, 89, 96, 98, 205
transcendental change 40, 53
treatment
  benefits in PDD 355, 364–5
  effectiveness studies 178
  rational 92–3
trust 68–9
Tsuang, M.T. 233
Turkheimer, E. 250
twin method 229–31
types/typification 33, 83, 205

U
underdetermination argument 14–15
units of observation 9
universal observation language 9, 10
US–UK Diagnostic Project 195

V
values in science 12, 13, 17, 22–3
Vienna Circle 192
violence 275–6

W
Whiggish historians 149, 150
Williams, J. 361
Wing, L. 333
Worboys, M. 291
Wright, S. and B. 334
Wundt, W. 153–4

Y
Yonkers, K. 353, 364

Z
Ziehen, T. 152, 158–60

The manufacturer's authorised representative in the EU for product safety is Oxford University Press España S.A. of el Parque Empresarial San Fernando de Henares, Avenida de Castilla, 2 – 28830 Madrid (www.oup.es/en or product.safety@oup.com). OUP España S.A. also acts as importer into Spain of products made by the manufacturer.

www.ingramcontent.com/pod-product-compliance
Ingram Content Group UK Ltd.
Pitfield, Milton Keynes, MK11 3LW, UK
UKHW042005230426
12048UKWH00009B/569